Dr. Jo's

Eat Out Healthy

MW00844025

"Dr. Jo lifts the lid on dining out, revealing her professional secrets for enjoying restaurant meals without the guilt. Her practical guide for eating out will help you make the healthiest choices at your favorite restaurants in order to maintain a healthy weight and optimal health."

- Sharon Palmer, RD, Editor of Environmental Nutrition and author of *The Plant-Powered Diet*

"Dr. Jo's Eat Out Healthy, is like a GPS for restaurants...it's here to help you effortlessly navigate around the array of menus we're faced with everyday."

- Bonnie Taub-Dix, MA, RD, CDN, author of *Read It Before You Eat It*

"Read this, eat that... Dr. Jo's book is a no-nonsense, simple and easy reference to help people make sense of how to make better food choices when they dine out! Her book is funny and practical."

- Dr. Felicia D. Stoler, DCN, MS, RD, FACSM, Host of TLC's show "Honey We're Killing the Kids" and author of *Living Skinny in Fat Genes*™

"Dr. Jo has done all the legwork to help you make the healthiest choices everytime you go out to eat. Not only will you find nutritional information for nearly 150 restaurants, the book is filled with practical tips for how to Eat Out AND Eat Healthy."

- Heidi McIndoo, RD, author of *When to Eat What*

"If you love to eat out (and 60 percent of Americans do), then purchase Dr. Jo's *Eat Out Healthy*. Packed with clear and valuable nutrition information, it is truly as good as it gets for a restaurant-lover's guide to making healthier food choices from the menu."

- Dr. Janet Bond Brill, PhD, RD, LDN, CSSD, Author of *CHOLESTEROL DOWN* and *Prevent a Second Heart Attack*

"This is the go-to resource for all things dining out. It's way more than a calorie counting book. It's packed with tips for making smart, informed choices in all types of restaurants and for all types of health concerns. You'll be able to estimate serving sizes, calories and more. This easy-to-use guide will quickly become a favorite."

- Jill Weisenberger, M.S, .R.D., C.D.E., author, *Diabetes Weight Loss Week by Week*

"Dr. Jo has done it again with another no-nonsense, contemporary guide to winding your way through the maze of restaurant meals. She takes readers by the hand and shows the way to healthy, lower-calorie choices that still allow them to enjoy the experience of dining out."

- Anne M. Fletcher, M.S., R.D., author, the *Thin for Life* books and *Weight Loss Confidential*

"Dr. Jo's Eat Out Healthy is a must-read for anyone with a hectic, on-the-go lifestyle who wants to "cut to the chase" and learn how to order the healthiest foods in any situation. Packed with practical, straightforward tips and useful and easy to understand information this book is fresh and innovative."

- Tammy Lakotos Shames, R.D. and Lyssie Lakotos, R.D. (The Nutrition Twins®), authors of *The Secret to Skinny*.

"Dining out is modern day fact of life, and Dr. Jo's easy to understand guide to doing it healthfully has advice to fit every personal need. Dr Jo's book is a must-read for anyone interested in pairing healthier eating with the convenience of eating out."

- Hillary M. Wright, MEd, RD, LDN, author of *The PCOS Diet Plan*

Dr. Jo's

Eat Out Healthy

Joanne "Dr. Jo" Lichten, PhD, RD

Nutrifit Publishing

Thanks to Elizabeth Piarote for the beautiful design of my cover. And, thanks to Maggie Cook-Newell, PhD, RD and Jill Rainford (my editors) and to Stephanie Prosonic (my software consultant).

And, I'm most appreciative of my husband and best friend, John, who kept me sane by dancing with me throughout the long ordeal of writing this book...ballroom, swing, and salsa!

Eat Out Healthy

Dr. Jo (Joanne V. Lichten R.D., Ph.D.)

Published by:
Nutrifit Publishing
contact@drjo.com
DrJo.com

Printed in USA

Publisher's Cataloging In Publication data:
Lichten, Joanne V.
Eat Out Healthy
p. cm.
ISBN: 1-880347-12-1: $19.95 (pbk.)
1. Nutrition - Handbooks, manuals, etc. 2. Restaurants - United States - Guidebooks. 3. Low-fat diet.

TX907.2   2012
613.2-dc20

Contents

PART 1

The Basics

Introduction

"What's the healthiest restaurant and what meal should I order?"

That's one of the most common questions I get at my speaking events. And I should know the answer. I've been writing about eating healthy in restaurants since 1991 (this is my fifth book on the topic, but there have been hundreds of articles).

Yet, the answer to that question is not quite as simple as it may seem. My responses often start with, "It depends" because it depends on what your taste buds are craving, what you mean by "healthy," and what else you've eaten already that day - or will be eating later. You do eat more than one meal a day, right?

Let me illustrate the point with this short quiz:

1. Which is a better choice - a hamburger or a grilled chicken sandwich?

2. Which has more sodium - soup or salad? Which one has more calories?

Let's start with the first question so you can see how complicated these questions really are. When you look at meat directly from the grocery store, that's an easy question. Ounce-for-ounce skin-less chicken breast is lower in fat and calories than the typical ground beef used in making a burger. But, at a restaurant, this is a more difficult question to answer.

For example, at Burger King®, the smallest hamburger is the WHOPPER JR®. As served, it contains 340 calories and 19g fat.

The grilled chicken sandwich (TENDERGRILL®) has 470 calories and 18g fat. Why is the chicken sandwich so much higher in calories? Both are prepared with mayonnaise so that doesn't explain the difference. If ordered without mayo, the WHOPPER JR® Sandwich drops to 260 calories and 10g fat while the TENDERGRILL® Chicken sandwich contains 360 calories and 7g fat. The grilled chicken sandwich is much higher in calories simply because it is just plain huge!

If you're watching calories and you're craving a burger (and have a tendency to eat everything you're served), the smaller burger has fewer calories and might be a better choice. Fat-wise, the grilled chicken sandwich has less total fat and saturated fat. What about sodium? The WHOPPER JR® has *half* the sodium of the TENDERGRILL®. So, which is the "better" choice? See what I mean? It really does depend on what you're craving and what you mean by healthy.

Now on to question #2, "Which has more sodium - soup or salad?" Ok, this question appears to be more straight forward. Soups are very salty, right? That is true, especially at restaurants where lower sodium soups are rarely available.

What about the salad? While unadulterated vegetables are very low in sodium, chefs often add cheese, croutons, olives, and other high sodium items to their salads. And that's before the salad dressing (which is notoriously high in sodium).

Consider the soup and salad offered at the Olive Garden®. One serving of Pasta e Fagioli soup contains 680mg sodium while one serving of the Garden-Fresh Salad with dressing contains 1930mg sodium. What! Yes, it's true. According to the nutrition information at OliveGarden.com, just one serving of salad has three times more sodium than a bowl of soup. (Three quarters of that sodium comes from the dressing, but the salad alone has 550mg sodium).

Which one has more calories - soup or salad? Surprisingly, the soup contains 130 calories and the salad (just one serving, mind you) has 350 calories. Have you ever ordered the All-You-Can-Eat Soup, Salad & Breadstick lunch? If you were to eat just a single serving of each, you'd be eating 630 calories! And, do you ever reach into the unlimited bowl for a second serving of salad? Another breadstick? Uh oh. For all those calories, fat, and sodium, you could have had a burger and fries!

Eating out healthy is not quite as simple as it seems. That's why I wrote *Dr. Jo's Eat Out Healthy*. I've done all the investigative work for you - and have examined the menus and nutritional information for nearly 150 restaurants. This book is chock-full of tips and strategies for all the different types of restaurants and cuisines, complete with nutritional information including calories, fat, carbohydrates and more - including the details for more than 150 of the most popular restaurants (representing a quarter of a million locations)!

Here we are back to the original question: what's the best restaurant and the healthiest item on the menu? The truth is, you can find many healthful options at just about every restaurant. You just need to know what to order, how to order it, and what portion is appropriate for your nutritional needs. So, turn the page and get started uncovering all the secrets for yourself.

Information in the front part of the book was obtained from USDA food composition tables, restaurant websites, recipe database analysis, food manufacturers, and scientific literature. The last part of the book contains nutrition information directly from the restaurants or the restaurant's website. For space considerations, when more than one item is listed, assume that these items are grouped because they are similar in values, and that the numbers represent averaged nutrition information.

Additional Tips

- Always consult with a Registered Dietitian and/or Medical doctor before making major changes in your eating style.

- Menu items, recipes, and nutritional information are always subject to change. Check with the restaurant before ordering.

- Nutritional information is provided for specific measures of food. Keep in mind that measurements such as teaspoons or tablespoons refer to level portions not *heaping* spoons!

- This book includes many abbreviations. Please refer to the key on the following page.

Abbreviations

c	cup	med	medium
cals	calories	mg	milligrams
carbs	carbohydrates	na	not available
CB	cheeseburger	oz	ounce
ch	cheese	PB	peanut butter
choc	chocolate	pkg	package
drsg	dressing	pkt	packet
ea	each	#	pound
fl oz	fluid oz	sce	sauce
g	gram	sl	slice
HB	hamburger	SW	sandwich
"	inch	Tbsp	Tablespoon
lg	large	tsp	teaspoon
<1	less than one	veggie	vegetable
mayo	mayonnaise	w/	with
		w/o	without

Nutrition & Health Recommendations

Whether you want to lose weight, lower your cholesterol, drop your blood pressure, or just eat healthier, this chapter has you covered. First, some sobering health statistics from CDC (Centers for Disease Control & Prevention) and the ADA (American Diabetes Association):

• Two thirds of all Americans are either overweight or obese

• Heart disease is the number one killer in the US

• One in three US adults have high blood pressure or high cholesterol - the two leading causes of heart disease

• Eight percent of the population has diabetes and another 25% have prediabetes

This book is so heavily focused on calories because excess calories, and the resulting excess weight, are major contributors for heart disease and diabetes. One of the two overriding recommendations set by the 2010 Dietary Guidelines suggests, "Maintain calorie balance over time to achieve and sustain a healthy weight." The other recommendation is to "Focus on consuming nutrient-dense foods and beverages" by cutting back on excess fat, sweets, sodas, refined (white) breads and pasta. Instead, increase fruits, vegetables, and non-fat dairy foods. This chapter covers the basics of these recommendations. The next page introduces your "nutritional budget" in a summary format, while the pages to follow provide the specifics behind these recommendations.

How Much Should I Be Eating?

To eat more healthfully, most of us don't need to count calories, grams of fat, or carbs. Many of us can benefit from using the guidelines in this chapter to simply evaluate the meals we eat or compare one meal against another. For example, finding out one of your favorite restaurant meals contains 60g fat doesn't mean much until you discover you only need 60g fat for the entire day!

The following chart offers you some insight into your daily nutritional needs. Read on to find the specifics behind these recommendations.

Women:	Calories	Fat (g)	Sat+Trans Fat (g)	Sodium (mg)	Carbohydrates (g)	Fiber (g)	Protein (g)
Weight Loss	1200	<40	<13	<2300	150	25	60
Sedentary	1800	<60	<20	<2300	225	25	90
Moderately Active	2000	<67	<22	<2300	250	25	100
Active	2200	<73	<24	<2300	275	25	110
Men:							
Weight Loss	1800	<60	<20	<2300	225	38	90
Sedentary	2300	<77	<26	<2300	290	38	115
Moderately Active	2500	<83	<28	<2300	315	38	125
Active	2800	<93	<31	<2300	350	38	140

Worried about Your Weight?

Considering the fact that two thirds of all Americans are overweight or obese (CDC), it's no surprise that about 25% are consciously dieting at any given time. Many others are simply trying to keep their weight in check.

I always recommend lifestyle changes instead of diets because they lead to a slow but permanent weight loss. It's a good idea to watch your weight because being overweight increases your risk for diabetes, heart disease, and stroke. How many calories should you be eating? While everyone's metabolism is different, the chart (primarily developed from the 2010 Dietary Guidelines), helps you estimate how many calories you might need in a day to maintain your weight based upon your needs and activity level.

After reading this book, it should be easier to choose lower calorie menu items. If you follow the tips presented throughout the book, and refer to specific information about all the major chain restaurants in the book's last section, you should be able to eat healthfully at any restaurant.

It's Just the Little Things

When people start putting on weight, they automatically think they're doing *everything* wrong. When in fact, it may be just a few small things that are packing on the pounds.

Even if you have more than a few extra pounds on your body, chances are, if you think back, you'll realize the weight came on relatively slowly. In fact, the average American adult is gaining a pound a year. (Ten pounds in a decade; 20 pounds over 20 years; sound familiar?)

Since a pound of fat contains 3500 calories, and there are 365 days in a year, it's easy to calculate that eating just 10 calories more than your body needs daily can add up to a pound of fat in a year's end (10 X 365 = 3650 calories). Just 10 extra calories a day will push the scale in the wrong direction!

Do you know what that means? If you're steadily gaining weight at a rate of just a pound a year, it could be due to inadvertently eating an extra small piece of hard candy, a nibble of a cookie, a sip of soda, or a thin smear of butter. And I mean just *one* of those extra things a day - not all of them!

Are you gaining more than a pound a year? Maybe 10 pounds over the past year? This can be explained by eating just 100 calories extra a day (100 X 365 days = 36,500 calories or 10 pounds!) There are 100 calories in a third of a doughnut, eight ounces of beer or soda, a tablespoon of salad dressing, fourteen chips, or ten French fries.

Dr. Jo's Eat Out Healthy will help you make wiser choices when dining out so you can stop (and then reverse) this creeping weight gain. It's loaded with numerous small changes you can undertake to make a major impact upon your weight while still satisfying your taste buds!

Focus on the Fat

Calories come from three basic nutrients: carbohydrates, proteins, and fats. Which is the best one to cut back on if you want to lose weight? Research indicates that it really doesn't matter. A weight loss can be induced by cutting back on any one of them.

Throughout this book, I will focus more on cutting back on fat than the other calorie-containing nutrients because:

• **Most restaurants add more fat to their food than you would at home.** Butter is poured onto steaks, chicken, and fish before being served. Even "steamed" vegetables have butter added.

• **The American Heart Association maintains that Americans consume too much fat,** especially dangerous saturated and trans fat (found in butter, fried foods, and baked goods). Restaurants typically use more of these unhealthy fats while preparing your food.

• **Fat has more than twice as many calories as carbohydrates or protein.** While carbohydrates and proteins have only four calories per gram, fats have a whopping nine calories per gram. This explains why a cup of white flour has 400 calories, a cup of sugar has 800 calories (pure carbohydrate), and a cup of oil (pure fat) has 2000 calories!

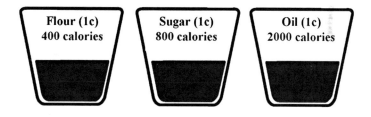

| **Flour (1c)** 400 calories | **Sugar (1c)** 800 calories | **Oil (1c)** 2000 calories |

• **Cutting out fat might be easier than cutting out the other nutrients.** Since fat has twice as many calories as carbohydrate or protein, you can reduce the calories faster (and still eat the same amount of food) by focusing on the fats, rather than the carbs. That's why the butter you spread on that very small piece of bread can easily double the calories!

Eat More, Lose Weight

While some people do well with simplistic advice to "Just eat half of what you're served," that just doesn't work for the many who like to eat larger portions! If you can't get filled up with small portions of foods, focus on the fat in your meal.

Years back, while dining out with a friend, we both ordered similar foods...until the dessert came. When I ordered a slice of cheesecake, she was irate, "It just isn't fair. We both eat the same foods and then you get to have cheesecake for dessert. It isn't fair that you have a better metabolism than me."

That was a bold accusation about me having a better metabolism than her, and I would venture that it isn't true. I know for a fact, that we didn't eat the same foods. Yes, we both had a drink. We both had a salad and just one breadstick. We both had fish, a potato, and broccoli. But that was where the similarity ended. Take a look at the nutritional breakdown of her meal versus mine:

My Friend's Meal

	Cals	Fat(g)
4oz Margarita	240	0
1 slice bread w/2t butter	160	11
Salad w/3Tbsp dressing	250	24
Loaded Baked Potato, sm	400	25
Fried Fish, 8oz	600	32
Tartar Sauce, 1/4c	320	36
Broccoli & cheese sauce	125	12
	2095	**140**

My Meal

	Cals	Fat(g)
4oz Wine	100	0
1 sl bread w/o butter	80	1
Salad w/1Tbsp dressing	105	8
Dry Baked Potato, sm	160	1
Broiled Fish, 8oz	250	5
Broccoli w/o butter	25	0
Cheesecake, lg slice	600	35
	1320	**49**

While we did eat similar foods, she selected versions that contained a lot more calories (mostly from fat) than my meal choices. Even with the addition of a rich dessert, I ended up eating a third fewer calories than she did.

That is just one example of how to cut calories; there are many other options. You may choose to cut back on your alcohol consumption. Or maybe you'll order an appetizer, instead of an entrée, or skip the bread and the potato just so you can enjoy another drink - or dessert. The choice is yours.

Simple mathematics makes a demonstrable case for controlling fat consumption. And, so do real life studies. The National

Weight Control Registry tracks more than 5000 people who lost at least 30 pounds and kept it off for a year or more. According to this database, a lowfat diet (23-24% of calories from fat) appears to be one of the major keys to keeping off the weight. By cutting back on fats, you can enjoy more real food and still lose weight.

Concerned about Heart Disease?

Since heart disease is the number one killer in the United States, many of us are concerned about our serum cholesterol levels. As mentioned earlier, one third of all Americans have a high serum cholesterol (over 200 mg/dL). Serum cholesterol is made up of both good cholesterol (HDL) and bad cholesterol (LDL and triglycerides). Research demonstrates that lowering your bad cholesterol levels can reduce your risk of developing heart disease.

According to the American Heart Association's guidelines, a heart-healthy diet consists of avoiding foods high in fat (especially saturated fat and trans fat) and cholesterol. These dietary components increase your risk of atherosclerosis (or the build-up of fatty deposits) in the inner walls of your arteries. Of course, maintaining an ideal body weight is also helpful.

Know Your Fats

The American Heart Association recommends limiting total fat intake to 25–35 percent of your total calories each day. Some dietary fats, though, are considered more unhealthy than others. The 2010 Dietary Guidelines recommend eating less than 10% of calories in the form of saturated fat, and limiting trans fat as much as possible. The American Heart Association recommends limiting saturated fat to less than 7% and trans fat to less than 1% of total daily calories. The daily recommendation table (in the beginning of this chapter) lists fat as 30% of calories from fat. The column listing saturated *plus* trans fat is calculated at 10% of the recommended calories. Think of these numbers as your recommended *maximum* fat and saturated/trans fat intakes.

Some people think that simply cutting back on their dietary cholesterol will lower their serum cholesterol level. While the

American Heart Association does recommend a reduction in dietary cholesterol to 300mg per day, focusing on fats is more important. This is because only 25% of the cholesterol in our bodies come from the foods we eat. The rest is produced within our bodies. To lower your cholesterol intake, reduce your intake of foods such as butter, lard, meat, cheese, and eggs. Notice, these are all animal products. Since cholesterol is manufactured in the liver (and only animal have livers), no plant foods contain cholesterol. Don't be confused by a vegetable oil whose label proclaims "no cholesterol." No vegetable oils have cholesterol. Furthermore, all oils contain the same amount of fat and calories (ounce-for-ounce) as butter or shortening. The only difference is the types of fat in each.

Remember, you want to limit your total fat intake by cutting back on the saturated fats and trans fats. Saturated fats are found in all animal meat, cheese, whole milk, stick margarine, and baked goods. While a small amount of trans fat occur naturally in some animal products, most trans fats come from hydrogenated fats. Hydrogenated fats are produced when food processing turns liquid vegetable oils into margarine and shortening. Thus, any products containing hydrogenated fats (especially baked goods and fried foods) tend to be higher in trans fats.

Over the past few years, food manufacturers and restaurants have been cutting back on their use of trans fats. Most of the large fast food restaurants have switched to "trans-free oil" for the fryer, but many of the independently-owned restaurants have not. You also should know that even when the nutrition information states "zero" for trans fat, your food may not be completely trans fat-free. The Food and Drug Administration (FDA) permits rounding values under 0.5g as "zero." The FDA has rounding rules for all nutrients, not just trans fat.

Since trans fats can raise serum cholesterol levels, and stick margarines contains trans fats, should we switch to butter? No. Butter is high in both saturated fat and cholesterol. Instead of using a stick margarine, switch to a tub margarine (with little or no trans fats). Or simply use a healthy liquid vegetable oil such as canola or olive oil. Most restaurants have these healthy options available - just ask.

What about sprays that are labeled as having zero calories per spray? It does have a few more calories, but the FDA allows products with less than 5 calories to be labeled as zero. This product is simply oil in a format that allows you to spray small quantities at a time. Most sprays are made with healthier oils, so go ahead and request that your omelet be prepared with the spray instead of butter.

What Foods Should I Eat? Avoid?

If you want to reduce your fat intake, especially the unhealthy saturated and trans fats, here are some suggestions for you to keep in mind when dining out:

• **Opt for egg substitutes** instead of whole eggs in your omelets and fritattas. Egg substitutes are made of egg whites. Since the high cholesterol egg yolk is removed, egg substitutes contain no cholesterol. Egg substitutes are also lower in saturated fat and calories. Of course you can always order egg whites.

• **Moderate the animal protein.** Beef, chicken, and turkey are all good sources of protein. Unfortunately, they also contain saturated fats and cholesterol. Therefore, the American Heart Association recommends that we eat no more than 6-8oz of animal protein *each day*. That's comparable to eating a piece of meat the size and thickness of a deck of cards at each meal. To limit your portions, select the smaller cuts on the menu, order pasta with meat instead of a meat entrée, or order a meat appetizer instead of an entrée.

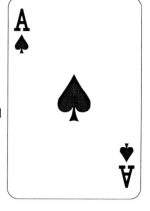

• **Slash the fried foods.** Fried meats and other foods contain at least double the amount of calories as the original food - all of which come from fat. So, order the meat grilled or roasted, skip the fries or onion rings, and ask for a fruit cup instead.

• **Cut the cheese.** Cheese is very high in fat (especially unhealthy saturated fat). Consider leaving off the extra topping of cheese.

- **Reach for the tub margarine instead of butter.** Even if butter is served at the table or used in the cooking, soft tub margarine and healthy vegetable oil is almost always available. The healthiest oils are canola and olive. But before you dip (or *soak*) your bread in olive oil, remember, that all oils still have the same number of calories. Every tablespoon of oil has 120 calories and 14g fat!

- **Leave off the butter completely.** To save fat calories, learn to enjoy your baked potato or toast prepared plainly. Ask for your "steamed" vegetables to be served without butter.

- **Load up on salsa and chutneys.** These fruit and/or vegetable-based sauces are much lower in calories than the fatty sauces.

- **Ask for the salad dressing on the side** so you can use less (or order an Italian or vinaigrette dressing). Flowing, liquid dressings tend to be lower in saturated fat, plus you tend to use less.

- **Request lowfat milk** (or better yet, nonfat) for your cereal or coffee beverages.

- **Skip the refried beans.** Substitute black beans or beans a la charra (bean soup) for the refried beans at a Mexican restaurant. Ask for plain rice instead of fried rice at an Asian restaurant.

- **Select broth-based soups** instead of the creamy varieties.

- **Order sorbet, lowfat frozen yogurt, or fresh fruit for dessert.** Most baked goods are very high in fat, especially the unhealthy fats. If you must have a fatty dessert, consider ordering a "mini dessert." These small-size portions are quickly becoming popular at many restaurants.

How Much Fat Could I Possibly be Eating?

Picture yourself placing an entire stick of butter on a slice of bread. Roll up that slice of bread and take a bite. Disgusting? Well, many Americans eat more fat than the equivalent of a stick of butter every day! For a visual, consider that each stick of butter (or margarine) has 88g fat.

Now let's compare that to some common restaurant meals:

• Three egg omelet with hashbrowns = 80g

• Large burger and fries = 73g

• Entrée salad with meat and dressing = 70g

• An individual-size cheese-only deep dish pizza = 120g fat

• A dinner order of baby back ribs, no sides = 80g

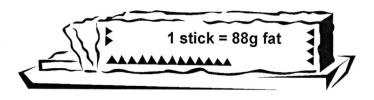

1 stick = 88g fat

Are you feeling queasy yet? Still think you couldn't possibly eat the equivalence of a stick of fat in just one meal?

Counting Carbohydrates?

Some people limit their intake of carbohydrates (carbs) as a way to lose weight. Others keep their carbs within a certain range to control their blood sugar levels. For health purposes, the Dietary Guidelines 2010 recommend carbohydrates to be kept to 45 - 65% of your total calories in a day. The table at the front of this chapter lists carbohydrate intakes of approximately 50% of total calories.

Most restaurants are loaded in carbohydrates, starting with the bread basket and ending with drinks and dessert. If you want to cut back on carbohydrates at your favorite restaurant, heed these suggestions:

• **Start with the obvious** - hand back the bread basket, choose diet beverages, and skip dessert.

• **Go topless!** Consider removing the top piece of bread or bun on your sandwich to cut the carbs in half.

• **Eat smaller portions.** Bagels are notoriously huge. Ask for sliced bread or an English muffin instead. Some carb counters pinch out the bagel innards and just eat the crust (or vice versa - eat only the innards).

• **Ask for steamed vegetables** instead of potatoes or rice.

• **Replace fried foods by requesting grilled or roasted meats instead.** Most fried meats are breaded first with carbohydrates such as bread crumbs, flour, or corn meal.

• **Get sliced tomatoes instead of hashbrowns** or homefries.

Focused on Fiber?

The National Academy of Sciences' Institute of Medicine recommends 25g of fiber (for women) to 38g of fiber (for men). Unfortunately, most restaurants seem to focus on the meats instead of fruits, vegetables, and whole grains - which are all good sources of fiber. But that doesn't mean you have to throw in the towel and give up trying to increase your fiber. Here are some ideas:

• **Split an entrée with a friend and then order an extra serving of veggies or a salad.** Keep in mind that dark green lettuce has more fiber than the usual pale-looking iceberg lettuce.

• **Get the baked potato instead of rice.** And don't be shy about eating the potato skin!

• **Order fruit instead of fruit juice.** You'll get more fiber with fewer calories when you get an orange rather than a tall glass of orange juice.

• **Opt for oatmeal.** It contains more fiber than most of the other typical breakfast choices. Ask for raisins or other fruit for your oatmeal, too.

• **Ask for fruit for dessert or as a substitute for fries.** Even if it's not on the menu, fresh fruit is often available.

• **Get the beans.** At the salad bar, load up on all different types of beans. Order black beans at the Mexican restaurant. BBQ restaurants will probably offer beans and maybe a bean salad, too.

• **Add nuts and seeds.** Nuts are not only a good source of fiber, they're rich in healthy monounsaturated fats, too.

• **Go vegetarian.** Veggie burgers are a higher fiber alternative to beef and chicken.

- **Request whole grain bread.** Though keep in mind that many darker breads may look like whole grain, but contain darkening molasses instead.

- **Ask if whole wheat pasta is available.** Some Italian restaurants are now offering this option.

Conscious of Sodium?

According to the American Heart Association, about 70% of all American adults have either high blood pressure (hypertension) or prehypertension. On average, the higher one's sodium intake, the higher the blood pressure. And, a body of literature suggests that lowering one's sodium intake can lower blood pressure.

According to the 2010 Dietary Guidelines, and as seen in the chart at the front of this chapter, most adults should be eating no more than 2300 mg sodium per day. But, individuals over the age of 51 and all African Americans should reduce their sodium intake to less than 1500mg (that's roughly half the adult population!) This recommendation also applies to those with hypertension, diabetes, or chronic kidney disease.

When people hear that a teaspoon of salt has 2400mg sodium, they often retort, "There's no way I'm getting that much." But, according to the CDC, we are consuming an average of 3400mg a day. Even if you never lift the salt shaker, you're still probably eating too much sodium. That's because most sodium is found in processed food. Nowadays, few restaurants prepare everything from scratch. And even when processed foods are used, restaurants often add even more salt (or other seasonings that contain salt) to the food they prepare.

Considering that many restaurant meals often contain more sodium than one should have in the entire day, here are some suggestions on how to keep the sodium low:

- **Tell the server you're watching your sodium.** Ask that your food be prepared without salt, MSG (monosodium glutamate), soy sauce, or seasoning salts.

- **Leave the salt shaker alone.** Or at least break the habit of salting *before* you taste the food.

- **Request grilled or baked foods rather than fried foods.** With grilled or baked foods the chef can often leave off the seasoning, whereas fried foods often are delivered to the restaurant pre-breaded and prefried!

- **Pick fresh meats** instead of processed cold cuts and sausage.

- **Avoid smoked & pickled foods**. Ask them not to serve that tempting pickle with your sandwich.

- **Skip the high sodium additions.** Order salads, burgers, tacos, omelets, and other foods without cheese, pickles, and olives.

- **Request unsalted butter or margarine.** Every little bit counts.

- **Request that all sauces and salad dressings be served on the side** and used sparingly. Use oil and vinegar (or just lemon) instead of bottled salad dressings.

- **Ask for fresh fruit instead of chip**s with your sandwich. If you want the fries, ask them not to salt them.

- **Enjoy yeast rolls or breads rather than biscuits or cornbread.** Yeast-raised breads are generally lower in sodium than those prepared with baking soda or baking powder.

- **Order fruit, low fat ice cream, frozen yogurt, or gelatin** instead of baked desserts.

Gluten Free Dining

Celiac disease is an inherited autoimmune disorder that affects more than 1% of all people. When a person who has celiac disease consumes gluten (a protein found in wheat, rye, barley, farina, and bulgur), the immune system responds by attacking the body and damaging the lining of the small intestine. Consequently, this inhibits the absorption of important nutrients into the body. Undiagnosed and untreated, celiac disease can lead to the development of other autoimmune disorders, as well as osteoporosis, infertility, neurological conditions and in rare cases, cancer.

To prevent health problems, people with celiac disease must follow strict dietary guidelines. Follow are some suggestions (from GlutenFreePassport.com) to keep in mind when dining out in restaurants.

- **Avoid products containing wheat, rye, barley, farina, and bulgar** such as breads, battering, croutons, pasta, dumplings, and most baked goods. Caution: some meats may not be breaded, but could be "flour dusted" before cooking. Ask.

- **Realize that cross-contamination can occur in restaurants,** especially in the deep fat fryer. Ask if the corn tortillas are fried in the same fryer as the wheat tortillas used for fried tortilla salad shells or chimichangas.

- **Ask for details.** Marinades and gravies, as well as broths and sauces using packaged bouillon, contain gluten. Other sources of gluten include salad dressing, malt vinegar, fish sauce, artificial potatoes, and imitation crabmeat. Ask if the hamburgers have bread crumbs added. Asian restaurants use both rice and noodle pasta - ask which is being used in your menu item. Even when ordering rice pasta, be sure that clean, fresh water is being used to prevent cross contamination.

- **Ask the chef to use a clean cutting board and knives, fresh oil, and a clean pan or pot.** Even small pieces of gluten can cause problems for people with celiac disease.

Some chain restaurants that offer gluten-free options include: Arby's, Bonefish Grill, Burger King, Carraba's Italian Grill, Chili's, Carino's Italian Grill, Carl's Jr., Chick-fil-A, Godfather's Pizza, Hardee's, Moe's Southwestern Grill, Outback Steakhouse, P.F. Chang's China Bistro, Red Robin, Romano's Macaroni Grill, Uno Chicago Grill, and Wendy's.

General Tips to Eat Out Healthy

Have you ever gone into a restaurant with all good intentions of eating healthfully, then found yourself ordering the usual? Wish you had more *willpower* to order healthier options? Stop waiting for willpower to magically appear! What you need to prevent overindulging is a plan. Just because restaurant meals tend to be heavier than your meals at home doesn't mean you have to "blow it." This chapter includes some practical tips and strategies that will help you stay in control.

Eat Your Pleasers; Skip Your Teasers

According to research, people who have successfully lost weight and kept it off continued to eat their favorite foods. You can too!

The secret is differentiating between what I have coined as your "pleasers" and your "teasers." Pleasers are the foods you really love. They are well worth all the calories. Come on, you know what your favorite foods are. For me, it's brownies and chocolate chip ice cream. Love 'em! Teasers are things that don't really taste good, but you eat them anyway. They could include so-so tasting bread or run-of-the-mill mints by the front door.

When you give yourself permission to enjoy your pleasers every now and then, you'll find it easier to avoid the teasers. That's because deprivation leads to rebound bingeing and weight gain. Once you've identified your pleasers, be sure to enjoy them! Of course, unless you have a fabulous metabolism, you may not be able to eat them *all* the time in *unlimited* quantities.

Stick to One Treat at a Time

If you want dessert, skip the soda. Craving a fried entrée? Then skip dessert. Remember, you can eat your pleasers when eating out - just not all at the same meal.

Have Fun

Eating is necessary for life and, therefore, should be pleasurable. There's no need to feel guilty about enjoying the foods you love in moderation. Remember, too, that dining out isn't just about the food. It's also about the atmosphere, the people you're with, and the break from cooking and cleaning. So, focus on these non-food aspects, too, and you will eat less and still feel satisfied.

Savor Every Bite

Are you a speed eater? Do you take big bites? Are you focused on putting food on your fork while you chew the previous bite? Do you swallow after just a few chews? What's the rush? Are you racing someone?

Fast eaters tend to eat more. Slow down and focus on savoring your food. Put your fork down between bites and don't swallow until all the flavor of the food is gone - and don't get the next forkful ready until after you swallow! These suggestions are even more significant when the food contains a lot of calories. So, if you have decided to spend the extra calories on your favorite dessert, take tiny nibbles and fully enjoy every bite!

Rethink "Getting Your Money's Worth"

No one wants to pay more for a meal than what it's worth. But when you're at an all-you-can-eat buffet (or at a restaurant that serves large portions), try not to focus on eating more than you need just to "get your money's worth" - unless you factor in the total cost of overeating. According to a 2008 bankrate.com article, weight loss programs cost anywhere from $13-$129 for every pound you want to lose. Case settled - you don't save money by eating more.

Make It "No Big Deal"

Dr. Jo's Eat Out Healthy is filled with nutrition information and tips for cutting back on calories, fat, and more. But please don't follow through on each and everyone of the suggestions, or your food will be totally unpalatable! Instead, focus on making only those changes that are "no big deal" to you. Establish your own priorities. This approach will allow you to enjoy eating out while keeping your waistline in check. You get to make your own rules based on your own priorities – and your own taste buds!

Speak to the Manager

At first glance, most menus appear to have just one or two healthier options - maybe a plain grilled chicken or a simple salad. Just seeing those same boring and repetitive menu items is enough for most of us to go back to our old ways. Don't give up!

Once you're provided with more details about the food offered, you'll realize there are plenty of additional healthful (and more exciting) options. But who to ask? Truthfully, the wait staff often isn't involved in the kitchen enough to fully answer your questions. And chefs are busy preparing the food. So, ask to speak to the manager. They know about portion sizes, how the food is prepared, and which substitutions are permitted.

Instead of approaching them in the middle of a busy time, speak to the manager *ahead of time*. After familiarizing yourself with the menu online, call during the slower times of 9 - 11 a.m. and 2 - 5 p.m. to ask questions. You may discover the restaurant is willing to offer smaller portions, flavorful lower calorie sauces, healthier side dish substitutes, or leaner cut of meats.

Take the Edge Off Your Hunger

Some people try to starve themselves during the day so they can "save" their calories for a large dinner meal. Usually this plan backfires. Arriving at the restaurant starving, they tend to order too much, eat too fast, and, subsequently, overeat.

Instead, eat smaller meals during the day - don't skip any meals. During the drive to the restaurant, take the edge off your hunger with a piece of fresh fruit and drink a full glass of water when you get there.

Fill up with broth-based soup or fresh fruit. Fresh fruit will fill your tummy without a lot of calories because of its fiber and high water content. At about 100 calories a cup (not bowl), soup will help curb your appetite. Choose from non-creamy soups such as bean, vegetable beef, chicken rice, and chicken noodle.

Make Peace with Your Plate

Remember the peace sign of the 1960s? Keep this modified version in mind when filling your plate at a buffet or salad bar. For a well-balanced meal, fill the bottom quarter of your plate with lean protein such as meat or beans, one side with healthful starches and grains (carbs), and the other side with fruits and veggies.

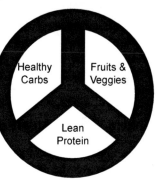

Split an Entree

Most full restaurant meals (from appetizers to dessert) have more calories than you need for an entire day! And, most entrées contain 1000 - 1500 calories. That's way more than you need for a single meal. So consider splitting an entrée with a friend. Then order an extra salad, a plate of steamed vegetables, or a baked potato so you both enjoy complete meals.

Order a la Carte

Order "a la carte" to get only what you want - without the extras that tempt you to overeat. For example, an enchilada plate at a Mexican restaurant often includes three enchiladas, rice, beans, sour cream, and guacamole - at close to 1500 calories. If you don't really like the rice, consider ordering a la carte to get just two enchiladas with a cup of black beans at under half the calories.

Make It Small

Some restaurants will allow you to order the "luncheon" portion at dinner for a discounted price. The luncheon portions are generally one half to three quarters the size of the dinner portions. These restaurants generally do not mention this fact on the menu (such as at the Olive Garden). You need to ask. Or just ask for a small plate to serve yourself from the larger serving.

Some restaurants specialize in "small plates" making it easier for you to pick a well-balanced meal. Buffet plates, bowls, and cups tend to be small. Use that to your advantage (you'll eat less per fill up) and consider just one serving, rather than going back for seconds.

Make a Meal of Appetizers

It's no surprise that most appetizers are fried; just one order could easily blow your fat allotment for the whole day! But if you are going to eat something fried, it's better to have an appetizer portion rather than an entrée portion, right? To complete the meal, add steamed veggies, and a slice of whole grain bread.

If you find some leaner appetizers such as pasta with a red sauce, shrimp cocktail, or beef strips on a skewer, consider making that your entrée. Appetizer-sized meat portions are often only 2-4oz, rather than the standard 8-10oz entrée size, so it's an easy way to control calories. Some foods, such as pasta in an Italian restaurant, are often offered in both entrée and appetizer portions.

Think Lean

When you order a full meal, meats and other protein sources are often the highest calorie item on your plate. Here are some suggestions to cut way back on the fat and calories.

• **Order the lean cuts of meat.** Leaner cuts of beef include filet, sirloin, or tenderloin steak. (The "prime" cuts of beef are the most heavily marbled, and therefore, highest in fat and calories). Choose the pork tenderloin, instead of higher fat pork chops. White chicken or turkey meat is the leanest.

• **Choose grilled, not fried.** Want boned-in chicken? Order the grilled chicken pieces, instead of fried. Also, ask your server if you can substitute grilled chicken for the fried chicken on the chicken sandwich or the chicken salad. If you're craving fish, select baked or broiled fish instead of pan-fried or deep fried.

• **Look for menu items that feature leaner ways to cook meats and vegetables:** broiling, roasting, char-grilling, grilling, poaching, stir-frying, boiling, and steaming. Avoid foods that are described as fried, crispy, creamy, buttery, pot pie, covered in gravy, Parmesan, au gratin or in a cheese sauce.

Limit the Fried Foods

Do you know that frying a food generally *doubles* the calories? But if you really love fried foods, try to balance your choices. If you order the fried fish, skip the fries and order a dry baked potato with it instead. Want fries? Then, choose the grilled chicken or blackened fish sandwich instead of the burger.

Make Special Requests

Don't think you have to order only what's on the menu. Most restaurants (from fast food restaurants to fine dining), allow you to request changes. Here are just a few ideas to get you thinking about how to save a few calories:

• **Ask for the bread to be prepared without butter or oil.** Many times, rolls and loaves are brushed with butter or oil.

• **Ask for the minimal amount of butter to be used during cooking and just before serving.** Most meats (such as steaks, grilled chicken, and fish) are finished with a brushing of clarified butter - or worse, butter is *poured* over the dish. Now you know why the meat shines and the fajitas sizzle!

• **Order "steamed" veggies without the added fat.** Yes, even steamed vegetables are often finished with a topping of butter, oil, cheese, or sauce.

• **Request your stir-fry to be prepared with less oil,** with broth, or even steamed.

Be Creative

Don't limit yourself to what's printed on the menu. If the restaurant offers fresh strawberries on the cheesecake, chances are they will serve you a bowl of fresh strawberries. And, if they make the Broccoli and Cheese Soup from scratch, they'll probably be willing to steam some broccoli if you ask. In addition, most restaurants have tomatoes on hand and will slice some up for you.

Vinegar is almost always available although rarely mentioned as a dressing option. Ask for some of the flavorful varieties such as red wine, balsamic, or tarragon vinegar. A squirt of lemon on your salad may also satisfy your palate. Picante sauce (at ten calories per tablespoon) makes a great low-calorie dressing or a topping for your baked potato. If you frequent a restaurant that doesn't serve a lower calorie dressing, consider bringing your own. Some food companies sell dressings in individual packets.

Ask for Simple Substitutes

If the menu states that fries are served with all sandwiches, ask if you can have a salad, steamed vegetables, or fruit cup instead. How about a baked potato instead of mashed potatoes? Or sliced tomatoes, instead of home fries, with your eggs?

Watch the Extras

Always read the description of the menu item to find out what's added. Take salads, for example. Many entrée-sized salads have over 1000 calories. To reduce the calories, take a look at the ingredients to find out what you can leave off. If you don't like olives, that would be a start. If you don't like the restaurant's croutons, leave them off too and save yourself another hundred calories.

Want Mexican Food? Do you really need the guacamole, sour cream, *and* the cheese? Leaving off any one of these ingredients might reduce the meal by 100 calories. Whatever you do, don't take off all the fun and the flavor! Just think about making a few "no big deal" changes to save some unnecessary calories.

Get It on the Side

Don't let the person in the kitchen determine how much salad dressing, sauce, or gravy you like and how many calories you need. Since most toppings are very high in fat, always ask for them on the side so *you* can decide how much to add. This is a good idea even when restaurants offer "low-calorie" dressings because most are not as low in calories as the ones you use at home.

Do the "Dip'N Stab"

After you order the sauces, dressings, and butters on the side, don't just pour them on. Dip your fork into the sauce and then into a piece of food. This way you get a taste with every bite. This is true not just for the salad dressing, but for the lemon butter sauce that comes on the fish, and the gravy that is added to chicken fried steak.

Skip the Salad

Yes, vegetables such as tomatoes, carrots, and peppers are chock full of healthy nutrients. Though dark green lettuces are very healthy, most salads are made of mostly iceberg lettuce, a vegetable with little nutritional value. I call it "crunchy water" because iceberg lettuce doesn't have much more than the nutritional equivalence of water. It's then covered with a lot of high-fat, high calorie dressing and other high-fat toppings which usually adds about 300 calories for just a small salad!

If you're eating salad just to help meet your daily veggie requirement, and you just can't eat it without drowning it in dressing, consider skipping it. You won't be missing many nutrients, and you'll save a lot of fat and calories.

Be Assertive

When ordering, be assertive about what changes you want. Emphasize key phrases such as *luncheon portion, on the side, half the sauce*, or *without butter*. Then, don't be afraid to send it back if it doesn't come the way you requested.

If that makes you uncomfortable, think about this: if you went to the store and asked for a size nine pair of shoes and they gave you a size twelve instead, wouldn't you send it back? Why should ordering food be any different?

It's OK to Play with your Food

If the food delivered to your table does not comply with your special request and you do not want to wait for another dish to be prepared, feel free to play with your food. Using your knife, wipe off the extra sauce or cheese, trim away the fat, or remove the skin off your chicken. Pour the sauce off your dinner plate and onto an empty bread plate. Use a paper napkin to blot away the extra fat on your slice of pizza. And go ahead and remove the top of the bun, if it's just too much bread.

Know Thyself

The average serving of fast food fries is 300-400 calories. And, let's face it, unless you're running marathons, those calories along with your sandwich is probably more than your body needs. Think about throwing half the fast food french fries away before you get to your table so there's no temptation to eat them all.

"Waste" is Better than "Waist"

Even when you can't take the extra food home, don't feel the need to "clean your plate." No matter what Mom told you, the starving children in Africa (or Asia or wherever she told you), won't benefit from your overeating. You can either *waste* it in the trash can or *waist* it around your middle. The choice is yours!

Bag It

Since most restaurants serve twice as much food as your body needs, it's best to ask for a doggie bag as soon as you get your dinner. Put half of the dinner in the doggie bag for tomorrow's lunch. "Out of sight, out of mind" really helps!

Studies conducted by Brian Wansink, Ph.D. (professor and Director of the Cornell Food & Brand Lab and author of *Mindless Eat-*

ing: Why We Eat More Than We Think) indicate the more we are served, the more we eat – and it is totally unconscious. Chances are you're eating more than you think when movie theatres serve popcorn in a bucket and restaurants serve food on platters instead of plates. So, bag up half!

Stand Up and Lose Weight

Have you ever stood up at the end of the meal and all of a sudden felt this uncomfortable, overfull sensation in your stomach? Since it takes 20 minutes for the stomach to tell the brain that it is full we often don't feel fullness until it is too late.

That's why it's so important to eat slowly so your brain has time to do its job. Or do as my daughter suggests, "Stand up and lose weight." Don't wait until the end of the meal to find out if you're full. Part way through the meal, stand up (maybe it's time to excuse yourself to the bathroom). How do you feel? Think about eating just until you feel "fine," not full or overstuffed. By that time, you've probably eaten more than your body needs.

Resist the Temptation

Does just *seeing* certain foods prompt you to eat? If so, remember the "Law of Proximity" and keep food reminders to a minimum. This may sound difficult in a restaurant, but here are some ideas:

- **Keep your distance.** Stay away from all-you-can-eat buffets or at least don't sit *next* to the buffet. And ask for a table away from the steady wait staff traffic bringing tempting dishes from the kitchen.

- **Take a taste.** To prevent nibbling on the free refill basket of bread or chips, take a few chips or a small roll and relinquish the rest to the server, or at least have it moved outside your reach.

- **Avoid temptation.** Hand the drink menu back to the server if they are not on your plan. And ask the server not to bring the dessert cart to the table. Do you really need the temptation?

Think Before You Drink

To quench your thirst (and help fill you up), always have a calorie-free beverage such as water, mineral water, club soda, unsweetened iced tea, diet soda, or hot tea or coffee nearby. For variety, make your own table-side diet lemonade by adding a few packets of sweetener to a glass of ice water with a lot of fresh-squeezed lemon.

Think before you order calorie-laden beverages such as sweet tea, fountain drinks, alcohol, and coffee beverages. Research shows that the body doesn't seem to register the calories in liquids. They fill you *out* without filling you *up*.

Create Closure

Most of us need a signal that the meal is over. For many of us, it's when the food is gone and the plate is empty. But since restaurants serve more than most of us need, using the empty plate as a signal is a sure prescription for weight gain. Other closure signals could include:

- **Out of sight.** If you're not taking your leftovers home, ask your server to remove your plate so you won't be tempted to keep nibbling.

- **Out of reach.** If the server is nowhere around, push your plate away, make your food unpalatable with excess salt or hot sauce, or place your napkin over the plate.

- **Make it hot.** Sip coffee or hot tea; use this activity as your signal that the meal is over.

- **Freshen your breath.** Bring a mint or piece of hard candy or gum to clear your palate.

- **Push away from the table.** Excuse yourself to the rest room and brush your teeth.

PART 2

Meal Specifics

Breakfast

Most of us are off and running in the morning, and that often means no time for breakfast. Perhaps you're thinking, "No problem. If I don't eat in the morning I'll have more calories to spend later in the day, right"?

WRONG! Research evidence indicates that people who skip breakfast eat larger meals later in the day when their bodies are the least active. In addition, skipping breakfast may actually lower your metabolic rate - which means you're burning fewer calories. Bottomline: breakfast skippers tend to be more overweight than those who eat breakfast.

When you skip breakfast, you are telling your body that you are still fasting from the night before. This will signal a lowering of your metabolism throughout the day. Breakfast literally means "Break Fast"– the meal that breaks your fast.

Our weekends can be equally disastrous if we sit down to a more leisurely BIG breakfast or brunch. These meals are often loaded in fat and calories. This might be alright if we were to "eat breakfast like a king, lunch like a prince, and dinner like a pauper." But how many of us eat dinner like a pauper? Most of us do not!

Even if it's just eaten once a week, the traditional large bacon, eggs, and biscuit meal can put on excessive unwanted pounds, due to the high caloric content of these foods. Check out this breakfast meal: bacon & cheese omelet with hashbrowns, one biscuit with butter and jam, and a small glass of orange juice.

Want to guess the calories? If you guessed 1300 calories, you're right. It also contains as much fat as an entire stick of butter!

What should you eat for breakfast? While some enjoy a fiber-rich bowl of oatmeal and fresh fruit, others prefer a protein-rich meal of eggs (egg substitutes are much leaner). Research demonstrates that both fiber and protein help to fill you up more than a refined carbohydrate-only meal such as pancakes. The rest of this chapter contains specific breakfast suggestions on how to cut back on calories while getting the morning energy boost you deserve.

Fruits & Fruit Juices

• **Fill up on fresh fruit.** Fresh fruits are virtually fat-free. They're also high in filling fiber and rich in vitamins and minerals. For a nutrient boost, think about ordering fresh fruit as a topping for pancakes or waffles, instead of the usual butter and syrup.

• **Dried fruit can be more caloric.** Dried fruit has exactly as many calories as the fruit they are derived from. So, a single raisin has as many calories as a grape. But because much of the water is removed, it is easier to eat more raisins than fresh grapes.

• **Fruit juice has as many calories as soda.** It's true. Ounce-for-ounce, fruit juice has the same amount of calories as most sugar-sweetened sodas. Sure, 100% fruit juice has more nutrients, but fluids don't fill us up like food does. If you are watching your weight, it's probably wiser to enjoy the high fiber benefits of fresh fruit instead of the fruit juice.

Cereal & Milk

• **Go with nonfat milk.** Request nonfat (or at least lowfat milk) as a stand alone beverage - or in your coffee drinks and cereal.

• **Limit the granola.** Sounds healthy, but most commercial varieties are loaded with fats and sugar, and may contain as much as 250 calories in a small ½ cup portion. Yikes!

• **Plain oatmeal is a great choice.** A serving contains 3g fiber to keep you satisfied all morning long. Birchermuesli is a cold cereal prepared with oats, fruits, nuts, and *cream*. Some restaurants use nonfat plain yogurt in its preparation so it is healthy, but most restaurants still prepare it in the traditional high-fat, Swiss manner using heavy cream or half & half. Ask before ordering this item.

• **Sugar has 16 calories per teaspoon.** Doesn't sound like too much? But if you eat just 16 calories a day *more* than your body needs, you'll put on an extra 1½ pounds each year! If you want to try your cereal without the sugar, remember that it may take a couple of weeks for your taste buds to make the adjustment. You could also choose to try a sugar substitute.

Breakfast Breads & Spreads

Nearly every breakfast includes some type of bread. Some are more caloric than others. Here are some suggestions to help you from blowing your calorie budget.

• **Stick with toast and English muffins.** Biscuits and croissants are significantly higher in fat and calories.

• **Bagels are really big.** Each one contains 350-450 calories. And, that's without any butter or cream cheese. Maybe just a half would be enough?

• **Order your toast "dry."** This way you can decide how much of the toppings to add and when you do, use them sparingly.

• **Vegetable oil is healthier than animal fat.** Soft margarine and vegetable oil have as many calories as butter, but butter contains unhealthy fats including cholesterol and saturated fats. Stick margarines contain unhealthy trans fat, while most spreadable margarines have negligible amounts. So stick with a vegetable oil or soft margarine. Like all other non-animal foods, vegetable margarine and oil contain no cholesterol.

• **Think jam or jelly.** A thin layer of jelly or jam has fewer calories and fat than a comparable portion of butter or margarine. And let's face it, chances are you're consuming plenty of fat in the rest of your breakfast.

• **Watch the cream cheese.** A thin, two tablespoon smear could add on 100 calories!

Breakfast Sandwiches

• **Choose an English muffin or a small wrap.** These are generally lower calorie choices than a croissant or biscuit. While bagels are lowfat, they're also big - which means more calories.

• **Try bacon or ham, instead of sausage.** When added to an egg sandwich, bacon or ham will save you more than 100 calories over a sausage addition. Yes, bacon is just as fatty as sausage but the portion size is much smaller.

Eggs

Eggs are a good source of protein. One egg has as much protein as an ounce of meat. While egg whites have no fat or cholesterol, an egg yolk contains 5g fat and 270 mg cholesterol. Keep these tips in mind:

• **Request egg substitutes instead of eggs.** Many restaurants will prepare your order with "egg whites only" or with egg substitutes (at about ⅓ calories and no fat), even if it is not on the menu! This includes omelets, frittatas, and possibly even French toast. Egg substitutes are colored and flavored egg whites. If you have not tried them recently, their taste has greatly improved over the years. Try them again!

• **Request a nonstick spray** (or "very little butter/oil"). Otherwise, cooks may use more than 100 calories of butter or oil to prepare your eggs. Most restaurants have the spray available for baking and will use it while preparing your meal.

Other Protein Sources

Protein helps to fill you up and stabilize your blood sugar. Remember to include a protein source at breakfast, not just lunch and dinner. You don't need much at each meal - only about as much as the size of a deck of cards, or the size and thickness of the palm of your hand (fingers not included).

• **Some meats have more fat than others.** For animal protein, keep in mind that ham, Canadian bacon, or smoked salmon are lower in fat than sausage. Bacon doesn't have much protein -

more than 70% of its calories come from fat! Though if you're satisfied with just a couple of strips of crispy bacon, that's under 100 calories. Keep in mind that all these breakfast meats are high in sodium.

• **Don't forget non-meat proteins.** Other breakfast proteins include beans, cottage cheese, aged cheese, or yogurt. Greek yogurt has twice as much protein as other yogurt. Select lowfat choices to cut calories.

Breakfast Potatoes and Alternatives

• **Big is better than shreds.** Even if they don't look it, breakfast potatoes are usually fried. If you must, consider ordering the larger cut home fries instead of the shredded hashbrowns. The smaller the pieces, the more fat will be absorbed.

• **Request sliced tomatoes instead of hashbrowns.** Tomatoes go great with eggs - and have negligible calories.

• **Think fruit.** Your server may also permit fresh fruit instead of potatoes - ask!

Pancakes, Waffles, & French Toast

• **Buttermilk pancakes are as caloric as sliced bread.** A slice of sandwich bread contains about 75 calories so a pancake about the same size has about 75 calories as well. But that pancake is actually as big as your plate, isn't it? Before you eat all three plate-size pancakes, count on 200-250 calories each.

• **Whole grain pancakes are more caloric.** Sure, they may contain more fiber. But whole grain pancakes are heavier and usually contain more fat (especially if they contain nuts) than the white variety. Consider that before you add the butter!

• **Belgian waffles are twice as tall as a pancake.** That means a waffle that looks the size of *three* slices or bread, probably contain the calories of *six* slices of bread. Oh, correction...make that six slices of *buttered* bread. Do you need to eat it all?

• **Ask for the nonstick spray.** Restaurants procure nonstick spray to prepare waffles, muffins, and other baked goods. Request the spray to be used for the pancakes and French toast as well.

- **Stay away from deep-fried French toast.** That is unless you can "afford" a breakfast with more than 1000 calories (and that's even before you add the syrup).

- **Go smaller.** Consider ordering a short stack of pancakes instead of the typical. And order the pancakes, waffles, or French toast without the added bacon or sausage. Smaller plate, smaller waist.

- **Request the French toast to be prepared with an egg substitute.** This substitution is not available for pancakes since the batter is usually prepared in advance.

- **Specify "no butter, powdered sugar, fruit toppings, or whipped cream on top."** These additions are what transform pancakes and waffles into nutritional disasters. Applesauce, sprinkled cinnamon, and fresh fruit make delicious, lower calorie toppings.

- **Use a minimal amount of butter and syrup.** Butter contains about 100 calories per tablespoon, and syrup has approximately 50 calories per tablespoon. In other words, the butter and syrup could easily *double* the calories of your pancakes! Most restaurants have diet syrup (about 10 calories per tablespoon). If your taste buds are not yet ready for the diet syrup, try mixing the regular and the diet together in a small bowl.

Nutrition Information

Fruit/Vegetable Juice, 6oz small (DOUBLE for 12oz large):	Calories	Fat (g)	Sat+Trans Fat (g)	Sodium (mg)	Carbohydrates (g)	Fiber (g)	Protein (g)
Apple Juice	85	0	0	15	21	0	0
Cranberry Juice	110	0	0	10	28	0	0
Grape Juice	120	0	0	5	30	0	0
Grapefruit Juice	70	0	0	0	17	0	0
Orange Juice	85	0	0	0	21	0	0
Prune Juice	130	0	0	10	32	2	0
Tomato Juice	40	0	0	490	10	2	0
Apple Juice, 7oz box	90	0	0	15	23	0	0
Fresh/Canned Fruit:							
Apple, whole medium	70	0	0	0	19	3	0
Apple, thick slice	15	0	0	0	4	<1	0
Applesauce, 2 Tbsp	25	0	0	10	6	<1	0
Applesauce, ½ cup	100	0	0	35	25	<1	0
Banana, 1 (7")	105	0	0	0	27	3	0

	Calories	Fat (g)	Sat+Trans Fat (g)	Sodium (mg)	Carbohydrates (g)	Fiber (g)	Protein (g)
Fresh/Canned Fruit (cont.):							
Banana/Strawberry Medley, ½ cup	110	1	0	5	22	2	0
Blueberries, ¼ cup	20	0	0	0	5	1	0
Cantaloupe, diced, ½ cup	25	0	0	15	7	1	0
Cantaloupe, 1 slice	10	0	0	5	3	<1	0
Fig, 1 fresh	40	0	0	0	10	2	0
Figs canned in heavy syrup, 3	85	<1	0	3	19	2	0
Fresh Fruit Chunks, ½ cup	60	0	0	2	15	2	0
Fruit Cocktail, heavy syrup, ½ cup	100	0	0	10	24	1	0
Glacéd Fruit, ¼ cup	50	0	0	5	12	0	0
Grapes, 25 small (1 cup)	60	0	0	0	16	<1	0
Grapefruit, ½ medium	60	0	0	0	16	6	0
Grapefruit, juice packed, ½ cup	45	0	0	10	11	<1	0
Honeydew, slice	15	0	0	10	11	1	0
Kiwi, 1 fresh	45	0	0	0	11	3	0
Mandarin Oranges in syrup, ½ cup	80	0	0	10	19	1	0
Mango, ½ cup sliced	55	0	0	0	14	2	0
Melon Balls, 1 cup	60	0	0	55	14	1	0
Nectarine, 1 medium	60	0	0	0	14	3	0
Orange, 1 medium	70	0	0	0	18	3	0
Peach, 1 medium fresh	40	0	0	0	9	2	0
Peaches, sliced & drained, ½ cup	100	0	0	10	24	1	0
Pears, 1 medium	100	0	0	0	26	5	0
Pears, ½ cup canned	60	0	0	5	16	2	0
Pineapple, slice	20	0	0	0	7	<1	0
Pineapple, ½ cup diced	35	0	0	0	10	1	0
Plum, 1 medium	30	0	0	0	8	1	0
Prunes, canned, 1	20	0	0	0	7	<1	0
Strawberries, 1	4	0	0	0	1	0	0
½ cup sliced	25	0	0	0	6	2	0
Tangerine, ea	50	0	0	0	13	2	0
Watermelon, diced, 1 cup	50	0	0	0	11	<1	0
Watermelon, 1 slice	10	0	0	0	2	0	0
Dried Fruit:							
Apricots, dried, 7 halves	60	0	0	0	15	2	0
Dates, dried, 3	70	0	0	0	17	2	0
Figs, dried, 2	90	0	0	5	20	3	0
Peaches, dried, 2 halves	60	0	0	0	15	2	0
Pears, dried, 2 halves	90	0	0	0	23	3	0
Prunes, dried, 3	60	0	0	0	15	2	0
Raisins, 2 Tbsp	60	0	0	0	15	<1	0

	Calories	Fat (g)	Sat+Trans Fat (g)	Sodium (mg)	Carbohydrates (g)	Fiber (g)	Protein (g)
Cold Cereals:							
Birchermuesli, ½ cup	175	13	2	210	13	3	4
Cheerios, 1 cup	110	2	0	215	22	4	3
Corn Flakes, 1 cup	100	0	0	200	24	<1	2
Granola, ½ cup	225	9	4	20	34	3	3
Raisin Bran, 1 cup	195	2	0	360	47	7	5
Shredded Wheat, minis, 1 cup	170	<1	0	5	41	6	4
Sweet Puff Cereal, 1 cup	120	1	0	150	26	<1	2
Wheat Flake Cereal, 1 cup	130	1	0	290	32	7	3
Hot Cereals:							
Oatmeal, ½ cup	75	1	0	190	13	2	3
Grits, unbuttered, ½ cup	75	<1	0	300	18	<1	2
Grits, ½ cup w/1 tsp margarine	120	6	<1	420	17	<1	2
Toppings:							
Sugar, 1 tsp	16	0	0	0	4	0	0
Brown Sugar, 1 Tbsp	32	0	0	5	8	0	0
Milk (1 cup):							
Whole Milk	150	8	5	120	12	0	8
2% Lowfat Milk	120	5	3	100	12	0	9
Nonfat or Skim Milk	90	0	0	100	12	0	9
Toast (1 slice w/o butter):							
Pumpernickel	80	1	0	215	15	2	2
Rye, deli slice	130	2	0	380	25	2	5
Sourdough, deli slice	130	2	0	290	25	3	5
Wheat	65	1	0	130	12	1	3
White	70	1	0	135	14	<1	2
Other Breakfast Breads (w/o spread):							
Bagel, medium-sized	220	2	0	380	43	2	9
large deli-sized	330	2	0	570	65	3	13
Biscuit, 3" diameter	250	11	7	675	31	1	5
large deli-sized	300	14	10	800	37	2	6
Croissant, medium	270	17	4	260	27	0	5
English muffin, standard	130	1	0	210	26	2	5
thick gourmet	195	2	0	320	39	2	7
Breakfast Sweets:							
Chocolate croissant	370	23	8	260	40	1	5
Cinnamon roll (medium fast-food-size)	225	10	2	230	31	2	3
large (mall-sized)	880	40	10	900	120	5	12

	Calories	Fat (g)	Sat+Trans Fat (g)	Sodium (mg)	Carbohydrates (g)	Fiber (g)	Protein (g)
Breakfast Sweets (cont.):							
Doughnut, cake (compact) or 5 holes	320	22	10	330	33	1	3
glazed, raised (fluffier) or 8 holes	260	14	6	250	31	1	3
raised and frosted	270	15	7	260	31	1	3
filled w/jelly or 8 holes	290	14	7	280	36	1	3
filled w/Bavarian crème	270	15	7	280	31	1	4
filled w/chocolate crème	370	21	10	370	42	1	4
frosted cake	370	24	11	400	33	1	3
Muffin, mini (1oz)	110	5	1	110	13	<1	2
tennis-ball-sized (3oz)	330	15	3	330	39	2	4
softball-sized (5oz)	550	25	5	550	65	3	9
Spreads:							
Butter, 1 tsp	35	4	3	25	0	0	0
Cream Cheese, 1 Tbsp	50	5	3	45	0	0	0
Honey, 1 tsp	20	0	0	0	6	0	0
Jelly, Jam, or Marmalade, 1 Tbsp	50	0	0	5	14	0	0
Margarine, soft,1 tsp	35	4	1	35	0	0	0
Eggs:							
Egg, poached or boiled, 1	75	5	2	100	0	0	7
Egg, fried, 1	120	11	3	100	0	0	7
Egg whites, 2	32	35	0	110	1	0	7
Scrambled Eggs w/butter (2), ½ cup	190	13	4	300	2	0	14
Egg Substitutes w/margarine, ½ cup	110	5	1	300	2	0	14
Egg Dishes:							
Eggs Benedict, 2 egg w/English muffin	860	56	23	1945	55	3	20
Vegetable Frittata w/2 eggs	250	22	6	300	5	0	15
Sausage Frittata w/2 eggs	325	33	9	600	0	0	21
Quiche Lorraine, ¹/₆ pie	525	41	19	220	25	1	20
Quiche Florentine, ¹/₆ pie	450	34	16	145	21	1	17
Quiche, ham & cheese, ¹/₆ pie	475	35	16	470	34	1	18
Omelets (3 egg):							
Plain	325	27	12	515	1	0	21
Bacon & Cheese	535	43	21	1435	5	0	31
Cheese	450	36	18	1060	5	0	29
Ham & Cheese	475	37	18	1385	6	0	35
Mushroom & Cheese	525	44	23	1115	6	0	30
Southwest w/sausage & cheese	600	47	21	1370	5	0	36

	Calories	Fat (g)	Sat+Trans Fat (g)	Sodium (mg)	Carbohydrates (g)	Fiber (g)	Protein (g)
Egg Sandwiches:							
Egg on Biscuit:	420	28	16	900	31	1	12
w/cheese	470	31	19	1130	33	1	17
w/bacon and cheese	530	36	20	1375	33	1	19
w/ham and cheese	500	32	19	1450	34	1	20
w/sausage and cheese	620	42	22	1435	33	1	21
Egg on Croissant:	450	34	13	480	27	0	12
w/cheese	500	37	16	710	29	0	17
w/bacon and cheese	560	42	17	960	30	0	19
w/ham and cheese	525	38	16	1035	30	0	20
w/sausage and cheese	650	48	19	1020	29	0	21
Egg on Large Deli Bagel:	510	19	9	790	65	3	20
w/cheese	630	28	15	1340	69	3	27
w/bacon and cheese	690	33	17	1590	70	3	29
w/ham and cheese	660	29	15	1660	70	3	32
w/sausage and cheese	780	40	18	1645	69	3	35
Egg on standard English Muffin:	310	18	9	430	26	2	12
w/cheese	360	21	12	660	28	2	17
w/bacon and cheese	420	26	13	910	28	2	20
w/ham and cheese	390	22	12	985	29	2	22
w/sausage and cheese	510	32	15	968	28	2	24
Breakfast Meats:							
Bacon, 1 slice	35	3	1	125	0	0	2
Canadian-style Bacon, 1 slice	45	2	<1	400	<1	0	6
Country Ham, 2oz	60	2	<1	750	<1	0	6
Smoked Salmon, 1oz	40	2	0	335	0	0	5
Sausage, 1oz patty	100	8	5	350	1	0	4
Sausage, link	52	5	2	105	<1	0	2
Breakfast Potatoes:							
Hashbrowns, ¾ cup	350	23	10	560	35	3	3
Home fries (bigger chunks), ¾ cup	250	18	8	400	20	2	3
Pancakes (4" diameter):							
Buttermilk Pancakes, 2oz	110	3	0	460	16	<1	3
Buckwheat Pancakes, 2½ oz	135	5	0	370	18	2	5
Wholegrain Nut Pancake, 2½ oz	160	7	0	390	18	2	6
Waffles:							
Toaster-size, 4" X 4" X ½"	100	3	<1	230	15	1	2
Regular Waffle, 4oz	300	15	1	460	31	3	7
Belgian Waffle, 6oz (7" round & thick)	400	20	2	900	59	2	10
Wholegrain Nut Belgium Waffle, 7"	460	25	3	1000	60	3	12

	Calories	Fat (g)	Sat+Trans Fat (g)	Sodium (mg)	Carbohydrates (g)	Fiber (g)	Protein (g)
French Toast:							
Regular-sized Bread, 1 slice	125	4	1	210	15	1	5
Thick-sized Bread, 1 slice	250	12	1	315	22	2	8
Deep-fried Toast Sticks, order	450	24	5	475	47	3	7
Sauces & Toppings:							
Applesauce, ¼ cup	50	0	0	2	3	<1	0
Butter, 1 Tbsp	110	12	8	75	0	0	0
Diet Syrup, ¼ cup	10	0	0	6	2	0	0
Fruit Flavored Syrup, ¼ cup	55	0	0	0	14	0	0
Fruit Topping, ¼ cup	100	0	0	11	25	0	0
Jelly, Jam, or Marmalade, 1 Tbsp	50	0	0	3	14	0	0
Maple Flavored Syrup, ¼ cup	200	0	0	65	49	0	0
Margarine, 1 Tbsp	100	11	2	100	0	0	0
Powdered Sugar, 1 Tbsp	30	0	0	0	8	0	0
Whipped Butter, 1 Tbsp	70	7	5	75	0	0	0
Whipped Margarine, 1 Tbsp	70	7	3	85	0	0	0
Powdered Sugar, 1 Tbsp	70	7	0	70	0	0	0
Whipped Cream, ¼ cup	105	11	7	10	1	0	0
Whipped Topping, ¼ cup	40	3	2	20	2	0	0

Pizza

I love pizza! And pizza can easily fit into a healthy eating program if you balance out the meal. Fill up with a green salad with minimal dressing (or grab a piece of fruit before the pizza arrives). Then, select your pizza wisely using these guidelines:

Crust

Pizza crust is generally low in fat and calories. Consisting of mostly flour, yeast, and water, pizza crust has approximately the same amount of fat and calories as white bread (ounce-for-ounce).

•**Choose pizzas cooked in the old-fashioned pizza ovens.** When using the old-fashioned pizza ovens, the pizza is simply placed on the floor of the oven and baked. The newer conveyor belt ovens (used by most pizza chains) use a higher temperature. With a higher temperature, the pizza will cook faster, but will require extra fat in the dough to do so. Thus, pizzas cooked in the conveyor belt ovens are generally higher in calories and fat than pizzas made in the old-fashioned pizza ovens. Hint: if you pinch the crust and oil oozes out (or leaves an oil spot on the box), it is not a lean crust.

•**Go with thin or regular crust pizza** rather than pan pizza (deep dish). If you're watching calories or carbs, you might want to select thin crust pizzas. It makes sense that pan pizzas have more calories than thin, or even regular crust pizza. But, interestingly, thin crust pizzas tend to have as much (or *more)* fat than the regular crust pizza! While thin and regular crust pizzas are cooked on a flat pan or screen, pan pizzas are cooked (or shall I say, "fried") in well-greased pans.

- **Leave the stuffed crust pizzas alone**...unless you're willing to stop at just one slice!

- **Don't eat the whole pizza!** For most of us, one, two or maybe three slices of pizza are adequate for our calorie needs. If you have a hard time stopping at just a few slices, buy a small enough pizza so there are no extra slices to tempt you.

Sauce

- **Tomato pizza sauce is low in fat**; the white cream sauce tends to be higher. Barbecue sauce is also low in calories, but contains additional sugar. Pesto sauce is one of the highest calorie sauces because it's almost pure oil.

- **Consider asking for "no oil on the crust."** Although not common in pizza parlors, some of the upscale restaurants brush the crust with oil before adding the sauce, or in place of the tomato sauce. Request that oil not be added if they use more than a thin brushing (you can tell because it leaves oil on the plate, your fingers, and more). Do you really need all that oil in addition to the fat in the cheese and meat toppings? No!

Cheese & Other Toppings

Nutritionally, pizza crust is about the same as white bread. What can make pizza fattening are the toppings and, of course, eating too many slices. Here are some general tips to guide you:

- **Cheese is high in fat.** Mozzarella cheese is the most frequently used cheese, but provolone and feta cheese are also used. Each of these cheeses contain about 6-8g fat per ounce; each pizza slice has roughly 1oz cheese.

- **Do not order extra (or double) cheese.** "Extra cheese" increases the calories by another 30 calories per slice (at least).

- **Dab your pizza with a paper napkin.** Feel free to blot off the melted fat that oozes from your pizza. Depending on the toppings, you can easily blot off 25-50 calories per slice. Every calorie counts!

• **Try pizza prepared "light on the cheese"** or even without cheese. If your favorite part of the pizza is the crust, consider requesting your pizza to be prepared "light on the cheese." You'll save about 50-60 calories a slice! Managers say that requesting less cheese has become a frequent request.

• **Add fruits and veggies.** Onions, mushrooms, green/red/ yellow peppers, broccoli, tomatoes, roasted pepper, spinach, and pineapple are healthful and low-calorie. Although they add 1-2g fat per pizza slice, olives are a smart choice because they contain a healthy type of fat (monounsaturated).

• **Choose the leanest protein toppings.** These include grilled chicken, ham, Canadian bacon, tuna, crabmeat, fresh fish, and shrimp. Each will add only 1-2g fat per slice. Hamburger meat will add a bit more. Piling on the high fat toppings such as pepperoni, bacon, sausage, and extra cheese can add another 100 calories per slice!

• **Watching sodium?** If so, limit the pepperoni, ham, sausage, olives, banana peppers, bacon, and jalapeno peppers. Each addition can add on another 60-190mg sodium per pizza slice.

Nutrition Information for Pizza by the Slice

Nutrition information for the most popular pizza restaurants can be found in Part 3 of this book. In the case that your favorite pizza restaurant is not featured, use the pictures on the next two pages to estimate the size of your slice. Then check out the chart on the last two pages of this chapter for estimated nutrition information.

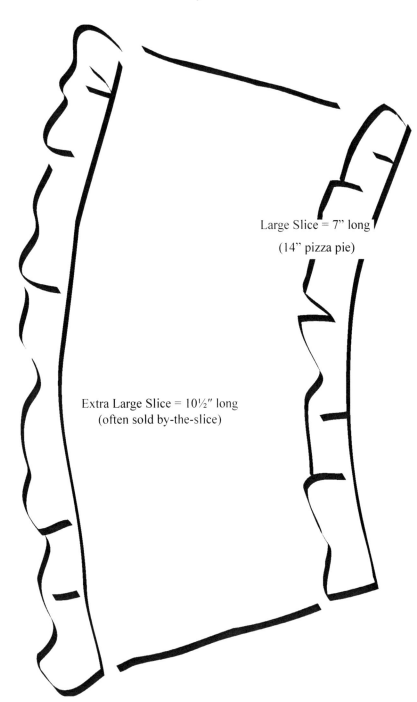

Large Slice = 7" long
(14" pizza pie)

Extra Large Slice = 10½″ long
(often sold by-the-slice)

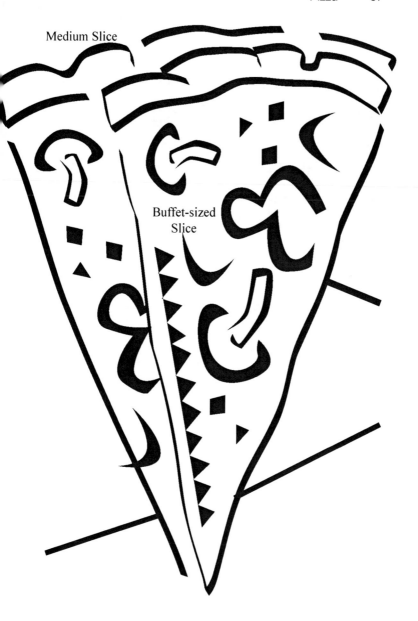

Medium Slice

Buffet-sized
Slice

Nutrition Information

	Calories	Fat (g)	Sat+Trans Fat (g)	Sodium (mg)	Carbohydrates (g)	Fiber (g)	Protein (g)
Buffet-Size Slice (thin crust):							
Cheese only or w/fruit/veggie toppings	120	6	2	280	12	<1	4
Ham & Pineapple (Hawaiian)	135	6	2	350	13	<1	6
Pepperoni	150	9	3	370	13	<1	6
Sausage	160	10	4	370	14	<1	6
Double Cheese	135	10	4	435	13	<1	5
Everything or more than 1 meat	170	10	4	435	13	<1	6
Buffet-Size Slice (regular crust):							
Cheese only or w/fruit/veggie toppings	155	6	2	350	20	1	6
Ham & Pineapple (Hawaiian)	170	6	2	420	21	1	7
Pepperoni	185	9	3	450	21	1	7
Sausage	195	10	4	450	21	1	7
Double Cheese	170	8	3	410	20	1	7
Everything or more than 1 meat	205	10	4	510	21	1	7
Medium Slice (thin crust):							
Cheese only or w/fruit/veggie toppings	185	11	5	280	16	1	6
Ham & Pineapple (Hawaiian)	200	11	5	330	17	0	7
Pepperoni	230	15	6	350	16	1	7
Sausage	225	16	6	350	17	1	7
Double Cheese	210	13	6	325	16	1	7
Everything or more than 1 meat	230	16	6	400	17	1	9
Medium Slice (regular crust):							
Cheese only or w/fruit/veggie toppings	220	9	4	560	26	1	8
Ham & Pineapple (Hawaiian)	240	9	4	660	28	1	9
Pepperoni	270	13	5	690	27	1	9
Sausage	280	13	6	690	28	1	9
Double Cheese	250	11	5	650	27	1	9
Everything or more than 1 meat	290	13	6	810	28	1	11
Large Slice (thin crust):							
Cheese only or w/fruit/veggie toppings	260	14	6	350	24	1	9
Ham & Pineapple (Hawaiian)	290	14	6	420	26	1	10
Pepperoni	315	21	8	450	26	2	10
Sausage	330	22	9	450	26	1	10
Double Cheese	290	18	7	410	25	1	10
Everything or more than 1 meat	350	24	9	500	26	1	12

	Calories	Fat (g)	Sat+Trans Fat (g)	Sodium (mg)	Carbohydrates (g)	Fiber (g)	Protein (g)
Large Slice (regular crust):							
Cheese only or w/fruit/veggie toppings	310	12	5	700	39	2	11
Ham & Pineapple (Hawaiian)	340	12	5	840	41	2	13
Pepperoni	370	18	7	890	41	3	13
Sausage	390	19	8	890	41	3	13
Double Cheese	340	15	6	820	40	2	13
Everything or more than 1 meat	410	20	8	1020	41	2	15
Large Slice (deep dish/pan):							
Cheese only or w/fruit/veggie toppings	350	16	7	810	41	3	14
Ham & Pineapple (Hawaiian)	375	16	7	950	43	3	16
Pepperoni	415	20	9	1000	43	4	16
Sausage	425	21	9	1000	43	3	16
Double Cheese	375	17	8	930	42	3	16
Everything or more than 1 meat	445	24	9	1130	43	3	18
Extra Large Slice (regular crust):							
Cheese only or w/fruit/veggie toppings	550	21	8	1230	68	4	20
Ham & Pineapple (Hawaiian)	590	21	8	1470	72	4	24
Pepperoni	650	30	12	1560	72	5	24
Sausage	685	33	13	1560	71	4	24
Double Cheese	600	25	11	1440	70	4	24
Everything or more than 1 meat	720	35	14	1790	70	4	28

Burgers & More

Yes, you really can eat healthy at a fast food restaurant, and grilled chicken sandwiches and salads are not your only options. There are veggie burgers, baked potatoes, chili, grilled chicken pieces with mashed potatoes, as well as subs filled with roast beef, turkey, and ham. And, yes, even a burger every now and then. Here are some specific suggestions:

Burgers & Other Fast Food Sandwiches

Burgers can fit into a healthy diet as long as you consider the portion size, the toppings, and, of course, how often you eat them.

- **Order the smallest burger available.** A plain, kid-sized burger on a bun (without any cheese or toppings) is about 250-300 calories. A plain ¼ pound burger weighs in at around 450 calories, a ⅓ pound burger starts at 600 calories and a ½ pound burger starts at 850 calories. Oh, and that triple patty burger? It's well in excess of 1000 calories!

- **Request the hamburger buns to be grilled without butter or oil.** While fast food restaurants may lightly spray the buns, many upscale burger restaurants liberally brush the buns with butter or oil before grilling them. At some restaurants, this practice can add up to an additional 100 calories. You won't miss the taste if you ask them to grill it dry.

- **Ask for the burger to be prepared well done.** The more you cook the burger, the less fat remains. And cooked meat is also safer than raw or rare meat.

- **Grilled chicken sandwiches or veggie burgers are also good options.** Keep in mind, though, that a *large* grilled chicken sandwich could have more calories than a *small* hamburger.

- **Limit the high-fat toppings.** Sure they add flavor, but each of these toppings adds on another 100 calories: sauteed mushrooms or onions, one slice of cheese, three crisp bacon slices, ¼ avocado, or a tablespoon of mayonnaise.

- **Use mustard instead of mayonnaise.** While some restaurants are offering lowfat mayonnaise, very few restaurants have the fat-free version. Choose mustard instead of mayonnaise for a flavorful, low-calorie option. Other lowfat dressings include salsa, picante sauce, ketchup, BBQ sauce, and fat-free salad dressing.

- **Select low-calorie toppings** including lettuce, tomato, and raw (not sauteed) onion.

- **Consider choosing turkey, roast beef, or ham sandwiches.** Most of us recognize turkey as a lean meat, but did you know roast beef and ham are often lean, too? The secret to selecting a lower calorie sandwich is to keep the sandwich small and use mustard or lowfat dressing instead of mayonnaise.

- **Choose a pita or wrap instead of a sandwich bun.** Some restaurants serve very large portions of bread which ends up boosting the calories of the sandwich in the 600-800 calorie range. Consider having the sandwich made into a wrap (if it's offered). The wrap is often lower in calories. Don't forget to choose lean meats and limited amounts of cheese and dressing. Grab 'n go offerings at airports often include wraps oozing with dressing. Feel free to ask for a freshly-made wrap without dressing.

- **Avoid fried chicken and fried fish sandwiches.** Sure, chicken and fish are healthier than ground beef, but not if they are fried! Chicken and fish sandwiches described as "crispy," are fried and often have twice as many calories and fat than a burger.

Other Fast Food Meals

- **Skinless, roasted chicken has less than half the fat and calories of fried chicken.** Fried chicken contains more fat than is readily apparent. Many fats, especially the saturated fats, solidify after cooking and don't look greasy. A wiser choice is to select roasted chicken and remove the skin (you will save another 80 calories).

- **Select grilled chicken salad with lowfat dressing** - and limit the toppings. If bacon, cheese, avocado, nuts, and salad dressing are added, they can more than double the calories. Decide what toppings you *must* have.

- **Broiled fish, roasted chicken, and turkey lunches are both lowfat and filling.** As an alternative to a sandwich, consider a full meal consisting of rice or potatoes, as well as vegetables. A full meal may contain fewer calories than a sandwich.

- **Ask for the stuffed potatoes to be prepared without butter.** Potatoes, by themselves, contain only negligible amounts of fat but are rich in vitamins, minerals, and fiber. If you are thinking of a huge, stuffed baked potato, keep the meal healthy by adding only lean meats, vegetables, and lowfat toppings. Specialty potato restaurants offer broth as an alternative to butter; they may also offer fat-free sour cream and cheese.

- **Act like a kid.** Fast food meals get bigger every year. Why not order a kid's meal instead? The calories are more in line with what most adults need. While the traditional kid's meal consisted of burger, fries, and soda, today's options are more expanded. Many fast food restaurants now allow juice or milk instead of soda, and fruit as a substitute for fries (at no additional cost). Take a look at the kid's meal choices at the end of this chapter.

French Fries & Onion Rings

Did you know that French fries and onion rings are more than 50% fat? Many people, focusing more on their wallet than their waist line, order a combination meal that includes a sandwich, medium or large fries, and a drink. Ways to address this less than ideal combination include:

- **Ask them to substitute a small bag of fries instead.** Most combo meals include "medium" fries (at a cost of nearly 400 calories). Request a *small* order instead for just 250 calories - fewer fries to tempt you, but probably enough to satisfy you.

- **Dump half the fast-food fries** into the trash can on the way to the table. You can't eat what isn't there to tempt you.

- **At full-service restaurants, ask for fewer to be served** so you are not tempted. Remember, each 5" fry contains 20 calories.

- **Don't "dress" your fries.** A "naked" side of fries has 300-600 calories. Don't dress them up with even more calories from cheese, chili, mayo, or even too much ketchup.

What's in your Fast Food Meal?

Before heading to a fast food chain restaurant, check Part 3 for nutrition information. If your favorite burger or fast food restaurant does not provide nutrition information, use the generic information on these next few pages.

Burgers on Buns:	Calories	Fat (g)	Sat+Trans Fat (g)	Sodium (mg)	Carbohydrates (g)	Fiber (g)	Protein (g)
Hamburger, plain, small/kid's	270	10	4	370	30	2	12
w/ketchup, mustard, pickles	275	10	4	590	32	2	12
Cheeseburger, small/kid's	330	15	6	620	33	2	15
w/ketchup, mustard, pickles	335	15	6	840	35	2	15
¼ Pound Burger, plain	465	19	8	570	43	2	25
w/ketchup, mustard, pickles	475	19	8	856	45	2	25
⅓ Pound Burger	615	25	11	760	60	3	36
w/ketchup, mustard, pickles	485	25	11	1200	65	3	36
½ Pound Burger	850	36	15	970	72	4	50
1 slice cheese, ADD:	60	5	3	250	1	0	5
1 slice bacon, ADD:	30	3	1	124	0	0	3
1 Tbsp mayo, ADD:	100	11	2	75	0	0	0
w/lettuce, tomato & onion, ADD:	20	0	0	5	5	1	0
Chicken Sandwiches on Buns:							
Grilled Chicken SW w/mayo, regular	420	15	3	1120	38	2	33
w/o mayo	310	5	1	1035	37	2	33
w/honey mustard	370	8	2	1050	42	2	33
Grilled Chicken Sandwich, large	510	19	4	1180	49	4	40
w/o mayo	400	7	2	1090	49	4	40
w/honey mustard	450	10	2	1200	53	4	40
BBQ Grilled Chicken Sandwich	375	4	1	1150	48	3	32
Fried Chicken Sandwich, small	410	17	5	1050	42	2	16
w/o mayo	300	10	3	900	41	2	16
Fried Chicken Sandwich, large	780	43	12	1730	73	4	32
w/o mayo	570	21	8	1540	73	4	31

Fish Sandwiches on Buns:	Calories	Fat (g)	Sat+Trans Fat (g)	Sodium (mg)	Carbohydrates (g)	Fiber (g)	Protein (g)
Grilled Fish Fillet SW w/tartar sauce	500	20	4	600	45	2	20
w/o tartar sauce	420	12	1	500	43	2	17
Fried Fish Fillet SW w/cheese, small	380	18	5	660	38	2	15
w/o tartar sauce	290	9	4	550	37	2	15
Fried Fish Fillet SW w/cheese, large	645	31	8	1285	70	4	25
w/o tartar sauce	475	13	5	1150	67	3	25
Other Fast Food Sandwiches on Buns:							
Hot Dog, regular plain	310	19	10	700	24	1	11
w/mustard and relish	310	19	10	850	24	1	11
Cheese Dog, regular	350	22	11	950	26	1	12
Chili Dog, regular	340	20	11	900	26	1	14
Chili & Cheese Dog, regular	380	23	11	1100	28	1	14
Corn Dog, regular	250	17	8	350	19	1	10
Foot Long Hot Dog or Sausage	625	28	16	1700	49	3	20
Roast Beef Sandwich, small	325	13	5	950	34	2	23
regular	420	22	10	1300	34	2	33
Gardenburger® on Bun, small, plain	350	8	2	885	53	6	22
medium-size on bun, plain	475	10	2	1200	72	8	33
steaksize on bun, plain	630	14	3	1565	92	12	43
Other Fast Foods:							
Buffalo Wing w/BBQ sauce, 1	75	5	1	165	4	0	5
boneless w/BBQ sauce, 1	90	5	1	400	9	0	5
Chicken Nugget, 1 piece	42	3	1	110	3	0	2
Chicken Strip, 1 strip	125	7	2	310	9	0	8
Fried Chicken, wing	140	9	3	350	4	0	11
breast	340	17	5	960	9	2	33
drumstick	140	8	3	340	3	0	11
thigh	350	27	8	870	7	1	16
Protein only:							
Hamburger Patty, kid's	115	8	4	30	0	0	8
¼ pound patty	230	15	7	65	0	0	18
⅓ pound patty	310	20	10	85	0	0	25
Gardenburger® Patty, small	120	4	<1	380	10	4	11
medium patty	165	5	<1	520	14	5	16
steaksize patty	240	8	1	720	20	8	22
Grilled Chicken Breast Filet	145	7	2	450	4	0	18
Small Hotdog w/o bun	180	16	7	620	1	0	5
Turkey Burger Patty	200	11	3	90	0	0	25

Toppings & Condiments:	Calories	Fat (g)	Sat+Trans Fat (g)	Sodium (mg)	Carbohydrates (g)	Fiber (g)	Protein (g)
Avocado, ¼	80	8	2	5	6	3	1
Bacon, 2 slices crisp	70	5	2	250	0	0	4
Cheese, American, fast food slice	60	5	3	250	1	0	5
Cheese, American 1oz	90	7	4	400	1	0	7
Cheddar Cheese, 1oz	115	9	6	175	0	0	7
Swiss Cheese, 1oz	110	8	5	75	0	0	7
Lettuce	2	0	0	1	0	0	0
Mushrooms, ¼ cup, sautéed	110	11	3	125	2	0	0
Onion, ¼" slice	16	0	0	1	4	0	0
Pickles, 2 slices	1	0	0	90	0	0	0
Tomato, 2 slices	10	0	0	3	2	<1	0

Condiments, 1 Tbsp* unless noted:

	Calories	Fat (g)	Sat+Trans Fat (g)	Sodium (mg)	Carbohydrates (g)	Fiber (g)	Protein (g)
Barbecue Sauce	15	0	0	90	4	0	0
Butter/Oil spread on bun	100	11	3	0	0	0	0
Chili Hot Dog Sauce	15	0	0	63	2	0	0
Honey Mustard Sauce	45	3	<1	75	5	0	0
Ketchup	15	0	0	165	4	0	0
Mayonnaise	110	11	2	75	0	0	0
Mustard, 1 tsp	10	0	0	90	0	0	0
Relish	14	0	0	165	4	0	0
Sauerkraut, 2 Tbsp	5	0	0	180	1	1	0
Sweet N'Sour Sauce	15	0	0	50	4	0	0
Tartar Sauce	80	8	2	110	2	0	0

* Your sandwich may have more or less

Fries & Onion Rings:

	Calories	Fat (g)	Sat+Trans Fat (g)	Sodium (mg)	Carbohydrates (g)	Fiber (g)	Protein (g)
Onion Rings, regular order	470	24	10	590	56	4	7
Onion Rings, each	80	6	1	150	8	1	1
Potato Puffs, each	15	<1	0	30	1	0	0
French Fries, small/junior	250	14	5	345	32	3	2
medium/regular	370	20	8	495	47	4	4
large	540	29	11	720	69	6	6
French Fries, 1 cup	155	8	2	170	15	1	2
Skinny French Fries, 1@2½" long	5	<1	0	8	1	0	0
20 @ 2½" long	100	5	2	75	14	1	1
Regular French Fries, 1@ 2½" long	10	<1	0	9	2	0	0
10 @ 2½" long	100	4	2	85	16	1	1
Battered French Fries, 1@2½" long	15	1	0	30	2	0	0
7 @ 2½" long	100	5	2	220	15	1	1
Steak Fries, 1 @ 2½" long	17	1	0	60	3	0	0
6 @ 2½" long	100	5	2	350	15	1	1

Nutrition Info: Kid Meals

(pick 1 from each category)

	Calories	Fat (g)	Sat+Trans Fat (g)	Sodium (mg)	Carbohydrates (g)	Fiber (g)	Protein (g)
ARBY'S®:							
1. Jr. Roast Beef	210	8	3	520	24	1	12
Chicken Tenders, 2	240	11	2	770	21	1	14
2. Curly Fries, kids	270	14	2	700	33	2	2
Potato Cakes, 2	260	15	2	400	28	2	2
Applesauce	80	0	0	10	21	2	0
3. Soda, small	180	0	0	5*	49	0	0
Capri Sun® Fruit Juice	80	0	0	25	21	0	0
1% Lowfat Chocolate Milk	160	2	2	200	28	0	8
2% Reduced-Fat White Milk	120	5	3	130	12	0	9
Nestle® Pure Life® Bottled Water	0	0	0	0	0	0	0
BURGER KING®:							
1. Hamburger	260	10	4	490	28	1	13
Cheeseburger	300	14	6	710	28	1	16
Chicken Tenders®, 4 piece	180	11	2	310	13	0	9
2. Fries, kids	220	11	3	340	28	2	2
BK® Apple Fries w/caramel sauce	70	<1	0	35	16	1	0
3. Soda, kid's	110	0	0	0	30	0	0
Fat-Free Milk	100	0	0	150	14	0	9
1% Lowfat Chocolate Milk	180	3	2	140	31	1	9
Minute Maid® Apple Juice	100	0	0	20	23	0	0
KFC®:							
1. Drumstick, original	120	7	2	310	3	0	11
extra crispy	150	10	2	360	5	0	12
spicy crispy	160	10	2	440	5	0	11
Extra Crispy Strip, 1	110	4	1	425	9	1	11
Popcorn Chicken, kids	260	17	4	690	12	1	15
2. Green Beans	25	0	0	260	4	2	1
Sweet Kernel Corn	100	<1	0	0	21	2	3
Mashed Potatoes w/gravy	120	4	1	530	19	1	2
Macaroni & Cheese	160	7	3	720	19	1	5
Potato Wedges	290	15	3	810	35	2	4
Sargento® Light Cheese	50	3	2	160	1	0	6
3. Soda, 16oz	180	0	0	35	49	0	0
Capri Sun® Roarin' Waters Tropical Fruit	30	0	0	15	8	0	0

Kids' meals aren't just for kids! At around 300-500 calories, they fit into most calorie budgets.

	Calories	Fat (g)	Sat+Trans Fat (g)	Sodium (mg)	Carbohydrates (g)	Fiber (g)	Protein (g)
McDONALD'S®:							
1. Hamburger	250	9	4	520	31	2	12
Cheeseburger	300	12	7	750	33	2	15
Chicken McNuggets	200	12	2	400	11	0	10
2. Fries, small	230	11	2	160	29	3	3
Apple Dippers w/low fat caramel dip	100	<1	0	35	23	0	0
3. Soda, child's	110	0	0	5	29	0	0
1% Lowfat Milk jug	100	3	2	125	12	0	8
1% Lowfat Chocolate Milk jug	170	3	2	150	26	1	9
Minute Maid® Apple Juice box	100	0	0	15	23	0	0
QUIZNO'S®:							
1. Toasty® Turkey (or Ham) & Cheese Sub	310	9	4	810	44	2	15
Cheesy Toasted Cheese Sub	330	11	6	580	43	2	13
Tasty Turkey or Ham Melt Sammie	200	7	3	585	26	1	11
Just Cheese Sammie	230	10	5	390	25	1	11
2. Chips or Chocolate Chip Cookie	na	na	na	na	na	na	na
3. Soda, small	na	na	na	na	na	na	na
SUBWAY®:							
1. Mini sub prepared w/o cheese, mayo, or oil:							
Veggie Delite®	150	2	0	210	29	3	6
Black Forest Ham	180	3	<1	470	30	3	10
Roast Beef	200	3	1	410	30	4	14
Turkey Breast	180	2	<1	460	30	3	10
2. Apple Slices	35	0	0	0	9	2	0
Baked Lay's®	130	2	0	200	23	2	2
Sunchips® Harvest Cheddar	210	9	2	240	29	3	4
3. Lowfat Milk	160	4	3	180	19	0	12
Chocolate Flavored Reduced-Fat Milk	300	8	5	300	43	<1	15
Juice Box	100	0	0	15	24	0	0
Soda, 16oz w/o ice	240	0	0	na	66	0	0
TACO BELL®:							
1. Crunchy Taco	170	10	4	330	12	3	8
Soft Taco, beef	200	9	4	540	19	3	10
Bean Burrito	370	10	4	980	56	10	13
Cheese Roll Up	190	9	5	450	18	2	9
2. Cinnamon Twists	170	7	0	200	26	1	1
3. Soda, 16oz	200	0	0	40	56	0	0

WENDY'S®:

	Calories	Fat (g)	Sat+Trans Fat (g)	Sodium (mg)	Carbohydrates (g)	Fiber (g)	Protein (g)
1. Chicken Nuggets, 4 piece	180	11	3	370	11	1	8
Hamburger, kid's	220	8	3	370	26	1	12
Cheeseburger, kids	260	11	5	570	26	1	14
Crispy Chicken Sandwich, kids	330	13	3	700	36	2	15
2. Fries, kids	230	11	3	250	30	3	3
Apple Slices	40	0	0	0	9	2	0
3. Soda, kids	100	0	0	0	26	0	0
TruMoo® Lowfat White Milk	100	3	2	125	12	0	8
TruMoo® Lowfat Chocolate Milk	140	3	2	170	22	0	7
Vanilla or Chocolate Frosty, small	255	7	5	120	42	0	6
Juicy Juice® Apple Juice	90	0	0	5	22	0	0

Subs & Sandwiches

A sandwich prepared at home is often a low-calorie meal. But in restaurants, large pieces of bread are over-stuffed with meat, cheese, and dressing – and served with high-calorie accompaniments. Making the wrong decisions can turn a healthy meal into a disaster. Consider, for example, Tuna Salad on a Croissant. This is easily 800 calories and 60g fat! Here are some tips to help you choose a healthier sandwich:

Bread

The key to selecting sandwich bread within your "calorie budget," is to pick a lowfat bread of an appropriate size.

• **Avoid flaky breads.** A croissant contains about 50% more calories than other breads of an equal size. The ingredient that causes a croissant to flake is the many, thin layers of butter or hydrogenated shortening. And, because these ingredients are solid at room temperature (rather than a *liquid* oil), croissants don't seem as fatty as a brownie, but they are. Remember, fat is fat - they all have the same number of calories. Instead of a croissant, choose sliced sandwich bread, French or Italian bread, bagels, pita bread, ciabatta, focaccia, or rolls.

• **Choose whole grain if possible.** Whole grains have more nutrients (including fiber) than refined white bread. While you can read the label at the grocery store (the first ingredient should read "whole wheat"), ingredient lists are not readily available at restaurants. Fortunately, some menus do highlight this feature.

Keep in mind that some manufacturers add molasses to make bread dark - so appearances can be misleading.

• **Size up the bread.** At home, a sandwich is typically prepared with two slices of regular sandwich bread (about 2oz or 150 calories). However, restaurant bread slices are often heftier. If the slices look the same as your bread at home, just fatter, that's 3oz (the equivalence of *three* slices of bread) or 225 calories for two slices. Most buns, ciabatta, lavash, crusty French bread rolls, or 6" subs also contain about the equivalence of three slices of bread. Is the bread wider, too? Then, you've got the equivalence of *four* slices of bread (300 calories). Deli bagels are often 4-5oz (or 350-450 calories).

• **Go for the pita or a smaller tortilla wrap.** They often contain as much calories as just two slices of bread - way less than most other deli options. There's no calorie advantage to ordering the very large tortilla instead of sandwich bread.

Meat, Cheese, & Other Fillings

Deli meat and cheese range widely from 30 to over 100 calories per ounce. Deli sandwiches also vary greatly in the portion size of meat. Some sandwiches contain as little as 1½oz meat (such as a 6" sub at Subway) to a whopping 8oz of meat and cheese found at some gourmet delis. When selecting your sandwich, consider these tips:

• **Choose sliced turkey, chicken, ham, or roast beef.** Specialty deli meats such as salami and sausage are at least twice as high in fat (especially saturated fat) and calories.

• **Use caution with mayo-mixed spreads** such as tuna, chicken, and egg salad. When mayonnaise is added to these leaner proteins, it can more than double the calories of your sandwich!

• **Skip the cheese.** Each slice of deli cheese adds about 100 calories per 1oz slice.

• **Keep meat portions to 3oz or less** (or the size of a deck of cards). If your sandwich contains more, consider splitting the sandwich with a friend and having an extra salad, cup of broth-based soup, or some fruit. In a restaurant that really piles on the meat, ask them to go "light on the meat." Or order just a half of a sandwich along with an extra slice of bread; split the meat between the two slices of bread to make a whole sandwich.

Condiments & Toppings

• **Get the dressing on the side** (except for mustard, fat-free mayonnaise, vinegar, and horseradish). You can always ask for the mayo or dressing to be added "light," but not everyone's idea of light is the same. Instead, get the dressing on the side so you can add them sparingly. Salad dressings have around 50-80 calories per tablespoon, mayonnaise has closer to 100, and oil has a whopping 120 calories per tablespoon! A thin smear of mayonnaise and a few shakes of oil to a 6" fast food sub can add more than 155 calories and 17g fat.

• **Sandwiches can be grilled without extra fat**, if you request.

Accompaniments

Most accompaniments (including potato salad, fries, and chips) are high in both calories and fat.

• **Request a low-calorie accompaniment.** If your sandwich is served with fries or chips, ask for a substitute such as salad, steamed vegetables, or fresh fruit. For more details, see the Soups & Salads chapter.

Sandwich Combos

Many sandwich restaurants are now offering combos in which you can select any two items. These options typically include a cup of soup, small salad, or a half sandwich. What's the healthiest combination? Here are some options:

• **Select a broth-based soup rather than cream-based.** Usually vegetable, bean, turkey noodle, or chicken rice are lower calorie options than creamy tomato, loaded potato, or cream of broccoli.

• **Pick your fat.** Both sandwiches and salads are loaded with hundreds of additional calories in the form of fat, so make some compromises. If you want pesto or mayonnaise on your sandwich, ask for the fat-free vinaigrette on the salad. Craving honey mustard dressing on the salad? Think about getting it on the side so you can control the amounts. Also, consider mustard instead of mayo on the sandwich.

Nutrition Information

Breads and More:

	Calories	Fat (g)	Sat+Trans Fat (g)	Sodium (mg)	Carbohydrates (g)	Fiber (g)	Protein (g)
Bagel, deli size	330	2	0	570	65	3	13
Sandwich Bread, white, 1 slice	75	1	0	135	15	<1	2
thicker slice, ¾"	115	2	0	205	22	1	3
deli-slice (large, rectangular)	150	2	0	270	30	1	4
Sandwich Bread, wheat, 1 slice	75	1	0	130	14	3	3
thicker slice, ¾"	115	2	0	195	21	4	5
deli-slice (large, rectangular)	150	2	0	260	28	6	6
Croissant, large sandwich-size	345	18	10	635	39	2	3
English Muffin, large sandwich-size	210	3	0	175	40	5	5
Focaccia bread, ½ of 9" round	450	10	1	1000	75	5	12
French Roll, 4" long	225	1	0	315	39	2	6
Pita Bread, 6½" round	165	1	0	320	33	2	5
wheat	170	2	0	340	35	5	6
Soft Bun, 4½" round	240	5	2	400	41	3	6
Sub Roll, white, 6" long	240	3	1	450	45	2	6
wheat	240	3	1	400	46	4	8

Deli Meat, per 1½oz:

	Calories	Fat (g)	Sat+Trans Fat (g)	Sodium (mg)	Carbohydrates (g)	Fiber (g)	Protein (g)
Bologna	135	12	6	500	1	0	4
Bratwurst, Brotwurst, or Braunschweiger							
Knockwurst or Mortadella	140	12	4	420	1	0	5
Chicken Breast or Turkey	45	<1	0	500	0	0	8
Corned Beef	60	3	2	570	0	0	7
Ham	60	3	1	560	2	0	5
Headcheese	80	6	2	460	0	0	4
Italian Sausage	150	12	4	520	2	0	8
Lox (Smoked Salmon)	50	2	1	850	0	0	8
Meatloaf	110	8	3	200	2	0	10
Pastrami, lean	45	1	<1	320	0	0	8
Proscuitto	100	5	2	1140	2	0	12
Roast Beef, lean	60	3	1	240	0	0	7
Salami, Pepperoni, Blood Sausage	160	14	5	500	0	0	10

Dr. Jo says

Most fast food restaurants prepare its subs with 1½oz deli meat and ½oz cheese. Casual restaurants use 2-3 times more. Count on nearly 8oz meat at gourmet delis.

	Calories	Fat (g)	Sat+Trans Fat (g)	Sodium (mg)	Carbohydrates (g)	Fiber (g)	Protein (g)
Spreadables:							
Chicken Salad, ½ cup	250	20	4	700	2	0	16
Egg Salad, ½ cup	290	28	5	230	0	0	10
Liver Pate (chicken), ¼ cup	105	7	2	200	3	0	10
goose liver, ¼ cup	240	23	8	360	2	0	6
Olive Salad Spread, 2 Tbsp	160	14	0	420	6	1	2
Tuna Salad, ½ cup	240	18	3	540	3	1	18
Cheese (per 1oz slice, unless specified):							
American, processed	90	7	4	400	1	0	6
Asiago	110	9	5	330	2	0	7
Cheddar or Pepperjack	120	9	6	180	0	0	7
Feta or Gorgonzola crumbles, 2 Tbsp	50	4	3	200	<1	0	3
Mozzarella	90	7	4	170	1	0	7
Provolone	100	8	5	250	0	0	7
Swiss	110	8	5	75	0	0	7
Condiments & Toppings (per 1 Tbsp, unless noted):							
Aioli Sauce (garlic oil)	100	10	2	0	0	0	0
Barbecue Sauce	30	0	0	180	7	0	0
Butter, whipped	70	8	5	70	0	0	0
Chutney	25	0	0	0	7	<1	0
Cream Cheese, 2 Tbsp soft	100	10	7	100	1	0	2
Dijonnaise	15	0	0	210	0	0	0
Dijon Mayonnaise	90	10	2	90	1	0	0
Guacamole	15	1	0	110	1	<1	0
Honey Mustard Sauce	35	<1	0	390	8	0	0
Horseradish Sauce, 1 tsp	10	1	<1	0	0	0	0
Ketchup	15	0	0	170	4	0	0
Margarine, whipped	70	8	2	100	0	0	0
Mayonnaise	100	11	2	80	0	0	0
reduced calorie	50	5	1	110	1	0	0
fat-free	10	<1	0	120	2	0	0
Mustard, 2 tsp	15	1	0	190	0	0	0
Oil, 1 tsp	45	5	1	0	0	0	0
Oil & Vinegar	70	8	2	0	<1	0	0
Pesto Sauce	80	7	2	120	1	<1	2
Picante Sauce	5	0	0	110	1	0	0
Ranch Dressing	70	7	1	200	0	0	0
Remoulade Sauce	80	8	2	110	0	0	0
Sour Cream/Cucumber Sauce	45	4	na	na	2	<1	0
Sundried Tomato Spread	50	3	<1	325	4	1	1
Thousand Island Dressing	60	5	1	130	2	0	0
Vinegar, 1 tsp	2	0	0	0	0	0	0

	Calories	Fat (g)	Sat+Trans Fat (g)	Sodium (mg)	Carbohydrates (g)	Fiber (g)	Protein (g)
Other Toppings:							
Avocado, 1/8	40	4	1	0	3	2	0
Bacon, 1 slice	35	3	1	130	0	0	2
Banana or Jalapeno Peppers	5	0	0	50	0	0	0
Cucumbers, Lettuce, Tomato, Onion	5	0	0	0	1	1	0
Olives, 1 Tbsp	10	1	0	80	<1	<1	0
Pickles, 1 deli slice	1	0	0	90	0	0	0
1 spear	5	0	0	310	1	<1	0
Salads (½ cup unless specified):							
Cole Slaw	170	12	2	210	14	2	1
Fresh Fruit Salad	60	0	0	0	15	1	0
Garden Salad	25	1	0	30	6	<1	0
Salad Dressing, 2 Tbsp	160	16	3	300	0	0	0
Lowfat Salad Dressing, 2 Tbsp	20	0	0	270	4	0	0
Macaroni Salad	295	26	3	400	15	1	3
Potato Salad	190	11	2	580	21	2	3
Crunchies:							
Baked Potato Chips, 1oz (12)	110	2	0	150	20	1	1
Baked Tortilla Chips, 1oz (10)	120	1	0	80	22	2	1
Pickle, 4" long	25	0	0	1730	6	2	1
Popcorn, 1 cup	55	4	3	40	6	1	1
Potato Chips, 20 regular or 12 ripple	150	10	3	180	15	1	2
Pretzels, 1oz (48 sticks)	110	0	0	530	23	1	1
Twisters (8) or Tiny Twists (18)	100	0	0	420	19	1	2
Thick Twists (4)	110	1	0	620	24	1	2
Tortilla Chips, 10	180	8	1	150	26	2	2

Appetizers and Small Plates

Appetizers were originally designed as small nibbles to pacify the appetite until the meal arrives. Unfortunately, today's appetizers combined with an average entrée will often meet your caloric need for the entire day! Therefore, consider the following options:

- **Order an appetizer instead of an entrée.** Add a salad or a side of veggies and perhaps a whole grain roll for a complete meal.

- **Pick a lean appetizer.** These include non-fried options such as shrimp cocktail, crabmeat cocktail, Thai (non-fried) spring rolls, chicken satays, sushi, sashimi, or steamed vegetable dumplings.

- **Choose two to three "Small Plates."** Like the traditional tapas found in Spain (and totally *unlike* most American fried appetizers), "Small Plates" are small portions of entrées. Instead of one entrée (and one taste), consider ordering two or three small plates with a variety of tantalizing tastes. Or share three or four small plates with a friend.

- **Ask for the appetizer portion.** If you're craving a fried entrée, ask if there is an appetizer portion (or half portion) available. Italian restaurants frequently offer appetizer portions of fried dishes, including Eggplant Parmagiana, which is sufficient for many appetites.

- **Limit the sauces** that are served with appetizers since they can often double the fat and calories. Order them on the side; dip your fork into the sauce and then into the food for a taste with every bite.

Nutrition Information

	Calories	Fat (g)	Sat+Trans Fat (g)	Sodium (mg)	Carbohydrates (g)	Fiber (g)	Protein (g)
Dippers:							
Artichoke, 1 medium cooked	60	0	0	115	13	6	3
butter sauce, 2 Tbsp	200	23	15	160	0	0	0
herb mayonnaise, 2 Tbsp	200	22	3	150	0	0	0
Artichoke Spinach Dip, 2 Tbsp	60	2	<1	200	5	2	1
Buffalo Wings dressed w/sauce, 1	75	5	1	165	3	0	5
Boneless Wings, 1	90	5	1	400	9	0	6
Blue cheese dressing, 2 Tbsp	155	16	3	335	3	0	0
Cheese Fondue, 1 tsp	13	1	<1	5	0	0	1
French bread, 1" cube	10	0	0	25	2	0	0
Chocolate Fondue, 1 tsp	25	2	1	1	3	0	0
White cake, 1" cube	20	1	0	20	3	0	0
Fruit, 1 chunk	10	0	0	0	3	0	0
Tortilla Chip, 6 large chips	140	6	1	110	19	1	3
Salsa, ¼ cup	20	0	0	360	4	0	0
Nachos w/cheese, 6 large chips	220	13	5	410	21	1	7
w/beans, cheese, salsa	290	16	6	810	31	2	9
w/beans, cheese, sour cream, guacamole	405	26	11	970	34	3	9
loaded with above, plus beef	495	31	13	1210	37	4	17
Potsticker, chicken, pan fried, 6	440	22	5	560	46	2	14
soy sauce, 2 Tbsp	15	0	0	2040	3	0	0
Fried Snacks:							
Calamari, fried, 3oz	210	12	3	260	7	0	16
Egg Roll, fried, 4"	200	12	4	490	16	2	8
Sweet and Sour Sauce, 2 Tbsp	55	0	0	70	14	0	0
Fried Mozzarella Sticks,	100	6	2	250	7	0	6
Marinara Sauce, ¼ cup	45	2	0	375	5	1	1
Fried Whole Onion	2000	160	48	4100	120	15	17
1 large onion ring	80	4	1	70	10	0	<1
Fried Zucchini/Mushrooms, ½ cup	180	10	3	400	19	1	3
1 fried mushroom	30	2	<1	22	2	0	0
Seafood:							
Ceviche, 3oz	95	1	0	75	0	0	22
Clams, raw, 3	60	3	0	60	2	0	7
Oysters Rockefeller, 3	300	25	15	500	11	0	7
Oysters, raw, 6	100	4	1	305	5	0	11
fried, 1	60	3	1	115	7	0	2
Shrimp Cocktail, 4 jumbo	135	2	0	300	0	0	21
Cocktail Sauce, 2 Tbsp	40	0	0	320	10	0	0

	Calories	Fat (g)	Sat+Trans Fat (g)	Sodium (mg)	Carbohydrates (g)	Fiber (g)	Protein (g)
Small Meals:							
Quesadilla, cheese-only, 10"	1090	70	26	1640	70	4	45
w/chicken and cheese	1240	80	24	2120	70	4	60
Marguerita Pizza, 12" (thin crust)	1100	50	25	1920	120	8	51
Munchies:							
Nuts, 1oz (about ¼ cup)	170	15	2	180	5	3	6
Olives, green, 1	10	1	0	110	<1	0	0
black, 1 large	5	<1	0	40	0	0	0
super colossal ripe, 1	12	1	0	135	1	0	0
Popcorn, 1 cup	55	4	3	100	6	1	1
Spreadables:							
Brushetta, 1 toast w/topping	100	7	1	na	9	0	0
Italian bread, 1 slice	55	<1	0	115	10	0	1
Melba Rounds, 4	45	0	0	100	9	1	1
Butter Crackers, 3	80	4	0	110	12	0	1
Tapenade (olive) topping, 1 Tbsp	25	3	0	175	1	0	0
Pate, chicken liver, 2 Tbsp	50	4	1	100	2	0	3
Pate, goose liver, 2 Tbsp	120	12	4	180	1	0	3
Caviar, 2 Tbsp	85	5	1	480	1	0	8
Veggies:							
Roasted Pepper, ½, oil-marinated	45	3	1	na	4	1	1
Stuffed Jalapeno, 1	75	4	2	245	7	1	2
Stuffed Mushrooms, 1 regular-size	70	4	1	150	7	1	1
Porcini, 1 large	150	10	3	400	15	1	2
Stuffed Potato Skins, 4 skins	520	34	15	500	40	4	13
Sour Cream, 2 Tbsp	60	5	4	10	1	0	0

Beverages

The human body is 60% water, so it's no surprise that many health authorities suggest we drink eight glasses of water a day. Do other liquids count? Yes - even coffee, tea, and soda.

Keep in mind though, that current research indicates that the body doesn't get full from liquid calories. In other words, a 300 calorie soda, coffee, or alcoholic drink won't fill you up as much as a 300 calorie sandwich. Therefore, if you *drink* many of your calories, you may be consuming more calories than you actually need. It may be best to save your calories for food, rather than a beverage. Yet, for many of us, water can get boring. So - what other beverages should you drink to keep your weight and health in check?

Most health experts recommend at least three servings of nonfat (or lowfat) dairy products to meet your calcium needs to build strong bones. Research has also linked a higher dairy intake with lower blood pressure - and, on average, the lower your blood pressure, the lower your risk of stroke. It's easy to get in your milk when dining out. Most restaurants now offer nonfat (or lowfat) milk as a solo beverage and for your coffee beverages.

While juice is often promoted as a healthier option to soda, keep in mind that it still contains the same number of calories (ounce-for-ounce) as soda. Yes, juice contains more nutrients than soda. Whole fruit is often more nutritious, though, because it contains fiber which is lacking in most juices.

Estimating the Calories in Your Beverage

How many calories are you drinking? It's easy to figure out the calories in your favorite beverage as long as you know the size of the cup and the calories per ounce (shown below on this beverage calorie-meter). Drinks contain anywhere from 0-125 calories per ounce:

Calorie-Meter (calories per fluid ounce):

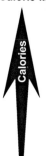

125	Crème de Menthe
100	Coffee Liqueurs
85	100 Proof Liqueurs
60	Manhattan, Martini
40	Nonalcoholic Eggnog, Table Wines
30	Ice Cream Shake, Sherry
25	Champagne, Dry White Wine, Frozen Yogurt Shakes
20	Whole Milk, Fruit Juice (Cranberry, Grape, Prune), Fruit Smoothies
17	Fruit Punch
15	2% Lowfat Milk, Fruit Juices (Apple, Grapefruit, Orange), Orange Sodas, Lemonade, Orange Breakfast Drinks
12	Regular Colas, 1% Lowfat Milk, Beer
10	Nonfat Milk & Buttermilk (made w/nonfat milk), Flavored Coffees, Sweetened Tea, Coffee w/cream & sugar
0	Water, Sparkling Waters w/o added sugar, Club Soda, Perrier, Diet Sodas, Unsweetened Tea & Coffee

Don't know the serving size of your favorite beverage? Here are some tips on guessing the cup size:

• **Soda**: Fast food restaurants usually offer several sizes including small (16oz), medium (22oz) and large (32oz). Children and senior sizes are generally 12oz. Sometimes the cup size is stamped on the bottom of the paper cup. Most other restaurants offer just one size and it's often as big as 32oz.

• **Coffee**: While an 8oz cup of coffee used to be standard, it's often now only available as a "senior size." The small is about 12oz, the medium contains 16oz and the large is about 22oz.

• **Shakes and Smoothies**: At a fast food restaurant, a small serving is often 12oz, while the medium and large are 16 and 22oz respectively. Smoothie shops generally have larger cups.

• **Alcohol**: Sizes vary greatly - depending on the drink. There's more detail on serving sizes later in this chapter.

Use the actual size drawing on the next page for comparison.

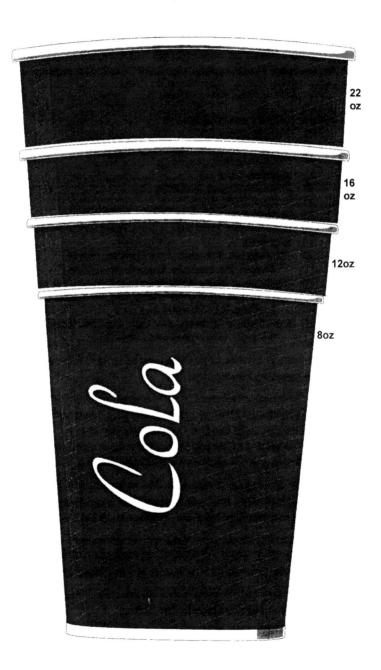

Cold Beverages

If you want something to drink other than water, but you're trying to cut back on your calories, try these tips:

• **Request nonfat or lowfat milk.** Most restaurants, including fast food restaurants, now offer the lower fat varieties - even if it's not on the menu. At just 80 calories a cup, nonfat milk offers a nutritional boost as a beverage, in your cereal, or in your hot beverage. Switching to a lower fat milk (recommended for people over the age of two) will help you reduce your saturated fat intake.

• **Rethink fruit juice.** While 100% fruit juices such as orange, grapefruit, prune, and tomato juice are powerfully packed with nutrition, most juices found in restaurants are either apple juice, a mix of juices containing mostly apple juice, or a fruit drink. Apple juice is not rich in many nutrients. Fruit cocktail, fruit drink, or fruit punch usually contains little if any real juice. Consider it like a soda, instead. Remember, fruit juices contain (ounce-for-ounce) as many calories as soda. Fresh fruit has far more nutritional value - and will fill you up more than juice.

• **Go diet.** While all sodas are fat-free, only the sugar-free sodas are calorie-free. A couple cans of soda (or a medium drink at a restaurant) has about 300 calories, or more than 19 teaspoons of sugar! While 300 calories a day may not sound like much, the calories have a cumulative effect. Over a full year you'd be consuming 109,500 calories from soda alone.

Dr. Jo says

If you're drinking just one medium-sized soda every day and switch to water or diet soda, you could theoretically lose up to 31 pounds in a year!

• **Adjust your sweetness threshold.** Some animal research has suggested that drinking non-caloric sweet beverages may increase one's desire for sweet tasting foods and drink. This prompting could cause you to consume more calories overall. While it's unclear whether this animal research correlates to humans, it makes sense to reach for beverages that are minimally sweetened. You might think about limiting the number of diet beverages you consume or diluting them with club soda. You could also mix fruit juices with 50% water or get used to the taste of coffee or tea, sans the sweetener.

• **Caution with shakes.** A large shake made with "real ice cream" could easily contain over 1000 calories! Instead, select a lowfat or fat-free shake. These lower fat versions still contain sugar, but about half the calories.

• **Consider caffeine.** Very few restaurants serve diet caffeine-free drinks - but ask. Sometimes the restaurant may provide caffeine-free iced tea or diet Sprite® or 7 Up®. Chick-fil-A® also offers a diet lemonade made with real lemons. And while not all root beer sodas are caffeine-free, A&W® Root Beer is.

How Much Caffeine Am I Consuming?

Caffeine is a stimulant which can ward off fatigue and improve your mood. Be careful, though, because too much caffeine can cause anxiety and heart palpitations and interfere with sleep. Coffee provides 75% of all the caffeine consumed in America. But caffeine is also found in tea, caffeinated fountain beverages, chocolate, and some medications. For most healthy adults, 200-300 mg caffeine per day is considered "safe." Children and pregnant women should consume less than 100 mg. How much caffeine are you consuming? Take a look:

Caffeine-Meter (mg caffeine per drink):

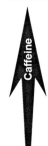

480	20oz Gourmet Coffee
320	16oz Gourmet Coffee
240	20oz Coffee, 12oz Gourmet Coffee or Triple Shot Espresso (or drinks made w/3 shots)
200	16oz Coffee
160	Double Shot Espresso (or drinks made w/2 shots), 12oz Coffee, 8oz Gourmet Coffee
100	8oz Coffee
80	1oz Espresso (or drinks made with a single shot), 12oz Tea (black or chai), 22oz medium-size Caffeinated Soda
50	12oz can Caffeinated Soda, 12oz Green Tea, 22oz Iced Tea
20	20oz Decaf Coffee, 1oz Dark Chocolate
10	8oz Decaf Coffee or 1oz Decaf Espresso (single shot), 1oz Milk Chocolate
5	8oz Chocolate Milk or Cocoa, 8oz Decaf Tea

Coffee & Other Hot Beverages

Current research indicates that coffee and tea may offer some health benefits. And, when prepared black, they have negligible calories. It is what you add to these drinks that can greatly impact your weight and waist! If your taste buds are asking for more to be added, consider these suggestions:

- **Request nonfat or lowfat milk** instead of whole milk or cream. Nearly every restaurant and coffee shop offer these lower fat alternatives for your coffee and espresso drinks. This won't make much difference if you're just adding a tablespoon or two (though every calorie adds up), but the savings is much greater for a mocha or latte.

- **Select a non-calorie sweetener.** There are sixteen calories in a teaspoon of sugar (or a packet). If you use just three a day, you could end up with an extra five pounds of fat each year. Can you afford the calories? When making a change, allow a few weeks for your taste buds to adjust.

- **Worried about the dangers?** There's no solid proof of risks associated with moderate consumption of non-caloric sweeteners. But there are known risks of consuming too many calories, especially empty calories from sugar. Researchers have uncovered definite risks associated with carrying around too much weight - including an increased risk of heart disease, high blood pressure, diabetes, and certain types of cancer. If you are still concerned about the safety of non-caloric sweeteners, cut out the sugar and sweeteners completely.

- **Give your taste buds time to adjust.** Any changes to your coffee or tea will initially affect the taste. Give your taste buds a couple of weeks to adjust to the new taste. Eventually, the new taste will taste better than the old, and be better for your health.

- **Think before you pump.** Flavored coffee beverages tend to have 50-150 more calories than the unflavored. Most coffee shops now offer sugar-free versions of the flavors with negligible calories. Cinnamon is a low calorie way to add sweetness.

- **Skip the squirt.** Some drinks, such as Cafe Mocha, are routinely prepared with the addition of whipping cream – be sure to ask how it's made! That ¼ cup squirt of whipping cream can add about 100 calories and 8g fat. Light whipped topping may also be available, and will save you some extraneous calories.

•**Caution with the chai.** Traditional Indian chai tea is a fairly low-calorie beverage consisting of boiled tea with the addition of spices and herbs (and a bit of milk and sugar). In most coffee shops, however, chai beverages are prepared with a lot more sugar and milk than you need. Expect a 16oz cup of chai, prepared with whole milk, to have more than 250 calories!

•**Go smaller.** If you can't break away from whole milk in your coffee drink, consider cutting back to a smaller cup than usual.

Alcoholic Beverages

Alcohol, a fermented carbohydrate, is more concentrated than other carbohydrates. It contains seven calories per gram, rather than four calories per gram for other carbohydrates. Sure, most alcoholic beverages are fat-free, but the calories from alcohol beverages can still be damaging to your weight! Here are some general guidelines for consuming alcoholic beverages:

•**Limit your alcohol consumption.** The American Heart Association recommends no more than one drink a day for women and two drinks a day for men. One drink is considered to be one beer, 1oz liquor, or 4oz wine. Drinking too much alcohol may lead to excess weight and can raise your triglyceride (bad fat) level in your blood. It can also lead to other health problems such as high blood pressure and heart failure.

•**Choose non-calorie beverages as mixers.** Choose the non-calorie beverages such as water, club soda, or a diet soda - alone or as an alcoholic mixer.

•**Save the high calorie specialty drinks for special occasions.** Many specialty alcoholic drinks have hundreds of calories per serving.

•**Dilute the calories.** Instead of drinking a shot, dilute the alcohol with diet soda, water, or club soda. A wine sparkler (wine mixed with club soda) will have almost half the calories of a premixed wine cooler.

•**Choose a lighter version.** Depending on your choice, a light beer might have 50 fewer calories than the regular; a Rum & Diet Coke will save you half the calories of a Rum & Coke.

•**Find another favorite.** Some speciality cocktails can have upwards of 500 calories in just one drink. Maybe it's time to find another favorite beverage!

Nutrition Information

Fruit/Vegetable Juices (6 fl oz):	Calories	Fat (g)	Sat+Trans Fat (g)	Sodium (mg)	Carbohydrates (g)	Fiber (g)	Protein (g)
Apple Juice	90	0	0	10	21	0	0
Cranberry Juice	110	0	0	10	28	0	0
Grape Juice	120	0	0	5	30	0	0
Grapefruit Juice	70	0	0	0	18	0	0
Orange Juice	90	0	0	0	21	0	0
Prune Juice	130	0	0	10	33	2	0
Tomato Juice	40	0	0	490	10	1	1
Fountain Drinks w/ice*							
Diet sodas, small 16oz	0	0	0	20	0	0	0
medium, 22oz	0	0	0	30	0	0	0
large, 32oz	0	0	0	45	0	0	0
PowerAde®, small 16oz	100	0	0	85	25	0	0
medium, 22oz	140	0	0	120	35	0	0
large, 32oz	200	0	0	190	50	0	0
Iced Tea, small, 16oz	120	0	0	5	30	0	0
medium, 22oz	170	0	0	10	42	0	0
large, 32oz	240	0	0	15	60	0	0
Coca Cola®, Pepsi®, Sprite®, Dr. Pepper®, 7Up®, Lemonade							
small, 16oz	150	0	0	10	38	0	0
medium, 22oz	220	0	0	15	55	0	0
large, 32oz	320	0	0	20	80	0	0
Root Beer, Punch, small 16oz	170	0	0	25	42	0	0
medium, 22oz	250	0	0	40	62	0	0
large, 32oz	350	0	0	50	88	0	0
Mountain Dew®, small 16oz	210	0	0	65	52	0	0
medium, 22oz	270	0	0	85	68	0	0
large, 32oz	420	0	0	130	105	0	0

*sodium varies w/local water content

	Calories	Fat (g)	Sat+Trans Fat (g)	Sodium (mg)	Carbohydrates (g)	Fiber (g)	Protein (g)
Milk (8oz):							
Nonfat Milk	80	0	0	105	12	0	8
Lowfat Milk	120	5	3	100	12	0	8
Whole Milk	150	8	5	100	12	0	8
Blended Beverages:							
Fruit only Smoothie, 22oz	275	<1	0	65	64	3	0
12oz	150	0	0	35	35	2	0
Fruit & Frozen Yogurt Smoothie, 12oz	300	4	2	90	60	1	2
16oz	400	5	3	120	80	2	2
Fruit & Nonfat Yogurt Smoothie, 12oz	210	<1	0	35	49	2	2
16oz	260	1	0	40	60	3	3
22oz	330	1	0	65	75	4	4
Fast Food Milk Shake, vanilla or strawberry							
12oz	410	9	6	200	74	0	9
16oz	545	12	8	265	100	0	12
22oz	745	17	11	375	139	0	17
Fast Food Milk Shake, chocolate							
12oz	430	10	6	200	79	0	9
16oz	560	13	8	265	105	0	12
22oz	775	18	12	375	140	0	17
Ice Cream Shake, vanilla or strawberry							
12oz, kids	380	12	8	190	63	0	11
14oz, small	530	19	13	260	80	0	14
20oz, medium	690	23	16	330	110	<1	18
28oz, large	880	29	21	450	140	<1	25
Ice Cream Shake, chocolate							
12oz, kids	460	16	10	210	73	2	12
14oz, small	610	23	16	280	90	2	15
20oz, medium	780	27	18	360	122	3	20
28oz, large	970	34	23	480	151	3	27
Icee®, 12oz	160	0	0	20	40	0	0
Coffee & Espresso:							
Coffee, black or decaf, 8oz	5	0	0	50	2	0	0
w/sugar	50	0	0	50	12	0	0
w/cream	55	5	3	52	2	0	0
w/cream and sugar	100	5	3	52	2	0	0
Espresso, 1 shot	5	0	0	10	1	0	0

Dr. Jo says

A 16oz iced espresso drink has the same nutrition as its 12oz hot drink version.

	Calories	Fat (g)	Sat+Trans Fat (g)	Sodium (mg)	Carbohydrates (g)	Fiber (g)	Protein (g)
Latte:							
Latte w/nonfat milk, 8oz	80	0	0	115	11	0	8
12oz	120	0	0	175	16	0	12
16oz	160	0	0	230	23	0	16
20oz	200	1	0	290	27	0	20
Latte w/lowfat milk, 8oz	120	4	3	115	11	0	8
12oz	180	6	4	175	17	0	12
16oz	240	7	4	230	23	0	16
20oz	300	9	5	290	28	0	20
Latte, w/whole milk, 8oz	145	7	4	115	11	0	8
12oz	215	10	6	175	17	0	12
16oz	270	14	8	230	23	0	16
20oz	360	17	10	290	28	0	20
Cappuccino:							
Cappuccino w/nonfat milk, 8oz	55	0	0	75	7	0	4
12oz	85	0	0	115	11	0	6
16oz	110	0	0	150	15	0	8
20oz	140	0	0	190	18	0	10
Cappuccino w/lowfat milk, 8oz	75	2	1	75	7	0	4
12oz	110	4	3	110	11	0	6
16oz	150	5	3	145	15	0	8
20oz	180	6	4	185	18	0	10
Cappuccino, w/whole milk, 8oz	95	5	3	70	7	0	4
12oz	120	7	4	105	11	0	6
16oz	150	8	5	140	15	0	8
20oz	210	12	7	175	18	0	10
Mocha (w/o whipping cream):							
Mocha, w/nonfat milk, 8oz	120	1	0	100	22	<1	6
12oz	180	2	<1	150	33	1	9
16oz	240	3	<1	200	44	1	12
20oz	300	4	<1	250	55	2	15
Mocha, w/lowfat milk, 8oz	130	4	3	105	22	<1	6
12oz	195	6	4	160	33	1	9
16oz	260	8	5	215	44	1	12
20oz	320	10	6	265	55	2	15
Mocha, w/whole milk, 8oz	150	6	4	100	22	1	6
12oz	230	9	6	150	33	1	9
16oz	290	12	8	200	44	1	12
20oz	380	15	11	250	55	2	15

	Calories	Fat (g)	Sat+Trans Fat (g)	Sodium (mg)	Carbohydrates (g)	Fiber (g)	Protein (g)
Other Hot Beverages:							
Tea, 1 bag	2	0	0	7	1	0	0
Hot Chocolate, pkg	120	2	1	190	23	1	0
made w/nonfat milk	180	2	1	265	31	1	6
made w/lowfat milk	210	6	3	265	32	1	6
made w/whole milk	235	8	5	285	32	1	6
Condiments (1 Tbsp, unless specified):							
Milk, nonfat	5	0	0	7	<1	0	<1
Milk, lowfat	8	0	0	8	<1	0	<1
Milk, whole	10	<1	0	8	<1	0	<1
Nondairy Lghtener, powered, 1 tsp	10	1	1	10	1	0	0
Half & Half	20	2	1	8	<1	0	0
Nondairy Lightener, liquid	22	1	0	0	2	0	0
Table Cream	30	3	2	6	<1	0	0
Sugar, 1 tsp	16	0	0	0	4	0	0
Honey, 1 tsp	21	0	0	0	6	0	0
Whipping Cream, whipped, ¼ cup	105	11	7	11	1	0	0
Whipped Topping, pressurized, ¼ cup	40	3	2	20	2	0	0
Flavored syrup, 2 Tbsp (1oz)	90	0	0	10	22	0	0
Alcoholic Beverages (12 fl oz):							
Light Beer	110	0	0	6	7	0	0
Beer, Dark Beer, Ale, Malt Liquors	160	0	0	10	13	0	0
Malt Beverages	240	0	0	300	36	0	0
Wine Cooler	170	0	0	29	20	0	0
Wine Spritzer	100	0	0	5	3	0	0
Liquors (such as whiskey, rum and vodka):							
80 Proof Liquor, 1oz shot	65	0	0	0	0	0	0
1½ oz jigger	95	0	0	0	0	0	0
100 Proof Liquor, 1oz shot	85	0	0	0	0	0	0
1½ oz jigger	125	0	0	0	0	0	0
Wine:							
Dry Wine, 6oz	150	0	0	10	4	0	0
Sweet Wine, 4oz	190	0	0	10	16	0	0
Sake, 4oz	160	0	0	10	4	0	0
Sangria, 8oz	160	0	0	15	16	0	0

	Calories	Fat (g)	Sat+Trans Fat (g)	Sodium (mg)	Carbohydrates (g)	Fiber (g)	Protein (g)
Mixed Drink, 8oz including ice:							
Daquiri, over ice or frozen	450	0	0	10	16	0	0
Margarita, over ice or frozen	400	0	0	10	25	0	0
Pina Colada	440	0	0	10	56	1	0
Gin & Tonic, Rum & Coke	220	0	0	10	13	0	0
Long Island Iced Tea	430	0	0	0	20	0	0
Cocktail, 3-4oz over ice:							
Bacardi Cocktail	150	0	0	0	12	0	0
Manhattan	220	0	0	0	3	0	0
Martini	240	0	0	0	2	0	0
Black Russian	275	0	0	0	12	0	0
Mint Julep	360	0	0	0	5	0	0
Whiskey Sour	300	0	0	40	35	0	0
Bloody Mary	160	0	0	550	6	0	0
Mai Tai	330	0	0	0	8	0	0
Tequila Sunrise	200	0	0	10	15	0	0
Cordial, 2oz:							
Cherry Brandy	150	0	0	2	19	0	0
Coffee	210	0	0	0	23	0	0
Coffee with Cream	210	6	na	60	12	0	0
Creme de Menthe	250	0	0	5	28	0	0
Grand Marnier, Triple Sec	160	0	0	0	13	0	0
Kirsch, Peppermint Snapps	170	0	0	0	15	0	0

Soups & Salads

Soup

You've just arrived at a restaurant and you're feeling famished. What can you order that will be served fast? Soups, if chosen wisely, can stave off your appetite (without increasing your waistline) until your main course arrives. Simply consider the following guidelines:

- **Choose broth-based soups.** Broth-based soups such as chicken rice or vegetable soup can help satiate your hunger so that you don't overeat during the rest of the meal. Unfortunately, all restaurant soups are high in sodium so be careful with the portion size.

- **Avoid cream-based soups.** They often have twice the calories of broth-based soups. Be sure to ask about the ingredients of the soup. While *creamy* soups at a salad bar or fast food restaurant are typically made with milk, upscale restaurants are likely to use a high-fat cream. Some restaurants are now serving healthy "cream" soups made with skim milk and pureed vegetables - so be sure to ask what makes the soup creamy.

- **Roux is deceiving.** Thick soups (such as gumbo, jambalaya, and baked potato soup) are often prepared with roux (a thickener made from fat and flour). Roux increases the caloric content of the soup much more than it appears. Do you *really* want to spend your full meal's allotment of calories on a bowl of soup?

• **Skip the garnish.** Some soups, especially in upscale restaurants, are "garnished" with a dollop of sour cream (50 calories and 5g fat) or a swirl of heavy cream (20 calories and 2g fat per teaspoon). The tortilla soup may have fried tortilla strips and avocado cubes added prior to being served. Baked potato soup might be topped with crumbled bacon. Unless you can afford all the extra calories, consider asking for your soup to be served plain or with all the toppings on the side - so you can decide which to indulge in.

• **Don't eat the bowl.** In some restaurants, soup is served in a bowl made of bread. Before you start nibbling on the "bowl," keep in mind that this bowl contains over 600 calories!

• **Select a cup, not a bowl.** A bowl of soup has 50-100% more calories than a cup.

• **Make soup your entree!** On the other hand, select a larger bowl of one of the lower calorie soups, add a slice of whole grain bread, and perhaps a side salad. This makes for a well-balanced meal that won't break the calorie bank!

Estimating the Calories in Your Soup

How many calories are in soup? It depends on what type of soup you choose and the portion size. Below is a listing of the calories per *cup*; higher calorie soups tend to also be higher in fat.

Calorie-Meter (per 8oz cup):

340	Thick Cheese Soup, Chili Con Carne w/o beans
300	Chili Con Carne w/beans, Butternut Squash, French Onion w/ toppings, Tomato Bisque
250	Thick Soups made with milk (ie. Baked Potato, Lobster Bisque, Broccoli & Cheese, New England Clam Chowder, Cheese)
200	Soups made with milk (ie. Tomato Soup, Cream of: Asparagus, Celery, Chicken, Mushroom, Potato, or Broccoli), Oyster Stew, Seafood Gumbo, Manhattan Clam Chowder, Tortilla Soup w/toppings, Vegetarian Chili w/beans (no meat), Bean Soup w/meat
180	Bouillabaisse (no rice), Pasta Fagioli, Split Pea w/ham, Bean Soup
160	Black Bean, Vegetarian
140	Lentil, Vegetarian
120	Chicken Noodle/Rice, Minestrone, Tomato (w/water)
100	Vegetable, Gazpacho

The previous information is for soups commonly found in fast food and fast casual restaurants; upscale restaurants typically serve a richer (and more caloric) soup. Note, too, the portion size in the previous chart is just 1 cup (8 fl oz). A small bowl (12oz) will have 50% more calories and a large bowl (16oz) will have *twice* as many as shown in the Calorie-Meter.

Salads

People watching their weight often have the misconception that all salads are low-calorie, lowfat meals. While raw vegetables *are* healthy, when laden with high-calorie toppings and dressings, an entree salad can contain far more calories than a hamburger and fries! Heed this advice:

• **Be picky.** Since entree salads at most casual restaurants contain 1000 calories or more, focus on which ingredients you can reduce or leave off. To drop the calories, request grilled chicken instead of fried, less cheese, or fewer nuts. You'll also save at least 100 calories if you ask for the croutons, cheese, or bacon to be completely left off.

• **Skip the shell.** Taco salads are frequently served in a fried tortilla shell (containing nearly 400 calories). Ask for your salad to be served in a plate or bowl instead.

• **Get the dressing on the side** so you can use less. Most salad dressings contain 60-80 calories per tablespoon. While a small salad may have just two or three tablespoons, large salads contain as much as ½ cup (or eight tablespoons)! You do the math. This could add up to 640 extra calories!

• **Choose a lower calorie dressing.** Since salad dressings are added moments prior to serving, it's no extra work for the kitchen staff to substitute it. Fat-free salad dressings typically have 5-30 calories per tablespoon and low-calorie dressings have about 30-50 calories per tablespoon. Restaurant servers sometimes confuse lowfat with fat-free when describing the salad dressing options. That's why it's a good idea to get in the habit of using all salad dressings sparingly. You could also try these options with minimal calories: picante sauce, salsa, lemon, and flavored vinegars (such as red wine, balsamic, or tarragon vinegar).

• **Watching carbs?** While *creamy* lowfat and fat-free dressings are lower in fat and calories, they are often two or three times higher in carbohydrates. The Italian or Vinaigrette lowfat dressings are not typically as high in carbohydrates.

• **Do the "dip 'n stab."** Instead of pouring on the dressing, dip your fork into the dressing and then into the salad for a taste with every bite. Trust me, you will use significantly less dressing and save yourself a lot of ancillary calories.

Salad Bar

Next time you're at the salad bar, consider the following suggestions:

• **Pile on the raw veggies, non-marinated beans, and fresh fruit.** These have the most nutritional value and are lowest in calories.

• **Add lean proteins** including grilled chicken, turkey, ham, broiled seafood, and cottage cheese. Protein helps fill you up and keep your energy up longer than just veggies alone.

• **Use minimal cheese.** Cheese is high in protein, but has as much fat (and calories) as fried chicken!

• **Watch the nuts and seeds.** Sure, they are chock-full of healthy monounsaturated fats, but consider that ¼ cup contains 200 calories. As a lower calorie alternative, add water chestnuts or raw jicama for some crunch.

• **Avoid mayo-mixed salads**. While *plain* pasta, cabbage, potatoes, chicken, and tuna fish are low in calories, the addition of mayonnaise (at 100 calories a tablespoon) will more than double the calories. Since three bean salad is often mixed with oil, be sure to drain it well.

• **Check out the size of the ladle.** Most salad dressing ladles will hold two tablespoons of dressing. Some hold four (which is ¼ cup)! How many ladles of salad dressing are you using?

Nutrition Information

Soups per 8oz cup:

	Calories	Fat (g)	Sat+Trans Fat (g)	Sodium (mg)	Carbohydrates (g)	Fiber (g)	Protein (g)
Baked Potato, w/cream & cheese	250	16	8	1000*	23	1	5
Bean Soup or Black Bean	180	2	0	1000*	31	16	10
w/ham	210	6	2	1000*	27	13	11
Bouillabaisse (seafood), w/out rice	200	8	2	1000*	6	<1	26
Broccoli & Cheese Soup	230	15	8	1000*	14	1	5
Butternut Squash, creamy	300	20	10	1000*	25	2	4
Cheese, thick, made w/cream	330	27	14	1000*	11	1	8
made w/milk	230	15	5	1000*	14	1	9
Chicken Noodle or Chicken Rice	120	3	1	1000*	19	1	4
Chili Con Carne, no beans	350	19	7	1000*	21	3	23
Chili Con Carne w/beans	300	14	6	1000*	30	9	15
Chili, vegetarian with beans, no meat	200	1	0	1000*	38	10	11
Clam Chowder, Manhattan	190	9	3	1000*	16	2	10
Clam or Fish Chowder, New England	250	15	6	1000*	20	1	6
Cream of Asparagus or Celery	180	9	3	1000*	18	1	6
Cream of Broccoli or Mushroom	200	15	5	1000*	16	1	6
Cream of Chicken	190	12	5	1000*	13	1	8
Cream of Potato or Vichyssoise	190	10	5	1000*	19	1	6
French Onion w/bread & cheese	300	17	10	1000*	25	2	12
w/out toppings	120	8	5	1000*	8	1	4
Gumbo w/rice, Seafood	200	8	2	1000*	19	3	12
Lentil, vegetarian	140	1	0	1000*	22	7	9
Lobster Bisque	250	15	7	1000*	15	1	13
Minestrone	130	2	0	1000*	24	4	4
Oyster Stew	180	14	7	1000*	10	0	4
Pasta Fagioli	160	6	1	1000*	22	1	4
Split Pea w/ham	190	6	2	1000*	26	5	8
Tomato, w/o milk or cream	120	3	0	1000*	20	1	3
Tomato, made w/milk	200	7	3	1000*	29	1	5
Tomato Bisque, cream-based	300	20	12	1000*	26	1	3
Tortilla Soup w/toppings	220	12	4	1000*	22	2	6
w/o toppings	120	6	1	1000*	10	1	6
Vegetable Soup or Gazpacho	100	1	0	1000*	17	2	6
Bread Bowl (fits 12oz soup)	625	6	0	960	120	8	24

*NOTE: Sodium content varies greatly depending on the recipe, ranging from 500-1400 mg/8oz cup. Most are in the range of 800-1000 mg per 8oz.

Dr. Jo says

Nutrition information above is per 8oz *cup*. Keep in mind that *bowls* range from 12-16oz.

SALAD: Vegetables:	Calories	Fat (g)	Sat+Trans Fat (g)	Sodium (mg)	Carbohydrates (g)	Fiber (g)	Protein (g)
Avocado, ¼	85	7	1	5	5	4	0
Green Peas, 2 Tbsp	15	0	0	70	3	<1	1
Jicama, ¼ cup	12	0	0	1	3	2	0
Lettuce, mixed variety, 1 cup	7	0	0	0	2	1	0
Olives, Black, 1	5	<1	0	40	0	0	0
Green, 1	10	1	0	110	0	0	0
Pickles, 2 slices	1	0	0	90	0	0	0
Pickle, 1 whole dill	23	0	0	1570	4	0	0
Sprouts, alfalfa, ¼ cup	2	0	0	0	0	0	0
Sprouts, beans, ¼ cup	15	0	0	3	2	0	0
Variety of Raw Veggies, 1 cup	25	0	0	5	4	1	2
Meats & Protein (2 Tbsp unless noted):							
Chopped Egg	30	2	<1	30	0	0	3
Whole Boiled Egg, 1	75	5	2	100	0	0	6
Cottage Cheese	25	1	1	100	1	0	4
Ham	25	1	0	250	0	0	3
Parmesan Cheese	70	5	3	210	0	0	7
Pepperoni, 6 thin slices	60	5	2	214	0	0	3
Shredded Cheese, cheddar	60	4	3	90	0	0	6
Salad Dressings (2 Tbsp or standard ladle, unless noted):							
Blue Cheese	160	16	3	300	1	0	<1
Caesar	120	12	2	250	2	0	1
French	160	16	3	260	5	0	0
Honey Mustard	150	14	2	200	7	0	0
fat-free	50	0	0	165	12	0	0
Italian	110	10	1	380	2	0	0
light or lowfat	50	4	1	410	3	0	0
fat-free	15	0	0	180	2	0	0
Lemon, ¼	4	0	0	0	0	0	0
Mayonnaise	200	23	3	150	0	0	0
Oil and Vinegar	140	16	2	0	0	0	0
Olive Oil, 1 Tbsp	120	14	2	0	0	0	0
Picante Sauce or Salsa	10	0	0	180	2	0	0
Ranch	150	16	2	250	2	0	0
light or lowfat	60	5	1	250	4	0	0
fat-free	30	0	0	350	8	0	0
Thousand Island	140	12	2	250	5	0	0
Vinaigrette	100	10	1	360	6	0	0
light or lowfat	45	2	0	310	7	0	0
Vinegar, 1 Tbsp	2	0	0	0	0	0	0

	Calories	Fat (g)	Sat+Trans Fat (g)	Sodium (mg)	Carbohydrates (g)	Fiber (g)	Protein (g)
Garnishes (2 Tbsp):							
Bacon Bits	50	2	0	200	3	0	4
Chickpeas (Garbanzo beans)	35	<1	0	75	5	2	2
Chow Mein Fried Noodles	30	2	0	25	3	0	0
Croutons	30	1	0	90	4	0	1
Granola	60	3	1	5	9	1	1
Kidney Beans	30	0	0	85	5	2	2
Nuts, unsalted	100	9	3	1	4	2	3
Raisins	60	0	0	0	15	<1	0
Sunflower Seeds	100	9	1	1	4	2	3
Water Chestnuts	15	0	0	2	4	1	0
Prepared Salads (¼ cup):							
Ambrosia w/coconut, marshmallows	75	3	3	170	12	<1	0
Banana Strawberry Medley	55	<1	0	3	11	1	0
Bean Salad	90	4	<1	250	8	2	6
Broccoli/Cauliflower/Ranch	80	8	1	200	5	1	0
Carrot Raisin Salad	95	6	1	185	10	1	0
Chicken Salad	150	10	2	300	4	1	11
Cole Slaw	80	6	1	100	7	1	0
Egg Salad	150	11	2	170	2	0	10
Fresh Fruit Salad	25	0	0	0	5	<1	0
Fruit Cocktail or Fruits in Sugar	50	0	0	0	15	<1	0
Macaroni, Pasta or Potato Salad	100	6	1	240	11	1	2
Marinated Mixed Vegetable Salad	60	4	<1	150	5	<1	1
Pea Salad	80	6	1	90	5	2	3
Tuna Salad	190	12	2	280	4	1	16
Waldorf Salad	110	10	1	60	3	1	1
Fresh Tossed Salads (1 cup):							
Caesar Salad w/dressing	170	13	2	550	9	1	5
w/o dressing	90	4	2	475	8	1	4
Chicken Caesar w/dressing	260	20	4	750	9	1	11
w/o dressing	140	7	3	450	8	1	11
Cobb Salad w/ dressing	200	16	4	500	7	1	7
w/o dressing	80	4	2	200	5	2	7
Garden Salad w/out dressing	25	0	0	0	5	1	1
w/shredded cheese	50	2	1	45	5	1	3
Greek Salad w/o dressing	60	4	1	170	3	<1	3
Oriental Grilled Chicken w/o dressing	160	8	1	260	9	4	12
Tomato & Mozzarella, w/o dressing	120	9	4	180	5	1	16
Spinach Salad w/dressing	240	18	4	500	8	2	10
w/o dressing	90	5	2	175	5	2	6

Breads & Spreads

Ooh, who can resist the smell and taste of freshly baked bread? I'm guessing very few based on the observation that nearly every full-service restaurant offers a basket upon being seated. Here are some suggestions on how to handle the temptation.

• **Go small.** A slice of sandwich bread or a *tiny* Parkerhouse roll weighs in at around 1oz and has just 75 calories. Most restaurant rolls and breadsticks are *twice* as big as these and therefore, have two times the calories.

• **Take a piece and ask for the rest of the bread to be taken away.** Don't torture yourself by staring at the bread basket all evening! You could also simply move it to the other end of the table.

• **Start low fat.** The higher the fat content of the bread, the more calories. Choose breads made with little fat such as pita, ciabatta, or yeast rolls. You can tell because they don't leave your fingers greasy like biscuits and croissants.

• **Ask for "no butter."** If the bread is typically served buttered, feel free to ask for your bread to be prepared without. It's an easy way to save a lot of calories!

• **Drizzle or dab - don't drench.** Butter and margarine each contain about 100 calories per tablespoon, so spread thinly. The same advice goes for oil - even olive oil. Sure, it's a healthy oil rich in monounsaturated fats. But like every other oil on the market, it contains 120 calories a tablespoon. So dip your bread into the oil instead of soaking it!

- **Choose margarine or oil over butter.** Like other non-animal foods, margarine and vegetable oil have no cholesterol – and they contain less of the unhealthy saturated fats. In the past, margarine contained high levels of the unhealthy trans fats. Most manufacturers have removed or reduced the trans fat content, especially from the soft tub formulations.

- **Muffins are loaded in calories.** Muffins have an undeserved healthy reputation - they are basically just unfrosted cake. But wouldn't a bran muffin be a better option than a cream-filled doughnut? Check the nutrition info at Dunkin Donuts. Yes, the bran muffin has more fiber (5g versus just 1g in the donut) but The Boston Kreme Donut has 360 calories and 16g fat while the Honey Bran Raisin Muffin has 490 calories and 15g fat.

Estimating Calories

To estimate the nutrition information for the breads you enjoy, two nuggets of information are necessary - calories per ounce and the weight of the bread in ounces. Interestingly, most breads fall within a fairly narrow range of calories per ounce.

Calorie-Meter (per ounce):

125 Biscuits, Plain Croissants
100 Muffins, Cornbread, Gingerbread, Chocolate Chip Bagel, and
       Buttered bread including breadsticks, dinner rolls, focaccia
75   Plain *unbuttered* bread including sandwich bread, rolls,
       breadsticks, French or Italian bread, pita, baguette, bagel,
       English muffin, lavash, focaccia, ciabatta

It's the portion size that often puts bread into the dangerous calorie range. The most accurate way to find the weight of a food is to use a postage scale, but how many of us drag our postage scale to the restaurant? These descriptions provide a good way to estimate portion size:

- **Bagels** - You can find mini (1oz) bagels and regular-size (2-3oz) bagels at most grocery stores. Watch out, though, because the gourmet bagels found in bagel shops are 4-5oz! At 75 calories an ounce for most varieties, that's more than 300 calories per bagel! A 4oz bagel is about 4" wide while the 5oz bagel is about 5" across.

- **Biscuits** - At 125 calories an ounce, biscuits are heavier and denser than plain bread. This density causes the portion size to be deceptively smaller than you may think. A 1oz biscuit is about the size of one of the "pop 'n serve" biscuits that come packed in a tube in the refrigerated section of the grocery store. These are not commonly served in restaurants though. Restaurant biscuits usually weigh at 2-3oz (or 250-325 calories).

- **Bread** - Compare bread slices at the restaurant with the familiar 1oz slice (75 calories) of ½″ thick sandwich bread at the grocery store. The thicker (¾″) slice, often referred to as "Texas Toast", weighs 1½oz and contains about 120 calories. Some restaurant breads are twice as thick as standard bread (2oz). A typical mini loaf of bread served in restaurants contains 3-5oz!

- **Breadsticks** - Restaurant breadsticks often come in two sizes. A 1oz breadstick is about 5½″ long and, therefore, contains about 75 calories unbuttered. A 1½oz breadstick (120 calories unbuttered) is 7½″ long and thicker.

- **Ciabatta** - a sandwich-size ciabatta roll (about 3½″ square) weighs nearly 4oz and contains about 280 calories. That 5" square ciabatta roll served in a bread basket may have 500 calories.

- **Cornbread and Gingerbread** - Portion sizes are about the same. A 1oz piece (100 calories) is 2″ X 1¾″ (1″ high) while a 2oz piece measures about 2″ X 3½″ (1″ high).

- **Croissants** - The 1oz dinner croissant is very small (just 3½″ long). A 3oz croissant is more sandwich-sized at 5½″ long.

- **English Muffin** - The standard size (1″ thick) found in most grocery stores and breakfast restaurants weighs in at 1½oz and contains just 120 calories. Upscale restaurants may also serve a 3oz gourmet English muffin which is only slightly larger in diameter, but denser and much thicker. This larger English muffin, sized for sandwiches, is twice as high in calories (about 230 calories).

- **Focaccio** - This flattened Italian bread is often used as a pizza crust, a sandwich bread, or served with oil for dipping. Because it's thick and dense, a small triangular slice (about 4″ long and 2½″ wide) weighs in at about 1oz (or 75 calories).

- **French or Italian Bread** - A 1oz slice (75 calories) of French or Italian bread is a 1½″ slice of a baguette (long, thin French bread) or a ¾″ slice of the regular French or Italian bread.

- **French Roll and Soft Rolls** - A dense crusty roll (about 3¾″ long) and a soft fluffy sub roll (6″ long) both weigh about 3oz and contain 225 calories.

- **Muffins** - Count on 100 calories for a golf-ball-sized muffin (1oz). Double that calorie count if it's the size of a racquetball (2oz). Triple it if it's tennis-ball-sized (3oz). Oh, and the ones as big as softballs? They're often 500 calories when they have flat tops, and may be as high as 700 calories if the top is overflowing.

- **Rolls** - A 1oz yeast roll is fluffy, yet quite small – about the size of the small "brown 'n serve" rolls found in the bread section of your local grocery store. Most restaurants serve rolls that are larger - about 1½-2oz in size and, therefore, 120-150 calories per serving.

Nutritional Information

Breads:	Calories	Fat (g)	Sat Fat (g)	Sodium (mg)	Carbohydrates (g)	Fiber (g)	Protein (g)
Bagel, 1oz (mini, 2½" diameter)	80	0	0	135	15	0	3
medium size	220	2	0	400	43	1	8
Bagel (large deli-size):							
Whole Wheat	280	2	0	450	54	4	10
Plain, Apple, Blueberry, Onion, Cinn. Raisin	300	2	0	540	60	3	10
Sesame or Poppy Seed	360	6	<1	660	64	5	13
Chocolate Chip	400	10	2	675	75	2	10
Biscuits, 1½ oz, 2½" square	190	8	2	400	17	<1	3
2oz, 3" round	250	11	2	533	22	1	5
Bread: thick slice sandwich	120	1	0	225	22	1	5
1" slice from small loaf, white	75	1	0	135	15	<1	3
1" slice from small loaf, wheat	60	1	0	130	12	2	3
Small white loaf, 4oz	280	5	0	640	52	2	11
Breadstick, 1oz plain	80	1	0	120	15	1	3
1oz buttered	115	5	3	160	15	1	3
1½ oz plain	120	2	0	180	22	2	4
1½ oz buttered	175	8	4	240	22	2	4
Ciabatta bread, sandwich square	270	2	1	500	55	2	10
large loaf served in bread basket	540	4	2	1000	110	4	20
Cornbread, 1oz (1¾" X 2" X 1")	90	3	1	480	15	1	2
1½ oz piece (2½" X 2" X 1")	135	5	1	720	19	2	3
2oz piece (3½" X 2" X 1")	180	6	2	960	26	2	4

	Calories	Fat (g)	Sat Fat (g)	Sodium (mg)	Carbohydrates (g)	Fiber (g)	Protein (g)
Breads (cont.):							
Crackers: Butter Crackers, 3	80	4	1	110	12	<1	2
Melba Toast, 2	20	0	0	45	4	0	<1
Saltine Cracker, 2	24	1	0	70	4	0	<1
Sesame Breadstick, 1	15	0	0	20	4	0	<1
Croissant, 1oz small roll	120	6	5	130	12	1	3
2oz large roll	235	12	8	260	22	1	5
3oz sandwich-sized	345	18	10	635	39	2	8
Focaccio Bread, 1oz	90	2	0	200	15	1	3
French Baguette, 1oz	70	1	0	110	15	1	3
French Roll, 2oz, 4" long	140	2	0	220	30	2	5
3oz, 6" long	210	3	0	470	38	2	8
Gingerbread, 1oz (1¾" X 2" X 1")	90	3	1	480	15	0	1
1½ oz piece (2½" X 2" X 1")	135	5	2	720	19	0	2
2oz piece (3½" X 2" X 1")	180	6	2	960	26	1	2
Italian Bread, 1oz	75	1	0	150	15	0	2
Spoon Bread, ½ cup	150	6	na	260	21	0	4
Yeast Roll, small, unbuttered, 1oz	80	2	0	140	15	<1	3
glazed w/butter	105	5	3	140	15	<1	3
Yeast Roll, large, unbuttered, 2oz	160	4	0	280	30	1	5
glazed w/butter	210	10	5	280	30	1	5
Spreads:							
Apple Butter, 1 Tbsp	20	0	0	0	4	0	0
Butter, 1 tsp	35	4	3	40	0	0	0
Country Gravy, ¼ cup	85	7	1	250	4	0	1
Cream Cheese, 2 Tbsp	100	10	7	85	0	0	2
lowfat, 2 Tbsp	50	4	2	150	0	0	2
Honey Butter, 1 Tbsp	90	8	4	35	4	0	0
Honey, 1 tsp	21	0	0	0	4	0	0
Jelly, Jams, or Preserves, 1 Tbsp	54	0	0	0	15	0	0
Margarine, 1 tsp	35	4	2	45	0	0	0
Olive Oil for dipping, 1 Tbsp	120	14	0	5	0	0	0
Whipped Butter, 1 Tbsp	70	7	5	65	0	0	0
Whipped Margarine, 1 Tbsp	70	7	4	70	0	0	0

Dr. Jo *says*

The measurements above are per *level* teaspoon or tablespoon. There are three teaspoons in a tablespoon.

Entrées, Sauces, & Sides

Entrées

Since most of the calories and fat grams in a single meal are found in the entrée, heed these general guidelines:

- **Limit the portion size.** If you're eating animal meat two or three times a day, you may want to limit your portions. Your heart health and weight will both benefit by limiting the portion to 3oz (especially if you like the fatty meat cuts) - this is about the size of a deck of cards. While you may be able to find a 3oz appetizer portion, lunch entrées are usually 6oz and dinner portions around 9oz. So split the entrée with a friend (and add more veggies to fill the plate) or request a "doggie bag" and take half the meal home.

- **Select leaner protein.** Fish, shellfish, chicken, and turkey tend to be leaner than ground beef and cheese. Pork tenderloin and leaner cuts of beef can still be fairly lean. Check out this comparison:

Calorie-Meter: Protein w/o added butter/oil:

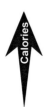

Sausage, Fried Steak, T-Bone, Porterhouse, Prime Rib
Fried Fish or Chicken, Cheese
Sirloin Steak (untrimmed) or Dark Chicken w/skin
Sirloin, Filet, Kabob, Medallions, Strip Steak (trimmed)
White Chicken w/skin, Pork Tenderloin
Skinless Roasted White Chicken
Grilled Bass, Salmon, Swordfish
Grilled Lobster, Scallops, Shrimp, Snapper, Tuna

- **Limit fried meats.** For the same size, fried meats twice as many calories as the baked, broiled, or grilled versions.

- **Trim off any visible meat fat and remove the poultry skin.** Leaner cuts of sirloin, trimmed of all visible fat, can be almost as low in fat and calories as chicken.

- **Avoid boned-in meats.** Much of the fat in a meat entrée is near the bone. So, order boneless chicken breast instead of boned-in chicken pieces, pork tenderloin rather than pork chops, and beef tenderloin instead of a T-Bone or order of ribs.

- **Request "no butter" on your protein before serving.** Steaks, fajitas, chicken, fish, and other protein sources are often brushed with oil during cooking to prevent sticking. On top of that, the chef often pours another tablespoon or two of clarified butter just before serving. Ask for it without the butter. (Now you know why the fajitas sizzle on your way to the table! Tell them you'd rather have "pretty thighs" than a "pretty piece of meat.")

- **Send the melted butter back.** Enjoy the sweet taste of lobster or crab legs without all that butter dip. Clarified butter contains 120 calories per tablespoon (and that small cup could easily contain four tablespoons)! Squeeze on fresh lemon instead.

- **Looking for a leaner steak? Look for "loin."** Beef sirloin and pork loin tend to be lean cuts of meat. Other lean cuts of beef include strip steak, filet, kabob, club steak, medallions, Delmonico, Kansas City, New York, and London broil. And oh yeah, skip the bacon that's typically wrapped around the Filet Mignon.

- **Avoid "Prime" cuts of beef.** Beef is graded upon the fat content. "Select" is the leanest and most difficult grade to find in restaurants. In the middle are "Choice" cuts, served in most restaurants. "Prime", the fattiest cut, is the grade typically served in upscale steakhouses. That extra fat contributes an additional 5-10% more calories and 10-25% more fat over the choice grade.

- **Order the "petite" size.** Portion sizes, when listed on the menu, are often in "raw" weights. Cooked portions will be about 25% less. Petite cuts of 7-8oz (raw) is more than enough protein for most of us. Keep in mind that since many upscale restaurants cut their own beef, they may be able to cut a steak any size you request.

• **Eat more fish and shellfish.** While their calories and fat varies widely, as a group, fish and shellfish generally comprise the leanest "protein" category. The American Heart Association recommends two servings of cold-water fish each week. These options include tuna, salmon, and herring. These fish are high in omega-3 fatty acids (a healthy unsaturated fat) which appears to lower serum cholesterol and triglycerides.

• **Request the use of a non-stick spray.** If you're dramatically cutting back on calories, you can ask for your protein to be stir-fried, pan-fried, or blackened with a non-stick spray. Restaurants stock the non-stick spray, not for diet purposes, but to prevent food from sticking to pans. Ounce-for-ounce, non-stick sprays have just as many calories as the oil it is derived from. But it is sprayed in such a thin layer that the non-stick spray adds on fewer calories (about 12 calories per five-second spray).

• **Watch the cholesterol.** The American Heart Association recommends dietary cholesterol be kept under 300mg per day. Variety cuts of beef, pork, and lamb (such as tongue, heart, or liver) are comparable in calories and fat grams to other meat cuts, but contain much higher amounts of cholesterol. While shellfish was once thought to be very high in cholesterol, the recent refinement of measuring procedures has demonstrated that it is not as high as was once thought. The cholesterol content of clams, mussels, oysters, scallops, Alaska king crab, and lobster are in the same range as chicken and beef. Shrimp and squid are higher in cholesterol, but they are so low in fat that they can still be included in a low fat/low cholesterol diet once or twice a week.

Sides

For better health, strive to eat smaller servings of animal protein, along with larger portions of grains, fruits and vegetables. The American Cancer Society suggests we eat at least five servings of fruits and vegetables and three servings of whole grains each day. When prepared without butter or oil, these foods are also low in calories and fat. Here are some more specific guidelines:

• **Split your entrée with a friend and order extra vegetables, starches, and/or a salad.** Ordered this way, the foods fill the plate as usual, but the meal is lower in fats and calories and it's usually just as filling.

• **Order double veggies.** Most restaurants serve a calorically dense meal in which large portions of meat and a "garnish" of vegetables are served. But you can order double the vegetables, and take half the meat home and make a meal for the next day.

• **Special order.** Vegetables aren't on the menu? Ask anyway. Restaurants often have broccoli, carrots, and tomatoes on hand.

• **Request vegetables "without butter."** If you don't, melted butter will undoubtedly be poured on top. (Yes, even on vegetables that are labeled as "steamed"!)

Calorie-Meter (per ¾ cup):

300	Refried beans
250	Buttered potatoes, rice, noodles, grits, polenta
225	French Fries
200	Buttered corn
180	Black beans or baked beans
170	Vegetables w/hollandaise sauce
150	Grilled or roasted low calorie vegetables, steamed rice
110	Low calorie vegetables with butter added
40	Steamed low calorie vegetables

• **Take charge.** If the vegetable arrives swimming in butter, drain the extra butter or cream sauce into your bread dish.

• **Think simple.** Get the plain baked potato instead of mashed, steamed squash instead of squash casserole, and steamed broccoli instead of broccoli & cheese. Gravies served by a quick service restaurant are typically not high in calories because they are usually prepared from lowfat gravy mixes. More upscale restaurants use meat drippings, butter, and/or cream to prepare gravies with far more calories and fat. Be careful!

• **Order the baked potato to be served "dry"** so you can control how many calories to add. A "dressed" potato can easily have double the calories of a plain potato. Salsa is a very low calorie topping whether it's plain or mixed with a little sour cream. Other leaner potato topping options include mustard or lowfat ranch dressing.

• **Size it up.** Every tennis ball-sized scoop of potato, rice, pasta, polenta, or grits has 100 calories (or 175 calories with butter). For potatoes, that's just a couple of tiny red potatoes. Most restaurants serve a 280 calorie potato (4.5″ X 2.5″). Oh, and that huge baked potato filled with barbecue meat and sauce?

Count on 500 calories "dry" and over 1200 calories with all the toppings.

• **Ask for a substitute for the fries.** The addition of French fries or onion rings can easily double the calories of your meal. In fact, count on an extra 450 calories and 25g fat. Consider asking for a lower calorie substitute (such as sliced tomatoes, fresh fruit, or salad with lowfat dressing). You could also split an order with a friend, or request that they only put a half order of the fried vegetable on your plate.

Butters, Sauces, & Toppings

Unless you requested otherwise, most entrées have butters, sauces, and toppings added - and most are high in both fat and calories. Here are some suggestions to keep your food flavorful without bulging in calories:

• **Skip the gloss.** Most chefs use oil to prepare meats, then brush (or pour) on another 100-200 calories of clarified butter to make the meat look pretty. Ask them to skip that final butter adornment.

Calorie-Meter (per 2 Tablespoons):

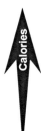

Calories	
240	Oil
200	Butter, margarine, mayonnaise, aioli sauce
140	Tartar sauce
120	Bearnaise sauce, cream sauce, pesto sauce
110	Vinaigrette
60	Sweet & Sour sauce, sour cream, cheese sauce
50	Chutney, Guacamole
40	Ketchup, Teriyaki sauce
30	Barbecue sauce, mustard, marinara sauce, relish, steak sauce
20	Worcestershire sauce
10	Salsa

• **Do the "dip 'n stab."** Since most sauces are either high in fat or high in sugar, ask for all sauces on the side so you can decide how much to use. Instead of pouring it on, dip your fork into the sauce and then into a piece of meat. You'll get the taste with every bite without as many calories.

• **Think fruits and veggies.** Most fruit and vegetable sauces are low in calories. These include salsa, marinara, chutney, black bean sauce, and sauces made from chicken stock and pureed vegetables.

Nutrition Information

ENTRÉES:

	Calories	Fat (g)	Sat Fat (g)	Sodium (mg)	Carbohydrates (g)	Fiber (g)	Protein (g)
Beef, per 3oz (unless indicated):							
Meatballs or Meat loaf, 3 oz	180	11	4	105	5	<1	15
six 1½" balls	400	25	9	630	11	1	33
Steaks: Sirloin, New York, Club, Delmonico,							
Tri-Tip, Strip, Kansas City, or Filet Mignon	200	12	5	50	0	0	23
trimmed	190	9	4	45	0	0	27
Corned Beef, trimmed	210	13	5	950	0	0	23
London Broil, Kabobs	210	13	5	20	0	0	23
trimmed	160	7	3	45	0	0	24
Pepper Steak, 3oz steak + veg.	225	18	8	100	2	<1	14
Rib Eye	225	14	6	45	0	0	25
Fajitas	250	17	7	500	4	0	21
trimmed	210	13	5	500	0	0	23
Split Back Rib meat w/BBQ sauce, 3oz	250	17	8	690	10	0	14
1 split back rib w/BBQ sauce	310	22	10	865	13	0	16
Chicken Fried Steak	270	19	8	500	16	0	9
Sausage	280	24	9	600	0	0	16
Prime Rib, Porterhouse, T-bone	290	23	9	50	0	0	21
trimmed	240	17	6	55	0	0	22
Ribs, per 3oz meat	300	24	8	15	0	0	21
1 rib w/BBQ sauce	175	11	4	400	3	0	16
Roast Beef, Pot Roast, Stew, Soup,							
or Stir Fry Meat	310	26	11	55	0	0	19
trimmed	170	8	3	30	0	0	25
Brisket	340	29	12	55	0	0	20
trimmed	190	8	3	45	0	0	30
Prime Rib	350	30	12	55	0	0	20
Short Ribs, per 3oz meat	400	36	15	45	0	0	19
1 short rib w/BBQ sauce	250	22	9	170	2	0	12
Pork (3oz):							
Pork Tenderloin	180	8	3	50	0	0	27
trimmed	140	4	2	50	0	0	26
Pork Ham	230	15	6	1000	0	0	24
trimmed	190	12	4	1000	0	0	21
Pork Chop	245	17	7	60	0	0	23
Pork Ribs	315	25	10	85	0	0	23

Dr. Jo says

Many appetizer or small plate portions contain 3oz meat. DOUBLE the information above for a typical 6oz lunch portion and TRIPLE for 9oz dinner portion.

	Calories	Fat (g)	Sat Fat (g)	Sodium (mg)	Carbohydrates (g)	Fiber (g)	Protein (g)
Chicken, per 3oz:							
Grilled Chicken Breast, no skin	150	4	1	600	0	0	29
Fried Chicken Breast Patty	250	12	6	630	18	1	18
Fried Chicken							
White w/skin	210	10	3	440	7	0	23
w/o skin or breading	165	5	1	140	0	0	30
Dark w/skin	245	15	5	600	5	0	23
w/o skin or breading	205	10	2	160	0	0	29
Roasted Chicken							
White w/skin	190	9	2	590	0	0	27
w/o skin	130	4	1	735	0	0	25
Dark w/skin (leg & thigh)	215	14	4	500	0	0	22
w/o skin	150	8	2	600	0	0	21
Chicken (per average piece):							
Fried Chicken							
drumstick (leg)	140	9	2	370	3	0	10
wing	130	8	3	385	3	0	11
breast	370	21	5	950	11	0	35
thigh	280	20	6	870	7	0	18
Chicken Pieces, 1 piece	42	3	1	110	3	0	3
Chicken Strips, 1	130	7	2	310	6	0	10
Buffalo Wings, 1	75	5	2	165	4	0	5
boneless wing, 1	90	5	2	400	9	0	3
Roasted Chicken							
Dark w/skin	300	18	5	500	0	0	35
w/o skin	210	10	4	725	0	0	30
Breast and wing w/skin	355	16	4	675	0	0	53
w/o skin	160	4	2	800	0	0	31
Chicken, Mixed Dishes (per 2 cups):							
Chicken and Dumplings	580	28	10	2500	60	4	22
Chicken Tetrazzini	730	39	14	1410	56	3	39
Other Poultry (3oz):							
Duck, w/skin	290	24	8	50	0	0	19
w/o skin	170	10	4	55	0	0	20
Goose w/skin	260	19	6	60	0	0	22
w/o skin	205	11	4	65	0	0	27
White Turkey w/skin	160	6	2	55	0	0	27
w/o skin	135	3	1	55	0	0	27
Dark Turkey w/skin	190	10	3	65	0	0	25
w/o skin	160	6	2	75	0	0	27

	Calories	Fat (g)	Sat Fat (g)	Sodium (mg)	Carbohydrates (g)	Fiber (g)	Protein (g)
Veal (3oz):							
Veal Sirloin Steak	170	9	4	70	0	0	22
Veal, roast or rib chop	215	14	5	75	0	0	21
Weiner Schnitzel, breaded w/sauce	320	21	7	550	17	0	16
Lamb (3oz):							
Leg of Lamb	210	13	5	55	0	0	23
Lamb Chops	260	20	8	65	0	0	21
Exotic Meats (3oz roasted, unless indicated):							
Snail	75	1	0	60	2	0	15
Frog Legs	90	<1	0	70	0	0	22
Turtle	135	6	1	125	0	0	21
Venison, roast or ground	135	3	1	45	0	0	27
Venison chop, 1	180	8	2	45	0	0	27
Reindeer	145	4	1	na	0	0	27
Beaver	180	6	2	50	0	0	32
Guinea Hen	180	7	2	75	0	0	29
w/o skin	125	3	1	80	0	0	25
Opossum	190	9	1	50	0	0	27
Muskrat	200	10	na	80	0	0	28
Pheasant, 3oz	205	11	3	45	0	0	27
breast, w/o skin	150	4	1	40	0	0	29
Quail, 3oz	220	14	4	60	0	0	24
breast, w/o skin	140	4	1	65	0	0	27
Rabbit	210	10	3	90	5	0	25
Raccoon	215	12	4	70	0	0	27
Squab (pigeon), 3oz	335	27	10	60	0	0	23
breast, w/o skin	150	5	1	65	0	0	26
Fish & Shellfish (3oz):							
Crayfish	75	1	0	85	0	0	16
w/Cajun seasoning	75	1	0	650	0	0	16
Shrimp	85	1	0	190	0	0	19
prepared w/butter	135	6	1	120	1	0	19
battered and fried	235	13	3	750	21	0	14
Lobster, Scallops, or Crab (Alaskan King, blue, dungeoness, & queen)							
plain	90	1	1	475	0	0	20
prepared w/butter	125	5	4	500	0	0	20
battered and fried	180	9	2	800	7	0	17
Catfish	90	3	<1	45	0	0	17
panfried	125	7	3	70	0	0	17
deep fried	240	15	4	180	11	0	16

Fish & Shellfish (3oz):

	Calories	Fat (g)	Sat Fat (g)	Sodium (mg)	Carbohydrates (g)	Fiber (g)	Protein (g)
Cod, Orange Roughy, Perch, Ling, Monkfish, Pike, Pollock, Pout, Sunfish, or Whiting							
raw, steamed	95	1	0	75	0	0	22
prepared w/butter	130	5	3	100	0	0	21
battered and fried	175	9	2	100	7	0	17
Oysters and Mussels	100	4	1	305	5	0	11
prepared w/butter	135	8	4	330	5	0	11
battered and fried	225	11	3	415	24	0	8
Mackerel, Tuna, Sea Bass, Snapper, Sheepshead, Smelt, Rockfish, or Wolfish							
raw, steamed	105	2	<1	75	0	0	22
prepared w/butter	140	6	3	100	0	0	22
battered and fried	210	10	2	120	7	0	21
Sea Trout, Sturgeon, Tilapia, Turbot	110	4	1	95	0	0	19
prepared w/butter	145	8	3	120	0	0	18
battered and fried	200	12	3	135	7	0	16
Octopus, Abalone	120	1	0	340	5	0	22
prepared w/butter	155	5	3	365	5	0	22
battered and fried	160	6	2	500	9	0	18
Squid	120	4	1	75	3	0	18
prepared w/butter	155	8	4	100	3	0	18
battered and fried	210	12	3	260	7	0	16
Crab, snow, leg	120	5	1	270	0	0	25
prepared w/butter	165	9	4	295	0	0	21
Clams	120	6	1	115	3	0	14
prepared w/butter	155	10	4	140	3	0	13
battered and fried	280	15	5	620	29	1	10
Bass (freshwater), Halibut, Salmon, Bluefish, Mullet, Spot, Swordfish or Tilefish							
raw, steamed	130	4	1	65	0	0	23
prepared w/butter	165	8	4	90	0	0	23
battered and fried	220	12	3	350	7	0	21
Cuttlefish	135	1	0	635	1	0	30
prepared w/butter	165	5	3	660	1	0	29
battered and fried	230	9	2	700	12	0	25
Carp, Rainbow Trout, or Cisco	140	7	2	140	0	0	19
prepared w/butter	175	11	4	165	0	0	19
battered and fried	225	13	3	155	9	0	18
Eel	200	12	3	55	0	0	23
battered and fried	275	20	4	90	6	0	18

Variety Cuts (3oz unless indicated):

	Calories	Fat (g)	Sat Fat (g)	Sodium (mg)	Carbohydrates (g)	Fiber (g)	Protein (g)
Tripe: beef	80	4	1	60	2	0	10
Lungs: beef, veal or lamb (braised)	100	3	1	50	0	0	18
Gizzards: turkey or chicken (simmered)	130	4	1	70	0	0	24
Kidney: beef or pork (braised)	135	4	2	80	0	0	25

	Calories	Fat (g)	Sat Fat (g)	Sodium (mg)	Carbohydrates (g)	Fiber (g)	Protein (g)
Variety Cuts (3oz unless indicated):							
Heart: beef, chicken, turkey (braised)	140	4	1	50	0	0	26
Liver: beef, chicken, veal, pork (pan fried)	200	10	2	80	8	0	20
Brains: beef or pork (pan fried)	175	14	3	150	0	0	12
Sweetbreads: lamb (cooked)	200	13	6	45	0	0	21
Feet: pork (simmered)	200	14	4	60	0	0	19
pickled	200	14	4	785	0	0	19
Pancreas: beef, pork, veal (braised)	210	12	4	50	0	0	26
Chitterlings: pork (battered and fried)	180	19	9	25	8	0	10
Tongue: beef, lamb, pork (braised)	235	17	7	70	0	0	21
pickled	235	17	7	885	0	0	21
Giblets: Chicken (fried)	235	11	3	95	4	0	23
Tail: pork (simmered)	335	30	11	20	0	0	16

SIDES

Most Vegetables, ¾ cup (broccoli, cabbage, carrots, cauliflower, green beans, greens, mushrooms, okra, onions, peppers, spinach, yellow/zucchini squash, tomatoes, turnips, or wax beans):

	Calories	Fat (g)	Sat Fat (g)	Sodium (mg)	Carbohydrates (g)	Fiber (g)	Protein (g)
Fresh, raw/steamed, w/o added fat	40	0	0	10	10	3	3
w/butter added	110	8	5	65	10	3	3
w/cheese sauce	115	7	2	480	15	3	6
w/Hollandaise sauce	170	14	8	120	12	3	3
grilled or roasted	150	12	1	210	10	3	3
sauteed w/bacon & drippings	135	10	5	225	6	3	4
canned, w/o added fat	40	0	0	600	10	3	3

Potatoes (per ¾ cup unless noted):

	Calories	Fat (g)	Sat Fat (g)	Sodium (mg)	Carbohydrates (g)	Fiber (g)	Protein (g)
Potato, Baked, medium 9oz (4.5" X 2.5")	280	0	0	20	65	6	6
1 Tbsp butter, ADD:	100	11	7	80	0	0	0
2 Tbsp sour cream, ADD:	60	5	4	10	1	0	0
2 Tbsp shredded cheese, ADD:	60	4	3	90	0	0	6
1 Tbsp crumbled bacon, ADD:	35	3	1	125	0	0	2
loaded w/ all above	535	23	15	327	66	6	14
Bacon bits, 2 Tbsp	50	2	na	205	3	0	4
Potato, Twice Baked, ½ medium	265	12	8	165	33	3	7
Potatoes, mashed w/butter	200	9	6	650	28	3	6
Home fries (chunks of potatoes, fried)	250	18	8	400	20	2	3
New Potatoes, buttered	140	3	1	120	24	3	4
Au Gratin	245	14	9	795	21	4	6
Scalloped Potatoes	160	7	4	615	20	4	5
French Fries, 1 cup	150	8	2	150	19	2	2
Potato Pancakes, one 4"	170	10	2	400	20	1	2
Sweet Potatoes, boiled	195	0	0	480	45	4	3
w/butter, marshmallows	300	3	2	150	60	4	3

	Calories	Fat (g)	Sat Fat (g)	Sodium (mg)	Carbohydrates (g)	Fiber (g)	Protein (g)
Other Sides (per ¾ cup unless noted):							
Avocado, ¼	60	5	1	0	3	2	0
Artichoke, steamed, 1	60	0	0	350	13	10	3
Beans, cooked whole, drained	240	6	2	700	35	10	13
Black Beans, whole	210	2	1	500	35	9	12
Boston Baked Beans	285	3	1	675	54	12	11
Refried Beans	300	15	5	240	33	8	11
Blackeyed Peas w/bacon or meat	180	5	1	600	22	6	11
Corn on the cob, 3" w/o butter	80	1	0	10	18	1	2
w/butter	115	5	2	40	18	1	2
Corn on the cob, 5" w/o butter	140	2	0	20	34	2	5
w/butter	205	13	5	75	34	2	5
Corn	160	0	0	525	34	5	5
w/butter	195	4	2	550	34	5	5
Couscous, plain	130	0	0	6	27	2	5
prepared w/oil	165	4	0	45	27	2	5
Green Bean casserole, ¾ cup	140	9	3	1065	12	2	2
Green Peas	95	0	0	400	17	7	5
w/butter	130	4	2	430	17	7	5
Mushrooms, ¼ cup sautéed in butter	110	11	5	125	2	2	0
Mushroom, 1 fried	30	2	0	22	2	0	0
Okra & Tomatoes	40	1	0	300	8	2	0
Okra, fried, ½ cup	90	6	1	60	7	1	0
Onion Rings, 1 large ring	80	4	1	70	10	0	0
Fried Whole Onion	2700	200	35	6400	195	15	20
Ratatouille, ¾ cup	75	4	0	200	11	2	0
Spinach Soufflé	180	13	6	575	6	1	4
Creamed Spinach, ¾ cup	280	23	15	580	12	4	6
Tomato, ½ broiled w/butter+cheese	80	6	4	350	6	1	3
Stewed Tomatoes	50	0	0	435	10	1	4
Yellow Squash Casserole	300	24	12	1300	21	3	0
Zucchini Marinara	60	3	0	310	8	2	0
Noodles or pasta, plain	160	1	0	2	31	2	6
buttered	225	9	5	55	31	2	6
Polenta, no butter, ½ cup	165	0	0	250	24	1	2
Fried Polenta, 2" round slice	110	4	0	130	17	0	1
Popovers, herbed, 1	190	11	5	150	18	<1	4
Red Beans w/rice, no meat	150	2	1	365	28	4	6
Red Beans w/rice, w/meat	230	10	4	400	24	3	11
Rice, steamed white	155	0	0	250	33	<1	3
Fried Rice	205	9	1	200	26	1	3
Mexican Rice	225	6	3	825	36	2	3
Rice Pilaf	160	6	2	750	24	1	3
Dirty Rice (w/sausage)	250	10	5	500	30	<1	10

	Calories	Fat (g)	Sat Fat (g)	Sodium (mg)	Carbohydrates (g)	Fiber (g)	Protein (g)
Other Sides (per ¾ cup unless noted):							
Risotto w/butter	205	5	3	280	33	<1	4
Risotto w/cheese	260	10	6	550	30	<1	10
Spaetzle, German noodles, plain	175	3	1	450	31	<1	3
Stuffing	200	9	1	600	25	2	2
Wild Rice	125	<1	0	5	26	2	4
Sauces, per 2 Tbsp (unless noted):							
Aioli Sauce (garlic mayonnaise)	195	21	3	5	0	0	0
Alfredo Sauce	75	7	5	180	0	0	3
Au Jus, canned broth	5	0	0	150	0	0	0
Au Jus, meat drippings	60	6	3	100	0	0	0
Barbecue	30	0	0	500	2	0	0
Béarnaise	120	12	7	220	3	0	0
Buerre Blanc	130	14	10	15	0	0	0
Bolognese, cream-based	50	4	1	45	2	0	1
tomato-based	30	2	1	145	3	0	0
Bordelaise	20	2	1	150	2	0	0
Brown Sauce	15	<1	0	30	2	0	0
Burgundy Wine Sauce	10	<1	0	5	1	0	0
Butter, salted	200	23	14	245	0	0	0
unsalted	200	23	14	4	0	0	0
Butter, 1 tsp (1 pat)	35	4	3	27	0	0	0
Butter, whipped, 1 Tbsp	70	7	5	75	0	0	0
Butter Wine Sauce	140	14	10	140	2	0	0
Caper Sauce	60	5	<1	265	3	0	0
Cheese or Mornay Sauce	60	4	2	180	3	0	3
Chili Cream Sauce	70	8	5	35	0	0	0
Chili Sauce	35	0	0	380	9	0	0
Chutney	55	0	0	0	14	0	0
Clarified Butter	240	28	2	0	0	0	0
Cocktail Sauce	40	0	0	320	10	0	0
Cranberry Sauce	50	0	0	10	13	0	0
Cream Sauce, thick	120	14	7	40	0	0	0
Cream Sauce, thin	50	4	2	180	1	0	0
Gravy, homemade	40	3	1	75	1	0	1
Gravy, canned	15	0	0	100	3	0	0
Guacamole	55	5	1	150	2	1	<1
Hollandaise	135	14	8	105	3	0	0
Horseradish, 1 Tbsp	6	0	0	15	1	0	0
Horseradish Sauce	60	6	4	20	1	0	0
Hot Sauce, 1 tsp	0	0	0	20	0	0	0
Ketchup	30	0	0	340	8	0	0
Lemon Butter Sauce	160	18	11	250	0	0	0

	Calories	Fat (g)	Sat Fat (g)	Sodium (mg)	Carbohydrates (g)	Fiber (g)	Protein (g)
Sauces, per 2 Tbsp (unless noted):							
Madeira	15	<1	0	30	0	0	0
Margarine, stick	200	23	4	200	0	0	0
whipped	140	20	3	170	0	0	0
Margarine, 1 tsp (1 pat)	35	4	2	45	0	0	0
Margarine, whipped, 1 Tbsp	70	7	2	85	0	0	0
Marinara	25	1	0	150	4	0	0
Mayonnaise	200	22	3	150	0	0	0
Meuniére	170	19	12	510	0	0	0
Mushroom Sauce	40	3	1	90	3	0	0
Mustard, 1 Tbsp	15	1	0	190	1	0	0
Mustard Sauce	45	3	2	200	3	0	0
Newburg	55	5	2	200	2	0	0
Oil	240	28	2	5	0	0	0
Orange Sauce	55	0	0	10	13	0	0
Oyster Sauce	55	4	0	150	5	0	0
Pesto	120	12	<1	280	3	0	1
Picante or Salsa	10	0	0	180	2	0	0
Relish, Corn	25	0	0	5	6	<1	0
Relish, Chow-Chow	35	0	0	160	8	<1	0
Relish, Cranberry Orange	60	0	0	11	16	0	0
Rémoulade Sauce	200	22	4	210	0	0	0
Salad Dressings, average	160	16	2	250	4	0	0
Sauce, green pepper chili (1 tsp)	1	0	0	1	0	0	0
Sour Cream	60	5	4	10	1	0	0
Soy Sauce, 1 tsp	3	0	0	340	0	0	0
reduced sodium, 1 tsp	3	0	0	170	0	0	0
Steak Sauce	30	0	0	200	4	0	0
Sweet and Sour Sauce	55	0	0	70	11	0	0
Sweet Pickle Relish	40	0	0	210	9	0	0
Tarragon Sauce	90	8	3	155	1	0	0
Tartar Sauce	140	14	2	200	3	0	0
Teriyaki Sauce	40	1	0	320	7	0	0
reduced sodium, 1 Tbsp	40	1	0	160	7	0	0
Tomato Coulis or Veracruz	40	2	0	100	4	0	0
Tomato Sauce	15	<1	0	20	3	0	0
Vinaigrette	100	10	1	10	0	0	0
White Sauce (thin), Béchamel, or Velouté	40	3	1	100	2	0	1
thick	60	4	1	100	2	0	2
Worcestershire	20	0	0	465	4	0	0

Ethnic Cuisines

Which ethnic cuisine offers the healthiest food? Actually, you can eat healthy at all different ethnic restaurants - as long as you know what to order and how to order it. This chapter offers tips and recommendations for dining out at Asian, Cajun & Creole, Italian, Indian, Mexican, and Middle Eastern restaurants.

Asian Cuisine

Traditional East and Southeast Asian cooking (including Chinese, Japanese, Thai, and Vietnamese) is considered "healthy" because small portions of meat are often combined with large amounts of lowfat vegetables, along with rice or noodles. Unfortunately, many Asian restaurants in North America now prepare their food "American-style" using large portions of meat. They are also known to add more oil than is absolutely necessary when stir-frying. The good news is that most Asian dishes are made-to-order so you can ask the cook to prepare your dish according to your dietary specifications. Here are some other tips:

- **Skip the buffet.** Have you ever noticed how buffet food literally "shines"? That's because foods featured on the buffet table are prepared with more oil to prevent sticking and drying in their pans. If you can afford the extra time, order from the menu. No time? Consider calling in your order ahead of time so it is ready when you arrive.

• **Avoid restaurants that serve their food too fast.** For speed in serving, some restaurants will cut up the meat and poultry in advance and deep-fry them (yes, deep-fry!) until the inside is cooked but the meat is not browned on the outside. When you order your meal, the individual orders are then stir-fried in the wok with *even more oil*. It is often difficult to determine whether the meat has been fried prior to being stir-fried because the color of the meat is the same. Be sure to ask how the meat is prepared.

• **Order steamed dumplings or fresh spring rolls.** Most restaurants offer a fried egg roll (sometimes called a spring roll). For a lower calorie appetizer or accompaniment, ask for steamed vegetable dumplings or a *non-fried* Thai spring roll (veggies and shrimp or crab meat wrapped in rice paper).

• **Fill up on soup.** Most Asian soups, although very high in sodium, are low in fat and calories. Select the Won Ton, Egg Drop (higher in cholesterol because of the egg), Hot & Sour, or Velvet Corn soup. Another good option is the Japanese Miso Hot Pot, often served family-style. The large bowl of broth-based soup contains udon (white) or soba (whole wheat) noodles, vegetables, and possibly shrimp or chicken.

• **Order steamed rice instead of fried rice.** It's almost always available for the asking - even if you see only fried rice on the buffet table. Brown rice is healthier than white rice, but not always offered. Boiled noodles are nutritionally similar to American wheat noodles and is a healthier choice than fried noodles.

• **Avoid "crispy."** Fried foods are often described as "crispy" on the menu. The frying process alone may double (or more) the calories of any meat or vegetable. That's why one piece of Japanese vegetable tempura contains 50 calories and 3g fat! Use caution at Dim Sum lunches since most of the items are fried.

• **Ask the chef to use as little oil as possible when stirfrying.** This is the most important request you should make at any Asian restaurant. Usually 1-2 tablespoons of oil (and sometimes lard) are used to stir-fry an entrée. That's 120-240 calories worth of fat. Some restaurants use even more!

• **More veggies, please.** Meat entrées have more calories than dishes that include vegetables. Beef, poultry, and seafood contain in the range of 120-520 calories per cup (or more if they are fried). On the other hand, most vegetables have only 50 calories or less per cup! Since your dish is made specifically for you, request more veggies than meat in any dish you select.

• **Use chopsticks.** It's difficult to eat quickly with chopsticks, especially if you are inexperienced. Eating slowly is beneficial because it will allow time for your stomach to signal your brain that you're full - before you get overstuffed.

• **Avoid sweet and sour entrées.** While sweet and sour sauce is high in sugar, that is not the biggest problem with it. The protein (chicken, beef, shrimp) is typically deep fat fried before the sugar-laden sauce is added. The same goes for Lemon Chicken and other fried and smothered dishes. Think before you order.

• **Caution with "House Specialties."** These higher priced items usually consist of large portions of meat, and little or no vegetables. This means that these dishes are higher in both fat and calories than mixed dishes. Of course, you can always special order the dishes as you like.

• **Rethink dishes with nuts.** Sure, nuts are filled with "healthy" monounsaturated fats. But a small handful of nuts (about ¼ cup) will add an extra 200 calories and 20g fat. And your dish could have even more than a ¼ cup! Water chestnuts (at just 20 calories per ¼ cup) are a great crunchy, low calorie alternative.

• **Order steamed foods with sauce on the side.** Some restaurant goers are choosing to order their food steamed. Of course, steamed foods will taste bland without the zing of traditional Asian flavors. As a remedy, mix the steamed foods with a pungent sauce such as plum sauce.

• **Four for dinner?** Order three dishes! It is common practice, in an Asian restaurant, to share your meal with others at your table. Consider ordering just three meals for a table of four. And, make sure at least one is vegetarian.

• **Order Chop Suey instead of Chow Mein.** Both dishes contain the same mixture of meat and vegetables. Chow Mein is topped with fattening fried noodles; Chop Suey is not.

• **Rethink tofu.** Tofu (a soft cheese made from soybeans) is high in protein, and moderate in both calories and fat - unless it's fried (like it is in most restaurants). And while tofu is known to soak up the flavor of the foods, it also soaks up a lot of oil. Sometimes a tofu dish can be as high in calories and fat as beef!

• **Ask for foods prepared without MSG** (Monosodium Glutamate). Some people are sensitive to this high-sodium flavor enhancer found in a shaker and certain ingredients (including some chicken broth). They report hot flashes, sweating, and headaches shortly after eating foods prepared with MSG. If sensitive, simply request that your food be prepared without it.

• **Pick lowfat sauces.** Most Asian sauces are low in fat, but high in sugar and/or sodium. If you are not restricting your sodium and sugar intake, these sauces are fairly low in calories and won't do a lot of damage on the scale: black bean sauce, hoisin, oyster, plum, and sweet and sour sauce.

• **Make your best guess.** Each Asian restaurant prepares its stir-fry dishes differently so it is difficult to list the exact calories per serving. Calorie count depends on three major factors: the amount of meat versus vegetables, whether nuts are added, and how much oil is used in stir-frying (an average is two tablespoons per dish). All-meat dishes will be higher in fat and calories than mixed or all-vegetable dishes. Generally speaking, here's how most Asian stir-fry dishes stack up:

Calorie-Meter: Asian Stir-Fry:

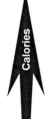

Beef w/nuts (Kung Pao Beef)
All Beef (Beef Sesame, Beef Orange Peel, Bejing Beef, Pepper Steak)
Chicken w/nuts (Kung Pao Chicken, Cashew Chicken)
Shrimp w/nuts (Shrimp with Candied Walnuts)
Fried Chicken or Pork (Sweet N Sour, Orange Peel, Honey Seared)
All Pork (Szechuan Pork)
Fried Tofu w/nuts (Vegetable & Tofu Kung Pao)
All Chicken (Sesame Chicken)
Fried Shrimp (Kung Pao Shrimp, Crispy Shrimp)
Fried Tofu w/vegetables
Beef w/vegetables (Beef N Broccoli)
Pork w/vegetables (Pork w/Green Beans)
Non-Fried Tofu w/vegetables
Chicken w/Vegetables (Moo Goo Gai Pan, Chicken w/Green Beans, Chicken Mandarin)
Shrimp w/vegetables (Shrimp Ginger Broccoli)
All Vegetable Dishes (Mixed Vegetables)

- **Use caution at hibachi Japanese Steakhouses.** At the hibachi grill, up to eight people sit around a flat grill to watch as the chef prepares all of the dinners at the same time. It's quite a show! Watch carefully and you will notice that a great deal of oil (and then butter) is added. Count on having more than two tablespoons in your serving alone. Since the dishes are prepared together, it will be difficult to request less oil. But you can always ask the chef to serve you before the final dollop of butter is added. Instead of adding rice to the food (which will sop up all the oil), use your fork or chopsticks to add the food (minus some of the high-fat, high-sodium sauce) to your rice. In addition, these meals are usually served with soup and salad. The orange Asian dressing is naturally low in calories and fat.

- **Drain the curry.** Thai curries are often made with coconut milk, which is very high in saturated fats. Instead of adding the rice to the curry, place the rice on a plate and add the curry "stuff" to it. Then add some, but not all, of the sauce.

- **Make a meal of sushi or negiri (raw fish and rice) and sashimi (raw fish only).** Queasy about eating raw fish? Sushi grade fish is frozen to destroy the parasites found in raw fish (though it should still be avoided by high risk individuals). But, no worries - not all sushi is raw. Sushi restaurants also offer cucumber rolls and American-style California rolls (cooked crab meat, avocado, and cucumber). You can also order scrambled egg, smoked or broiled eel, smoked salmon, boiled shrimp, crab, fried tofu, or grilled squid or octopus sushi. Enjoy the low-calorie wasabi (Japanese hot "horseradish" that looks like green paste) and request low-sodium soy sauce for dipping - it's often available for the asking.

- **Stick with the "rolls," instead of "cones."** Temaki (hand-rolled cones of sushi rice, fish, and vegetables wrapped in seaweed) are quite large and often topped with a high-fat sauce. Stick with the sushi rolls instead.

- **Caution at Dim Sum restaurants.** Dim Sum consists of small bite-sized foods. While some are steamed or baked, many are fried. Count on at least 100 calories in every piece.

- **Enjoy the fortune cookie.** It has just 30 calories.

Nutrition Information

	Calories	Fat (g)	Sat+Trans Fat (g)	Sodium (mg)	Carbohydrates (g)	Fiber (g)	Protein (g)
Appetizers (sauce not included):							
Egg Foo Yong, 2 – 1oz patties	210	16	8	na	7	0	10
Egg Roll, fried, 4"	200	12	4	490	16	2	8
Fried Beef/Chicken/Pork Dumpling, 1	80	5	2	150	6	0	4
Fried Pork & Shrimp Wonton, 1	45	2	0	100	3	0	4
Cream Cheese Ragoon, 1	65	3	2	60	8	<1	2
Shrimp Balls, 1	170	16	3	1450	2	0	5
Shrimp Toast, 2 small pieces	180	15	2	220	8	1	3
Spareribs, 2-3	340	20	3	1000	11	0	29
Steamed Vegetable Dumplings, 1	45	0	0	170	6	0	4
Thai Spring Roll w/shrimp (non-fried)	105	0	0	na	22	1	4
Crab Wontons, 2	190	13	3	250	13	1	6
Edamame, ½ cup	100	5	0	70	9	1	9
Soups (1 cup):							
Egg Drop	50	3	0	1000	2	0	4
Hot and Sour	75	2	<1	1000	8	2	6
Velvet Corn made w/broth, not cream	165	5	2	1000	23	2	7
Won Ton Soup w/4 won tons	180	8	2	1000	16	1	9
Chinese Noodle	200	9	3	1000	23	1	6
Rice & Noodles:							
Brown Rice, 1 cup	215	2	0	10	45	4	5
Crispy Chow Mein Noodles, ½ cup	120	7	1	100	13	1	1
Fried Rice, 1 cup	300	12	2	700	43	1	3
Glutinous Steamed White Rice, 1 cup	170	0	0	10	37	2	3
Oriental Noodles, ½ cup	95	1	0	na	21	1	1
Pad Thai (fried noodles w/shrimp), 2 cups	705	31	6	1085	88	5	19
Beef & Pork Entrées (1 cup unless noted):							
Chop Suey, Beef or Pork	220	12	3	na	14	2	16
Stir-fried Beef or Pork w/vegetables	325	23	6	na	13	2	17
Pepper Steak, 4oz	340	21	5	na	5	1	30
Beef or Pork w/vegetables	360	28	7	na	8	1	19
Mongolian Beef w/green onions/rice noodles	375	24	6	na	17	2	22
Oriental Noodles w/beef or pork & sauce	385	25	6	na	18	1	20
Shredded Pork w/Garlic or Peking Sauce	390	28	5	na	8	0	25
Beef or Pork w/cabbage & bok choy	395	30	7	na	7	1	24
Szechuan Beef or Pork	400	28	7	na	5	0	28
Twice Cooked Pork	420	29	7	na	10	0	28
Pork in Hoisin Sauce	450	30	8	na	17	0	28
Sweet & Sour Beef or Pork	515	35	9	na	30	0	20
Cashew Beef or Kung Pao Beef	580	49	10	na	14	1	22

	Calories	Fat (g)	Sat+Trans Fat (g)	Sodium (mg)	Carbohydrates (g)	Fiber (g)	Protein (g)
Fish & Shellfish (1 cup unless noted):							
Shrimp w/Snow Peas	165	10	4	na	7	2	12
Shrimp Chop Suey	180	10	2	na	11	2	12
Szechuan noodles w/scallops & veggies	280	16	4	na	20	2	14
Shrimp w/Cashews	460	38	8	na	5	1	24
Sweet & Sour Shrimp	495	38	8	na	16	0	22
Shrimp Fried Rice, 2 cups	770	33	7	885	85	3	34
Chicken Entrées (1 cup unless noted):							
Chicken Chop Suey	180	9	1	na	14	2	15
Moo Goo Gai Pan (chicken & vegetables)	190	9	1	na	14	2	13
Chicken & Snow Peas	200	12	3	na	7	2	14
Noodles w/chicken/veg/Szechuan sauce	290	17	2	na	21	2	13
Chicken Teriyaki, 1 quarter piece	335	16	2	na	6	0	39
Almond or Cashew Chicken	495	40	8	na	12	1	22
Kung Pao Chicken or General Tsao's	520	45	7	na	5	1	23
Sweet & Sour Chicken	550	39	8	na	28	0	22
Green Curry Chicken, 2 cups	650	45	8	750	28	1	33
all the "stuff "w/half the curry "soup"	405	24	4	550	16	1	31
Lemon Chicken	575	44	7	na	19	0	22
Vegetable (½ cup):							
Water Chestnuts	35	<1	0	5	9	2	0
Snow Pea/Mushroom/Bamboo Shoots	40	2	0	na	5	2	1
Chop Suey, vegetable	45	3	0	na	4	1	1
Bok Choy, oriental style	55	4	1	na	4	1	1
Stir-Fried Broccoli or String Beans	70	5	1	na	6	2	1
Szechuan-Style Eggplant	135	11	2	na	6	2	3
Tofu, ½ cup pieces raw firm	185	11	2	20	2	2	20
Szechuan noodles/cabbage/snow peas	195	11	2	na	19	2	5
Tofu, ½ cup pieces fried	275	21	3	20	2	2	20
Japanese Hibachi Meals (w/o rice):							
Vegetable Hibachi w/2 jumbo shrimp	385	30	6	1560	14	4	15
Steak Hibachi	725	52	25	1350	15	0	46
Chicken Hibachi	635	41	20	1540	15	0	48

Dr. Jo says

While much of the nutrition information listed on these pages is per *one* cup, most entrées tend to be *two* cups or more!

	Calories	Fat (g)	Sat+Trans Fat (g)	Sodium (mg)	Carbohydrates (g)	Fiber (g)	Protein (g)
Sauces & Oils (2 Tbsp unless noted):							
Soy Sauce, 1 tsp	2	0	0	340	0	0	0
reduced sodium, 1 tsp	2	0	0	170	0	0	0
Teriyaki Sauce, 1 Tbsp	15	0	0	690	3	0	0
reduced sodium, 1 Tbsp	15	0	0	320	3	0	0
Sesame Soy Dip, 1 Tbsp	30	2	0	500	1	0	0
Chinese BBQ Sauce	45	0	0	570	11	0	0
Sweet & Sour Sauce	55	0	0	70	14	0	0
Mustard Sauce	60	6	2	na	0	0	0
Plum or Duck Sauce	60	0	0	190	13	0	0
Sesame Oil or Vegetable Oil, 1 Tbsp	120	14	2	0	0	0	0
Sushi (per average piece):							
Cucumber Roll	30	0	0	10	5	0	1
California Roll	40	2	0	10	5	0	1
Sushi w/Shrimp or Snapper	35	0	0	5	4	0	5
Sushi w/Clam	40	<1	0	20	4	0	5
Sushi w/Salmon Roe (caviar)	50	2	0	170	4	0	5
Sushi w/salmon, mackerel, tuna or omelet	55	1	0	5	4	0	6
Sushi w/fried eel	70	3	0	10	4	0	7
Negiri w/shrimp or snapper	60	0	0	10	6	0	9
Negiri w/clam	65	<1	0	30	6	0	9
Negiri w/salmon roe (caviar)	80	3	0	275	6	0	7
Negiri w/salmon, mackerel, tuna or omelet	65	1	0	5	6	0	8
Negiri w/fried eel	95	4	0	15	6	0	9
Sashimi (tuna or salmon only, no rice)	35	1	0	20	0	0	7
Desserts:							
Fortune Cookie, 1	30	0	0	22	7	0	0
Lychee fruit in syrup, ½ cup	60	0	0	1	15	0	0

Cajun & Creole Cuisine

Cajun-style cuisine (originating from the Acadian French immigrants living in Louisiana) and Creole foods (born from the West Indies) is spicy and flavorful. To stay within your calorie budget while eating at these types of restaurants, follow these guidelines:

• **Appetizers can be entrées.** Boiled shrimp and crawfish are lowfat and low-calorie appetizers, but you can select either of these as a lean, filling entrée.

• **Go for red.** Choose the red sauce for dipping (and for your Po Boy sandwich). This flavorful sauce is much lower in calories than tartar sauce or the butter sauces.

• **Consider the sprinkle.** While Cajun and Creole foods do not have to be high in sodium, restaurants often rely on high-sodium seasoning salts (280 mg sodium per ½ teaspoon). Ask for a lower sodium option such as naturally low-sodium vegetables, herbs, and spices.

• **Skip the salad.** Most salads consist of iceberg lettuce doused with high-fat dressing. Iceberg lettuce ("crunchy water") is not nearly as nutritious as dark green leaves. You could easily get 300-500 calories in a side salad - and very little nutritional value. If you're eating salad just to get in a vegetable serving, skip it!

• **Ask what's in the salad.** For the more complex Cajun salads, you may want to omit some of the high-fat ingredients such as cheese, olives, and croutons (especially if they are simply "teasers" for you).

• **Keep it unadulterated.** Sure, fish is most often a lean protein, but only if it's prepared simply. So avoid the cod cakes, stuffed fish, and seafood salads that are prepared with hundreds of extraneous calories of mayonnaise, butter, and high fat salad dressings. Or keep these to an appetizer portion.

• **Go grilled or broiled.** If your taste buds are craving sauteed or blackened protein, ask the chef to use as little oil or butter as possible. Blackened chicken or fish is lower in fat than blackened beef.

• **Skip the crispy.** Fried fish has about twice as many calories as an equivalent portion of grilled or broiled fish. Plus, the fried portions tend to be much larger. That could make the difference between a lean 300 calorie fish portion - or one that's 800 calories or more! If you must have some crispy fried fish, consider having a fried fish appetizer instead of an entrée. The traditionally-fried Po Boy sandwich can often be prepared with broiled or grilled fish instead, if you ask.

• **Order the butter and sauces on the side.** A large serving of crab or lobster may have under 300 calories, but just one tiny dipping cup of melted butter adds another 400 calories.

Instead, dip your fork into the sauce and then into the fish – for a taste with each bite. Even if the vegetables are described as "steamed," keep in mind they are often doused with butter - order them without.

• **Roux can ruin a waistline.** Foods prepared with roux (a mixture of melted fat and flour used to thicken items such as étouffés and gumbo) contain more fat than they appear - and thus, more calories!

• **Maybe not the muffaletta.** This huge, frisbee-sized sandwich includes more than a pound of fatty meats and cheese - plus a full cup of the signature olive spread intended to fully saturate the bread. Eat just a half, and you've probably consumed more than your day's calorie needs!

• **Request plain rice instead of dirty rice**, which is prepared with a variety of meats including chicken liver, gizzards, sausage, and pork. Red beans and rice may be a lowfat choice, though if meat is added, the calories increase greatly.

• **No one-pounders!** Baked potatoes often weigh in at a pound (or about 400 calories without any toppings)! So, think twice before you add much butter.

Nutrition Information

Appetizers (3oz unless noted):	Calories	Fat (g)	Sat+Trans Fat (g)	Sodium (mg)	Carbohydrates (g)	Fiber (g)	Protein (g)
Alligator, fried	260	16	2	500	15	0	15
Calamari, fried	210	12	3	260	7	0	16
Coconut Shrimp, fried	320	19	8	755	23	0	14
Crabcake, 1	160	10	2	500	5	0	12
Crayfish, Boiled w/Cajun seasoning	70	1	0	650	0	0	14
fried, 3oz	200	8	4	500	18	1	14
Onion Rings, 1 large ring	80	4	1	70	10	0	0
Oysters, raw, 6	100	4	1	305	5	0	11
Baked w/butter & cheese, 3	330	24	15	500	11	<1	17
Shrimp, boiled, 6	135	2	0	300	0	0	21

Entrées w/o accompaniments or toppings: (9oz portion unless noted)							
Blackened Fish	460	28	12	1250	0	0	51
Chargrilled Fish	420	24	10	360	0	0	51
Crayfish Étouffeé, 2 cups w/o rice	590	40	22	1880	22	3	36
Jambalaya, chicken/sausage w/rice, 2c	600	19	4	740	56	3	30

	Calories	Fat (g)	Sat+Trans Fat (g)	Sodium (mg)	Carbohydrates (g)	Fiber (g)	Protein (g)
Entrées w/o accompaniments or toppings:							
(9oz portion unless noted)							
Oysters, Fried	675	33	9	1245	72	0	24
Seafood Platter, Fried w/hushpuppies, no fries	945	48	10	2350	69	1	66
Broiled Platter, w/o hushpuppies or fries	520	21	11	820	1	0	81
Shrimp, Fried	705	39	9	2250	63	0	42
Shrimp Creole w/rice, 2 cups	620	25	4	740	60	3	35
Soft Shell Crab, Fried	540	27	6	2400	21	0	51
Sides:							
Dirty Rice (w/sausage), ¾ cups	250	10	5	500	30	<1	10
French Fries, 2 cups	500	28	10	690	64	6	4
Gumbo, seafood/sausage, 2 cups w/o rice	460	27	10	1200	22	4	30
Hominy, ¾ cup	100	3	0	250	15	3	2
Hushpuppy, 1	60	3	<1	200	9	1	1
Red Beans w/rice, no meat, ¾ cup	150	2	1	365	28	4	6
prepared w/meat	230	10	4	400	24	3	11
White Rice, 1 cup	170	0	0	300	37	2	3
Buttermilk Biscuits, 3" round	250	11	7	675	31	1	5
Cornbread, 2½" X 2"	135	5	1	720	19	2	3
Muffaletta, ½ large sandwich w/o olive spread, unless noted:							
Turkey & Cheese w/o spread	715	23	18	2983	68	2	59
w/1c olive spread	1840	145	35	4119	75	6	59
Original (mortadella/ham/salami/cheese)	1200	73	31	3940	70	3	58
w/1c olive spread	2325	195	48	5075	77	6	58
Po Boy Sandwiches, 6":							
w/Fried Seafood & tartar sauce	985	54	4	1587	73	4	25
w/Grilled Seafood & cocktail sauce	628	12	2	1888	68	3	29
Sauces and Toppings:							
Crabmeat & Butter Meat/Fish Topping	270	26	2	240	0	0	8
Red Cocktail Sauce, 2 Tbsp	40	0	0	320	10	0	0
Tartar Sauce, 2 Tbsp	140	14	2	200	3	0	0
Desserts:							
Beignets, 3 small (2" square)	360	22	10	500	44	1	3
honey, 2 Tbsp	130	0	0	1	35	0	0
Bread Pudding, 1 cup w/bourbon sauce	540	22	14	512	74	1	12
Pralines, 1 piece	185	10	3	40	23	1	1
Sweet Potato Pecan Pie, ⅙	570	32	8	310	55	2	4

Indian Cuisine

Restaurants in North America often serve food from all over India. Some of these foods include basmati rice and dals (beans and legumes) of the north, sweet and sour food from the west, coconut and chilis popular in the south, and fish from the east. Vegetarian dishes are also common. Here are some tips for eating out Indian-style:

- **Avoid the buffet.** Like any other buffets, Indian buffets are an invitation to eat too much. Order a la carte whenever possible.

- **Skip the fried appetizers** including Samosa (fried vegetable turnover), Papadum (fried lentil wafers), Alu ki Tikki (deep fried potato patties), Pakoras (deep-fried chick pea flour fritters), and Tikki Ki Chaat (fried potato patty served with spicy mashed chick peas.

- **Opt for these lower fat appetizers** - Dahl Rasam (pepper soup with lentils), Mulligatawny (lentil and vegetable soup), Alu Chat (diced potatoes, chopped tomatoes and cucumber), or Chole (hot chick pea curry to be eaten with bread).

- **Order family-style.** If you try to order a well-balanced meal, you'll find yourself with too much food. Instead, share three dishes at your table of four. Choose two vegetable options and a meat dish - or one vegetable, one bean, and one meat dish.

- **Choose tandoori or tikka dishes.** Tandoori and tikka chicken, fish, and lamb are marinated in spices and grilled in the clay oven. Tikka dishes have cream sauce added, but you can ask for it to be prepared without.

- **Pick another lower fat protein entrée.** These include Kebobs (skewered chunks of meat); Alu Chole (chick peas cooked with tomatoes and potatoes); Chicken, Fish, or Beef Vandaloo (cooked with potatoes and hot spices); Chicken or Fish Masala (cooked with spices and a thick curry sauce made of yogurt); and Shrimp or Lamb Bhuna (cooked with onions and tomatoes).

- **Avoid dishes cooked in a cream sauce.** Names such as korma or makhani/malai are giveaways. Chicken or Lamb Saag is also cooked with spinach in a spicy curry sauce, but you can ask for it to be prepared without the cream.

- **Select lowfat vegetable dishes** such as Chana (spicy chick peas) and Saag Alu (sauteed curry made with greens and potatoes).

- **Watch the ghee** (clarified butter). It's often used in the cooking preparation and brushed on the bread (naan or roti). Like butter, it is high in saturated fat and cholesterol. Ask the chef to use as little as possible - or ask for vegetable oil to be used instead.

- **Ask for roti** (unleavened flatbread made with whole wheat flour) rather than naan (large leavened flatbread prepared with ghee). Other high-fat breads to avoid include poori (fried circles of bread) or paratha (fried bread often stuffed with potatoes or meat).

- **No cream, please.** Heavy cream is often used in Indian cooking. Ask for the dal/bean soups to be served without added cream. Spinach saag, cauliflower, mixed vegetables, and eggplant are some of most popular vegetable options. Ask the waiter to have the vegetables cooked without cream. Curries are often made with cream but can also be prepared without it, if requested.

- **Plain steamed basmati rice (Pullao) comes with most entrées.** Therefore, there's no need to order additional Biryani (rice pilaf) - just watch the portion size.

- **No need to avoid the protein-rich calcium.** Dahi (plain yogurt) and Paneer (fresh cottage cheese) are used in Indian cooking. While whole milk is commonly used, lowfat milk is becoming more popular. Feel free to use Raita (yogurt with grated cucumbers, onions, and spices) as a sauce - it's only 25 calories per ¼ cup.

- **Jazz it up.** For extra flavor, enjoy fat-free condiments that are typically served with your meal such as cilantro chutney, tamarind chutney, and vegetable relish. Chutney consists of crushed fruits and/or vegetables. You may want to avoid the Papad (fried thin cracker made from lentils, chick pea, and rice flour) that is also often served.

- **Enjoy the chai.** Indian chai is simply tea infused with spices, and mixed with little milk and sugar. This is different from the typical American chai that's loaded with added sugar (and calories).

Italian Cuisine

Pasta sounds fattening, but it really doesn't have to be. Just follow these tips:

• **Think before you order.** Before diving into the salad and bread (since they can contain as much calories as a full meal), consider what else you want to order.

• **Dip, don't drench.** Olive oil is known as a healthy oil because it's rich in monounsaturated fats. But keep in mind that like other oils, it still has 120 calories per tablespoon. Use it sparingly. While Bruschetta sounds healthy (diced tomatoes spread on toasted Italian bread slices), oftentimes it is prepared with a lot of oil - and calories.

• **Get the salad dressing on the side,** even when the salad is served family-style. Just one serving of dressed salad at the Olive Garden contains 350 calories - and no, I'm not talking about the large bowl. Also, don't be confused about the term "Vinaigrette." I know it sounds light, but it's still Italian dressing at 75 calories per tablespoon. Try using a flavored vinegar (such as balsamic vinegar) for a zing of zero-calorie flavor.

• **Fill up with lowfat soups.** Minestrone, Bean, or Pasta Fagiolo soups are rich in vegetables and beans. These lowfat soups are much healthier options than appetizers of carpaccio or prosciutto ham. Those processed meats are nearly all fat, and then often get drizzled with olive oil.

• **Order a luncheon or appetizer portion.** Many Italian restaurants will serve you the small portion even if it's not mentioned on the menu. This is an especially good idea if you're a fan of Chicken, Veal, or Eggplant Parmigiana. The appetizer portions will be more in line with your calorie budget.

• **Size matters.** Each ½ cup portion of pasta (about the size of a tennis ball) contains about 100 calories. Unfortunately, many restaurants serve about 4 cup portions. It's then covered with sauce, and possibly cheese. Some Italian restaurants offer family-style portions of up to 8 cups of pasta.

• **Want a specialty pasta?** Sometimes whole wheat pasta is available - the calories are the same, but with a boost of fiber.

Homemade pasta may contain eggs which will add about 50 mg cholesterol per cup and a few grams of fat as well. Some restaurants offer dried pastas (made without egg) for patrons who are closely monitoring their cholesterol. Gluten-free pasta may also be available.

• **Stick with the red.** Check out the nutrition information on the next page. Marinara, pomodoro, puttanesca, and other red sauces are the lowest calorie choices. Sauces rich in cream and meat are higher in calories. These include creamy tomato, meat sauce, Alfredo, or carbonara sauce. If the menu states a particular sauce, you can always substitute a healthier sauce. For example, order Pasta Primavera with marinara sauce instead of the typical Alfredo or cream sauce. Although Pesto is prepared with healthy ingredients such as olive oil, pine nuts, and basil (plus cheese), it remains a very high-calorie sauce. You can ask the chef to use the pesto sauce sparingly.

Calorie-Meter: 2 cups Pasta with sauce listed below:

750	Carbonara sauce
720	Alfredo sauce
670	Pesto or Meat sauce
630	White Clam, Creamy Tomato, or cream-based Bolognese sauce
590	Tomato-based Bolognese sauce
550	Red Clam, Puttanesca, or Vodka Cream sauce
510	Marinara or Pomodoro sauce

• **Lighten up.** If you want cream sauce, ask them to use half the usual amount. The dish will still be flavorful, but oh so much lighter on the palate - and on the waistline.

• **Hold the oil.** Request for the meat to be steamed or grilled instead of sautéed or fried (even if the menu suggests otherwise). Upscale Italian restaurants (including Romano's Macaroni Grill) cook the vegetables and meat with oil before adding it to the pasta. The chef will gladly saute these in broth or wine instead if you ask. Once you cover the dish with sauce, you probably won't even notice the difference!

• **Pasta might be a better choice than meat.** Pasta with or without meat typically contains fewer calories than all-meat entrées. Parmigiana (breaded and fried) items have twice as many calories as the non-fried versions!

- **Cut the cheese - or at least use less.** Cheese has as many calories (ounce-for-ounce) as fried chicken. Instead of selecting pasta stuffed with cheese, choose pasta with a sprinkling of cheese.

- **Chicken, seafood, and veal are the leanest protein** - as long as they are not fried. Strips of beef are higher. The meats best avoided, due to their high fat and calorie content, is ground beef (and meatballs), cheese dishes, Pancetta (Italian bacon) and sausage.

- **Order "no sauce."** When ordering a side order of pasta, consider asking for no sauce to be added. Instead, use the sauce from the meat entrée to mix with the pasta.

Nutrition Information

	Calories	Fat (g)	Sat+Trans Fat (g)	Sodium (mg)	Carbohydrates (g)	Fiber (g)	Protein (g)
Appetizers:							
Brushetta, 1 toast w/topping	100	7	1	na	9	0	0
Pasta (1 cup):							
Pasta, no sauce or oil	210	1	0	5	42	2	8
Pasta Primavera w/tomato sauce	260	6	0	500	52	4	11
Pasta Primavera w/Alfredo sauce	510	29	18	725	50	2	16
Pasta Sauces (½ cup):							
Marinara Sauce	85	4	0	750	9	2	3
Pomodoro Tomato Sauce	100	5	0	270	11	2	3
Red Clam Sauce	120	8	2	240	6	1	7
Puttanesca Sauce	140	10	2	605	10	2	4
Vodka Cream Sauce	140	10	5	710	10	0	2
Bolognese Sauce, tomato-based meat sauce	170	11	4	585	7	2	10
Spinach, Mushrooms, & Cream	220	19	10	160	5	2	7
Bolognese Sauce, cream-based meat sauce	220	19	5	180	6	1	11
White Clam Sauce	200	17	5	600	2	0	8
Creamy Tomato Sauce	210	17	6	313	5	2	6
Meat Sauce (chunky w/meat)	250	16	7	300	4	1	22
Alfredo Sauce	300	28	18	720	8	0	8
Carbonara Sauce	330	30	15	770	0	0	15
Pesto Sauce	480	46	2	1120	10	2	6
Cheeses:							
Parmesan or Romano, 2 Tbsp	70	5	3	220	0	0	6
Mozzarella, 1oz	90	7	4	165	1	0	6
Feta Cheese, 2 Tbsp	50	4	3	200	1	0	3

	Calories	Fat (g)	Sat+Trans Fat (g)	Sodium (mg)	Carbohydrates (g)	Fiber (g)	Protein (g)
Accompaniments:							
Gnocchi Dumplings, 1 cup potato	270	13	8	141	33	2	5
Meatballs, 1 @ 2" diameter	80	6	2	300	2	0	5
Polenta, creamy, ½ cup	220	10	0	180	33	1	2
Fried Polenta, 2" round slice	110	4	0	130	17	0	1
Polenta Pasticciata, w/sauce	350	22	13	400	32	2	6
Prosciutto, Italian ham, 1oz	80	6	2	800	1	0	6
Risotto w/ butter, ½ cup	170	7	1	280	23	<1	5
Roasted Potatoes, ½ cup	170	11	2	300	16	2	2
Entrées:							
Cannelloni Florentine, 4 stuffed noodles	750	47	9	1000	59	6	24
Chicken Cacciatore, 6oz chicken	400	21	7	na	18	2	35
Chicken Parmesan, 6oz w/sauce	675	43	18	na	28	2	44
Chicken or Veal Scallopini, 6oz w/sauce	645	48	25	625	11	1	40
Chicken Tetrazzini, 1 cup	365	20	7	700	28	2	19
Eggplant Parmesan, 3" X 4" or 1 cup	380	22	9	1180	34	6	12
Chicken Fettuccine Alfredo, 1½ cups	900	58	24	770	67	4	28
Lasagna, traditional, 3" X 3"	390	16	7	1020	40	3	22
w/meat & cream sauce, 3" X 4"	685	45	23	538	36	2	28
Manicotti, 2 stuffed	675	42	21	1835	42	3	30
Ravioli, Cheese, 1 cup	340	10	4	220	38	3	25
w/red tomato sauce	430	14	4	490	47	3	28
w/Alfredo sauce	750	48	22	1180	49	3	32
Ravioli, Beef or Chicken, 1 cup	300	9	3	350	38	2	16
w/red sauce	370	14	3	620	44	3	19
w/Alfredo sauce	600	37	21	1310	45	2	24
Tortellini, meat & cheese, 1 cup	440	12	4	560	53	2	27
w/red sauce	530	17	4	830	61	3	31
w/Alfredo sauce	750	39	22	1520	63	2	33
Sauces for Entrées (2 Tbsp):							
Butter Wine Sauce	140	14	10	140	0	0	0
Cream Sauce, thin	50	4	2	180	1	0	0
Cream Sauce, thick	120	14	7	40	0	0	0
Lemon Butter Sauce	160	18	11	250	0	0	0
Meuneire Sauce	170	19	12	510	0	0	0
Tomato Sauce	15	<1	0	20	3	0	0
Desserts (others can be found in the Desserts chapter):							
Stuffed Cannoli, one 5"	250	10	6	100	30	1	8
Pirouline, 3 thin rolled/filled cookies	200	9	5	25	27	<1	2
Fruit Sorbet, ½ cup	120	0	0	0	31	0	0

Mexican Cuisine

If you like hot, spicy foods, Mexican restaurants may top your list of favorite ethnic cuisines. Yet most health-conscious individuals think Mexican restaurants are definitely off the list of acceptable restaurants. Good news - lean choices are available if you heed these suggestions:

• **Be selective.** Are you eating the chips, rice, beans, *and* the tortillas? That's a lot of carbs, fat, and calories! Which accompaniments do you really enjoy (your pleasers), and which do you eat simply because they are there (the teasers)?

• **Skip the fat.** Some upscale restaurants may offer baked chips or fresh corn tortillas with salsa instead of fried chips. At about 25 calories per chip, it's easy to consume hundreds of calories worth of chips before your entrée even arrives.

• **Stay in control.** You might want to decide how many chips or tortillas fit into your calorie and fat budget. Count out the chips you have allotted yourself and ask the server to remove the rest. You could also move the chips out of your reach so you don't unconsciously keep eating them.

• **Pile on the pico.** Pico de gallo, picante sauce, and salsa have a lot of flavor and nutrients for negligible calories. These are leaner choices than guacamole or sour cream (110 calories per ¼ cup). Sure, guacamole is rich in healthy fats, but it is calorie-ladened with fat nonetheless.

• **Share the nachos.** It's tempting to make nachos your meal but just 6 loaded chips can contain 500 calories!

• **Enjoy ceviche as an entrée.** Ceviche is fish "cooked" with lemons or limes (not with heat) and flavored with onions and jalapeno so it's lowfat, and low-calorie.

• **Choose corn tortillas over flour tortillas.** If you think you don't like the taste of corn tortillas, find a restaurant that makes their own. You just might like them better than the higher calorie flour tortillas.

• **Go for the simple beans.** Black beans are the leanest. Request charro or borracho beans (pinto bean soup) instead of the high fat refried beans (since most restaurants are still preparing it with unhealthy lard). Because the bean soup is prepared with bacon or other fat, it's best to use a fork to eat just the beans and leave the broth (and added fat) in the bowl.

• **Ask about the tortilla soup.** Tortilla soup is often prepared from a simple lowfat vegetable soup. The added bacon, cheese, avocado, and strips of fried tortilla are what contribute most of the calories and fat. Since they are added just before serving, you can ask for some or all of these components to be omitted.

• **Beans help to dilute the calories of beef.** Enjoy chili (made with beans) rather than chili con carne (beans with meat). Ask what toppings are added (such as sour cream and cheese); you can ask for them to be omitted as well.

• **Ask what's in the salad.** While lettuce and tomato are low in fat, most other additions are not. In fact, at many restaurants the Taco Salad is the highest calorie item on the menu! Ask yourself what components (such as cheese, sour cream, or avocado) you can do without. Select the chicken fajita salad over the beef fajita salad. Both are healthier options than the taco salad, which is prepared with ground beef.

• **No dressing on the salad.** Use the picante sauce or pico de gallo for a low-calorie, spicy dressing instead. If you want to tone down the spiciness, try mixing equal amounts of sour cream and picante sauce for a dressing with less than 20 calories per tablespoon.

• **Skip the temptation.** Most meals contain 1500-2000 calories. Order "a la carte" to get just the items you're craving and no more. Think about ordering a single chicken fajita (or two) or chicken tacos al carbon as a lean entrée. Depending on the size, each will contain 1-2oz meat. Pile on the lettuce, tomatoes, and onions for a filling meal. Less food translates into fewer temptations.

• **Ask for high-calorie items to be left off the plate** – especially if you tend to eat them just because they are there, rather than because you like them. The higher calorie accompaniments include refried beans, Mexican rice, guacamole, sour cream, and cheese.

• **Trim the meat.** This extra step will save at least 20 calories an ounce. That's more than 100 calories in a typical serving!

- **Choose leaner protein.** This includes grilled chicken, shrimp, or fish rather than beef. Select strips of beef instead of ground beef. Ground beef and fatty beef can be twice as fattening as chicken pieces, shrimp, or fish.

- **Not too much cheese.** Yes, ground beef is high in calories but cheese has as many calories and as much fat (ounce-for-ounce) as fried chicken! So, if you have a choice between an enchilada made with cheese or ground beef, pick the ground beef (or stick with chicken for the leanest variety).

- **Corn over flour.** Flour tortillas are prepared with fat, while corn tortillas are not. Plus, flour tortillas tend to be larger than the ones made with corn. The end result? A corn tortilla has 50 calories while the smallest flour tortillas contain 100.

- **Soft flour versus crispy corn?** It may sound counterintuitive, but crispy corn tacos (even though they are fried) may still end up with fewer calories and fat grams than non-fried (larger) soft flour tortilla tacos or burritos. Therefore, Chalupas or Tostadas (flat, fried corn tortilla topped with beans, meat and/or cheese) would probably be a lower calorie option than a large burrito.

- **Don't eat the salad shell.** Taco salads and fajita salads are often served in a fried flour tortilla shell. It's tempting to nibble away at the shell. Request that the salad be served on a plate for a savings of more than 400 calories!

- **Skip the sizzle.** Have you ever noticed the sizzle and smoke as fajitas are served? After the fajitas are placed on that hot cast iron pan, clarified butter is often poured on top just before leaving the kitchen. Ask for the fajitas to be served without the butter. Go ahead and request raw peppers and onions instead of the usual sautéed green peppers and onions. This is a very flavorful and crunchy topping with far fewer calories.

- **Request lower calorie entrées** (preferably prepared with chicken, fish, or shrimp). These options could include Fajitas, Tacos al Carbon or Soft Tacos (fajitas sold per taco), Camarones de Hacha (shrimp sauteed in red or green tomato sauce) or Arroz con Pollo (chicken and rice).

• **Watch the size.** Soft Burritos (chicken, beef, or beans/cheese wrapped inside a large flour tortilla) can easily exceed 1000 calories. Ask for two Chicken Enchiladas instead of the usual three. In restaurants where cheese is used liberally, you may want to ask for your dish to be prepared "light on the cheese."

• **Avoid high-fat dishes.** Chili Rellenos (breaded, stuffed, and fried peppers) and Chimichanga (fried burrito) are not only fried, they are often covered with a cheese sauce. Other high-fat dishes to be avoided include Flauta con crema (crisp tortilla stuffed with beef or chicken and covered with a cream sauce) and Beef or Chicken Mole (meat covered with a spicy sauce which often includes nuts and chocolate).

• **Opt for flan instead of sopapillas.** Flan, a baked custard made with egg and whole milk, is usually served in a small portion. Sopapillas (fried flour dough sprinkled with sugar and cinnamon) are high-calorie so share an order with friends.

Nutrition Information

	Calories	Fat (g)	Sat+Trans Fat (g)	Sodium (mg)	Carbohydrates (g)	Fiber (g)	Protein (g)
Soups (1 cup):							
Tortilla Soup w/avocado, tortilla strips	220	12	4	na	22	2	6
Gazpacho Soup	100	1	0	na	17	2	5
Black Bean Soup	180	2	0	1000	31	16	10
Chili (beans only)	200	1	0	na	38	10	11
Chili con Carne (beans and meat)	300	14	6	na	30	9	15
Chili con Carne, no beans	350	19	7	na	21	3	23
Chips and Tortillas:							
Tortilla Chip, 6 large chips	140	6	1	110	19	1	3
Salsa, ¼ cup	20	0	0	360	4	0	0
Nachos w/cheese, 6 large chips	220	13	5	410	21	1	7
w/beans, cheese, salsa	290	16	6	810	31	2	9
w/beans, cheese, sour cream, guacamole	405	26	11	970	34	3	9
loaded with above, plus beef	495	31	13	1210	37	4	17
Corn Tortilla, 6" diameter	60	<1	0	30	12	2	2
Tostada Chip, crispy, 4½"	50	3	<1	50	7	0	1
Taco Shell, crispy, 5"	60	3	<1	50	8	1	1
Taco Shell, crispy, large, 6"	110	6	1	130	14	2	3
Flour Tortilla, small, 6" diameter	100	3	<1	200	16	1	3
medium, 8"	150	5	1	350	22	1	4
large, 10"	225	8	1	450	30	2	6
Fried Flour Tortilla, 8"	220	11	3	350	22	1	4
10"	325	16	4	450	35	2	6

	Calories	Fat (g)	Sat+Trans Fat (g)	Sodium (mg)	Carbohydrates (g)	Fiber (g)	Protein (g)
Rice & Beans (¾ cup):							
Mexican Rice	225	6	3	825	36	2	3
Refried Beans	300	15	5	240	33	8	11
Beans, cooked whole, drained	240	6	2	700	35	10	13
Black Beans, whole	210	2	1	500	35	9	12
Toppings:							
Avocado, ¼	60	5	1	0	3	2	<1
Avocado + Salsa Verde, 2 Tbsp	45	3	<1	80	4	2	0
Cheddar Cheese, 2 Tbsp shredded	60	4	3	90	0	0	6
Enchilada Sauce (red, green), 2 Tbsp	15	1	0	130	3	1	0
Cheese Sauce (Queso), 2 Tbsp	80	7	4	300	2	0	4
Guacamole, ¼ cup	110	10	2	300	4	2	1
Hot Sauce, 1 tsp	0	0	0	20	0	0	0
Jalapeño, 1	20	0	0	3	3	0	0
Mole Sauce, 2 Tbsp	40	3	1	200	2	0	0
Olives, ea	5	<1	0	40	0	0	0
Pico de Gallo, 2 Tbsp	15	1	0	150	3	1	0
Salsa or Picante Sauce, 2 Tbsp	10	0	0	180	2	0	0
Sour Cream, 2 Tbsp	60	5	4	10	1	0	0
Salads w/3oz meat & cheese, sour cream, avocado (w/o fried bowl or dressing):							
Chicken Fajita Salad	365	22	9	880	10	5	31
Chicken Taco Salad w/tortilla strips	435	25	15	850	18	6	33
Beef Fajita Salad	440	31	14	800	10	5	30
Taco Salad, w/chili meat	545	35	14	1240	24	7	32
Fried Taco Shell Bowl only	420	30	8	250	32	3	6
Meats (3oz unless noted):							
Shrimp, marinated/grilled (12 medium)	135	5	1	120	1	0	30
Chicken Breast Fajita Meat, white	150	4	1	600	0	0	29
Chicken Fajita Meat, dark	180	8	2	600	0	0	22
Beef Fajita Meat, trimmed	210	13	5	500	0	0	23
Beef Fajita Meat, untrimmed	250	17	7	500	0	0	21
Beef Taco Meat, ¼ cup	175	9	3	480	6	1	17
Cheddar or Jack Cheese, ¼ cup	120	9	6	180	0	0	7
Chorizo (Mexican sausage)	315	30	11	600	3	0	6

A 3oz portion is about the size of a deck of cards.

Entrées:

	Calories	Fat (g)	Sat+Trans Fat (g)	Sodium (mg)	Carbohydrates (g)	Fiber (g)	Protein (g)
Arroz Con Pollo, 2 cups	530	22	8	1200	48	3	35
Beef Fajita							
1½ oz, trimmed, in 6" flour tortilla	205	9	3	450	16	1	15
2oz, trimmed, in 8" flour tortilla	290	14	5	700	22	1	19
Burrito (Soft), Bean & Cheese, 6"	340	9	4	1100	52	7	13
Beef Burrito, 1	430	19	9	1100	48	4	17
Chicken Burrito, 1	575	26	12	1800	60	4	25
Beef Fajita Burrito, 1	610	30	13	1800	60	4	25
Chicken Fajita							
1½ oz white meat in 6" flour tortilla	180	6	1	500	16	1	16
2oz white meat in a 8" flour tortilla	260	10	2	700	22	1	20
Enchiladas, Chicken, 2	545	32	13	1800	37	5	27
Cheese, 2	630	44	23	1700	33	5	26
Beef, 2	610	41	17	1400	32	5	28
Shrimp Fajita							
6 marinated shrimp in 6" flour tortilla	170	8	1	260	16	1	10
8 marinated shrimp in 8" flour tortilla	230	9	2	430	22	1	15
Quesadilla, cheese only, 10"	1090	70	26	1640	70	4	45
w/chicken	1240	80	24	2120	70	4	60
Taco w/beef & cheese, 2 small	395	27	10	870	22	2	16
Tamales, 4	350	17	4	500	33	3	16
Taquito w/shredded beef, 5	350	12	3	500	37	3	23
Tostada: bean/cheese, 3@4½" diameter	465	23	11	630	29	1	35

Desserts:

	Calories	Fat (g)	Sat+Trans Fat (g)	Sodium (mg)	Carbohydrates (g)	Fiber (g)	Protein (g)
Flan, ½ cup w/caramel topping	290	8	4	110	45	0	7
Fruit-Filled Chimichanga w/caramel topping	490	29	10	600	86	1	6
Sopapilla, one 3" piece	190	10	2	100	23	0	2
Honey, 1 Tbsp	65	0	0	0	17	0	0

Middle Eastern

Middle Eastern cuisine includes foods which are native to Greece, Syria, Lebanon, Iran, Iraq, Turkey, Armenia, and surrounding areas. Some of the staples common to this region include eggplant, olives, olive oil, legumes, yogurt, dates, figs, lamb, plain yogurt (commonly homemade with whole milk), and tahini or sesame seed butter. Frequently used spices are parsley, mint, cilantro, and oregano. Following are some general guidelines for healthful eating at Middle Eastern restaurants.

- **Avoid fried foods.** These include falafel (mashed fava beans and chick peas), calamari (fried squid), and kasseri casserole (fried Kasseri cheese served with lemon & butter sauce).

- **Request "no oil" to be added on top of the dishes.** While you may not be able to avoid the olive oil that is frequently used in the preparation, you can ask for "no oil to be added" on top of many of the dishes prior to serving. Think about making this special request when ordering hummus (mashed chick peas) and babba ganoush (mashed eggplant).

- **Request tomato sauce** rather than lemon & butter sauce or cream sauce.

- **Start off light.** If you're looking for an appetizer, choose these lower fat starters: hummus, baba ghanoush, Greek salad (with the dressing on the side), tabouli (cracked wheat mixed with parsley, tomatoes, and spicy dressing), or lentil soup.

- **Stay away these high-fat appetizers and salads**. These include Avgolemono soup (traditional Greek soup made with chicken broth, rice, vegetables, lemon, eggs, and often whole milk and butter), fish roe dip (made from fish eggs), Spanikopita (spinach & feta cheese pie layered with phyllo dough and a lot of fat), and taramolsalata (caviar blended with olive oil and lemon juice).

- **Get the pita bread plain.** Much of the pita bread is grilled in butter or oil. If you're picking some other high-fat foods, you may want to ask for your pita bread plain.

- **Share entrées.** You'll get plenty of food if you order just three dishes for a table of four. Make at least one of the dishes a vegetable dish.

- **Choose chicken rather than beef or lamb.** For example, select a chicken pita sandwich rather than gyros made with beef and lamb.

- **Select meat dishes rather than casseroles.** Casseroles are typically prepared with ground meat and have high-fat sauces.

- **Ask for cream and other high-fat sauces on the side.** When you have a choice, remember that tomato sauces are leaner than cream sauces. Unfortunately, casseroles are made in advance and their sauces can't be substituted. Enjoy the yogurt-based Tzatziki sauce - it contains just 30 calories per ¼ cup.

• **Choose lower fat entrées.** These include chicken in pita bread, dolma (grape leaves stuffed with rice and meat), lah me june (Armenian pizza topped with ground meat), kafta (grilled ground beef with spices), Sheik el Mahski (baked eggplant stuffed with ground lamb and pine nuts), Shish Kebobs, and souvlaki (marinated, grilled fish, or chicken).

• **Limit higher fat entrées.** Higher fat menu items include gyros (pita bread stuffed with thinly cut beef or lamb), kibbeh (fried cracked wheat, meat, sautéed onions, and pine nuts), moussaka (casserole of layered eggplant, lamb, and cheese topped with a white sauce), spanikopita (spinach and feta cheese pie made with phyllo dough), pasticchio (baked macaroni with ground beef and eggs, topped with a creamy sauce), omelets (typically filled with feta cheese and sausage), and loukanika (sausage).

• **Dilute the calories.** A meal of mostly meat, in any restaurant, will be high in calories and low in fiber. It's best to choose a smaller portion of meat (or share an entrée) and order steamed vegetables and a carbohydrate-rich food such as couscous, steamed rice, or rice pilaf.

• **Make dessert simple.** Choose fresh fruit or rice pudding (rizogalo) instead of baklava (a rich dessert of layered phyllo dough, butter, honey, and nuts). If you really must have a piece of baklava, make it small or share it with others.

Nutrition Information

Appetizers, Soups, & Salads:	Calories	Fat (g)	Sat+Trans Fat (g)	Sodium (mg)	Carbohydrates (g)	Fiber (g)	Protein (g)
Avgolemono (egg & lemon soup), 1 cup	130	5	2	500	14	0	7
prepared w/milk instead of broth	214	11	6	575	19	0	10
Baba Ghannoush, ¼ cup	80	6	1	5	7	3	1
w/oil on top	120	10	2	5	7	3	1
Cucumber Soup, 1 cup	195	13	5	85	13	2	6
Falafel Patty, 1 fried	150	13	2	50	5	0	3
Fattoush, 2 cups w/dressing	175	10	2	115	18	2	3
Greek Salad w/olive & feta, 2c w/o dressing	240	9	3	550	25	4	11
Lemon/herb dressing, 2 Tbsp	155	16	2	335	2	0	0
Hummus, ¼ cup	100	5	1	300	12	3	3
w/oil on top	140	11	2	300	10	3	3
Lentil Soup, vegetarian, 8 oz	140	1	0	1000	22	7	9
Pine Nuts, 1oz or ¼ cup	180	17	3	20	5	3	3
Stuffed Eggplant, ⅛ eggplant or 1 slice	135	8	4	345	10	3	6

	Calories	Fat (g)	Sat+Trans Fat (g)	Sodium (mg)	Carbohydrates (g)	Fiber (g)	Protein (g)
Appetizers, Soups, & Salads (cont.):							
Tabouli Salad, ½ cup	130	7	1	400	13	3	4
Tahini (sesame butter), 1 Tbsp	90	8	1	20	3	0	0
Yogurt/Cucumber Salad, ½ cup	70	3	2	30	8	3	2
Entrées:							
Baked Chicken, ¼ Greek Style w/potatoes,							
onions, lemon sauce	550	35	9	na	29	2	30
Gyro, chicken on 6" pita w/feta & sauce	480	28	6	1700	37	2	17
Gyro, beef/lamb, 6" pita w/feta & sauce	650	46	15	1500	37	2	17
Dolmades, 3 (stuffed grape leaves)	200	14	2	92	15	1	3
w/ground beef or lamb	290	21	5	120	14	1	11
Greek-style Lamb w/orzo, 4oz lamb	540	22	9	1075	54	3	31
Kibbeh, 1 cup	450	18	4	na	28	3	44
Lamb chops, 2 w/lemon sauce	400	18	6	na	3	0	50
Moussaka, 4" X 4"	460	30	8	900	24	7	25
Sheik el Mahshi, 2 cups eggplant casserole	525	41	19	1245	26	10	13
Shish Kebab, 1 skewer w/3oz beef	265	14	7	110	9	2	25
Shish Kebab, 1 skewer w/3oz chicken	215	8	4	120	9	2	27
Accompaniments:							
Couscous, plain, ¾ cup	130	0	0	5	27	2	5
Couscous, prepared w/oil, ¾ cup	165	4	0	45	27	2	5
Lemon & Egg Sauce, 2 Tbsp	25	2	<1	30	2	0	0
Lentils & Rice, ¾ cup	175	5	<1	475	27	5	7
Pita Bread, white, 6½" diameter	165	1	0	320	33	2	6
wheat	170	2	0	340	35	5	4
Rice, plain, ¾ cup	155	0	0	250	33	<1	6
Rice Pilaf w/veggies, ¾ cup	160	6	0	750	24	1	3
Tzataki Sauce (yogurt/cuke), ¼ cup	30	2	1	15	3	<1	1
Desserts:							
Baklava, 2" X 2"	440	30	10	300	33	2	10
Figs in syrup, 3 figs & 3 walnuts	250	8	1	10	42	5	3
Yogurt, plain w/whole milk, ¼ cup	40	2	1	30	3	0	2

Sweets & Treats

Are your taste buds craving something more? Want to splurge? Since most desserts are very high in fat and calories, here are some strategies to help you satisfy those cravings without undoing all the good things you do for your body.

Fresh Fruit

- **Choose fresh fruit.** It may not sound very exciting, but a beautiful dish of perfectly ripe fruit might be just what you need to satisfy your sweet tooth.

- **Fresh fruit not on the dessert menu?** Look closely. Are fresh strawberries served on the cheesecake? Does the restaurant offer mango salsa with the mahi mahi? If so, there's fresh fruit in the kitchen and they will probably serve you a dish, if you ask.

- **Ask for it to be served "without cream or other toppings."** Especially in upscale restaurants, fruit is dressed with whipping cream, powdered sugar, and/or possibly a cookie. A dollop of whipped cream could easily add 100 calories to a low calorie dish of fruit. It might be less tempting to ask to leave these off.

Frozen Yogurt, Soft-Serve, Ice Cream, & Sorbets

What about something creamy to end a meal? Other than fruit, a small serving of frozen yogurt, ice cream, or sorbet can be one of the lowest calorie desserts out there. But the selections available vary greatly! A scoop of no-sugar-added frozen yogurt at Baskin Robbins has just 90 calories while there are more than 1000 calories in a large custom creation at Cold Stone Creamery. Here are some suggestions to making your dessert fit into your plan:

• **Try sorbet, sherbet, or ice.** Each has 100-130 calories per ½ cup scoop. While ice and sorbet don't usually contain milk (and, therefore, may be acceptable for a person who has lactose intolerance), sherbet does.

• **Ask your taste buds.** Fat-free frozen yogurt, or no-sugar-added lowfat ice cream, has less than half as many calories as regular ice cream. Would you rather eat more of the lowfat dessert, or would you be more satisfied with a smaller portion of the high-fat stuff? Only your taste buds can answer that question.

• **Select frozen yogurt instead of soft serve.** While they both look the same dispensed from the machines, they are very different nutritionally. The self-serve machine in restaurants (unless it's clearly labeled as frozen yogurt) is probably soft serve. Soft serve is ice cream, and it contains about 50% more calories than frozen yogurt.

Calorie-Meter (per ½ cup or 4 fl oz serving):

250	Ice Cream or Custard Mixer
180	Soft Serve (ice cream) or Lowfat Ice Cream
150	Lowfat No-Sugar-Added Ice Cream
125	Lowfat Frozen Yogurt or Sherbet
100	Nonfat Soft Frozen Yogurt, Ice, or Sorbet

• **Order it served in a cup or small cone.** The small cake cone (25 calories) or sugar cone (45 calories) has fewer calories than the large waffle cones or bowls (160 calories). Those waffle cones dipped in chocolate contain more than 300 calories (nuts and sprinkles add even more calories). In addition, the larger cones hold more ice cream, meaning even more calories to tempt you!

• **Rethink mixers.** Cold Stone Creamery and similar ice cream shops are known for their voluminous servings of ice cream blended with candies and other toppings. Count on close to 400 calories for a small mixer and more than 1000 calories for a large mixer (not counting the waffle dish or cone).

• **Watch the toppings, too.** Fresh fruit is the healthiest topping. Most other toppings will add another 100 calories on a small cup. A large hot fudge sundae with whipped cream could easily have more than 1000 calories.

Estimating Calories in Frozen Desserts

• **Know your portion size.** Oftentimes nutrition information is provided per ½ cup portion, but no information is provided for the portion size that's actually served. Compare your scoop to the size of ½ cup measuring cup at home - or about the size of a tennis ball.

• **Don't confuse weight ounces with fluid ounces.** Some places, such as workplace cafeterias and frozen yogurt shops, sell soft serve and frozen yogurt by the weight on a scale (that's *weight* ounces). But nutritional information is provided per *fluid* ounce (how much space it holds in a measuring cup). While weight ounces and fluid ounces are the same for most liquids (such as milk, juice, and soda), they are *not* the same for frozen desserts. These desserts are pumped with air during the freezing process and can often increase in volume up to 50%. If you serve yourself an 8oz soft-serve frozen yogurt containing 100 calories per 4 fl oz, how many calories are in your cup of yogurt? No, not 200 calories. It's actually 300 calories! Of course, you can always rely on the measuring cup or visualize a tennis ball to estimate your portion size. If you know the weight of your frozen dessert, however, simply add another 50% to the *weight* ounces in order to find the *fluid* ounces. So, 8 *weight* oz on the scale is the same as 12 *fluid* oz.

Baked Desserts

• **Pick your pleasure.** There's no shortage of sweets and treats to choose from, so make sure you select something you really, really love. If you choose one of your pleasers, then the dessert will be worth the calories! Only you can decide.

• **Savor every bite.** Eat your dessert slowly and don't feel guilty!

• **Share.** Order one dessert and several forks so everyone at the table can share. Our taste buds are the most sensitive in the first few bites; that's when a sweet and rich dessert offers the most satisfaction. Since most desserts have anywhere from 300 to over 1000 calories per restaurant serving, a few bites may be all our waistlines can handle too.

• **Plan ahead**. When the dessert arrives, cut it into a piece that fits into your calorie budget - and then totally enjoy it. You may need to smoosh the rest to make it non-tempting.

• **Customize.** Ask the wait staff to serve you just a thin piece. Yes, they will do that. Of course, you'll still have to pay the full price, but you've saved yourself the temptation of more calories.

• **Don't rule out fast-food desserts.** Casual restaurants are notorious for serving huge desserts containing over 1000 calories. Yet, most fast-food restaurants still serve moderate portions of about 300 calories.

• **Choose one of the lower fat desserts.** Angel food and sponge cakes, as well as reduced-fat brownies and muffins may be offered. While these lowfat and fat-free baked goods often have significantly less fat than their regular fat counterparts, the calories may be still fairly high. That's because lowfat desserts are often higher in sugar and served in very large portions. Don't take this as an opportunity to overindulge. Check the calorie information first, if it's available!

• **Skip the crust.** Most of the fat and calories in pies, cobblers, and turnovers come from the crust. The fruit filling, while high in sugar, is relatively low in calories. So, if you're not a big fan of the crust, don't feel guilty about leaving it behind. You'll save more than half the calories.

• **Think sugar-free**. Sometimes the sugar-free varieties can save you some calories. With pie, it's only a 50-80 calorie savings over the regular. The reason why it's not any lower in calories is because 40% of the pies' calories come from the fat in the crust. But, of course, every little bit counts!

• **Muffins are very misleading.** As mentioned earlier, a muffin often has more calories than a doughnut. While it's true that muffins are not fried, they contain a lot of oil in the recipe. While the muffin may even have fewer calories *per ounce* than doughnuts, they often weigh more. An average doughnut is about half the weight of a 4-6oz muffin.

Calculating the Calories & Fat in Baked Goods

While large chain restaurants provide nutrition information, it's difficult to find it for small independent bakeries. So how do you find out the number of calories and fat grams in your favorite dessert? It's really quite easy to estimate. You can calculate the calories of any desserts as long as you know the weight of the item (place it on a postage or food scale) and the calories per ounce using this chart:

Calorie-Meter (calories per oz):

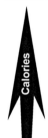

160	Shortbread
135	Almond & Chocolate Almond Biscotti, Brownie, Cake Doughnuts, Chocolate Croissant, rich Cookies (chocolate chip, peanut butter), Pound Cake, Macaroons, Peanut Butter Brownie
125	Cookies (butter, oatmeal, sugar)
120	Plain & Almond Croissant, Chocolate Cream-Filled Doughnuts, heavy Cakes (Italian Cream Cake, Carrot Cake)
110	Cheesecake, Coffeecake, Cinnamon Rolls & Danish, Scones, Gingerbread, Madeleine, Sweet Cheese Croissant, Pecan Pie, Muffins (chocolate chip, lemon poppy seed)
100	Plain Biscotti, Fritters, Glazed Fritters, most Cakes/Cupcakes (plain or frosted), Muffins (fruit or grain), Yeast Doughnuts (including glazed, frosted, crème & jelly filled), Fruit Tarts & Turnovers, Pies (Boston Cream, Buttermilk, German Chocolate, Chocolate Cream)
80	Tiramisu, Angel Food Cake, Sponge Cake, Lowfat Muffins, Pies (Fruit pies including Lemon & Lime, Coconut Custard, Mincemeat)
60	Pies (Banana Custard, Banana Cream, Custard, Pumpkin)

Don't have a scale? Here are some tips to help you estimate your portion size:

• **Brownie** - As you can see above, nearly every brownie has 135 calories an ounce, even the peanut butter or nut varieties. A 1" thick brownie measuring 2" X 2" weighs about 3oz. Most restaurant brownies are 2-3 times bigger!

• **Cake** - Both frosted and unfrosted pieces of cake contain about 100-120 calories per ounce. Count on 300 calories for a very small piece and double for a larger one. A piece of unfrosted slice of cake will contain 100-150 fewer calories than a equal size of frosted piece simply because it weighs less.

- **Cheesecake** - Most varieties contain about 110 calories an ounce. A thin 1½″ slice (similar to a slice found in your grocery freezer or fast food restaurant) weighs about 3oz while large thick slices may contain as much as 10oz.

- **Cinnamon Rolls** - Similar to cakes, cinnamon rolls have about 110 calories an ounce, but they are much denser. The mini rolls weigh about 3oz, while large cinnamon rolls at the mall are 7-8oz.

- **Cookies** - It doesn't really matter which flavor you pick. Most cookies contain 125-135 calories an ounce (shortbread cookies are a bit higher). It's hard to find a 1oz "mini" cookie (about 2″ across). Cookies found in convenience stores and fast food restaurants typically weigh about 3oz.

- **Doughnuts** - Dense "cake" doughnuts contain about 135 calories an ounce, while fluffy "yeast or raised" doughnuts average about 100 calories an ounce. This is not the only difference. Cake doughnuts look smaller, but they actually weigh more than larger, raised doughnuts. Therefore, a raised doughnut typically contains about 250 calories, while a cake doughnut contains about 100 calories more.

- **Muffins** - Most muffins, like cakes, contain about 100-110 calories an ounce. Because they are dense though, they often contain more calories than you think. A 1oz bite-size muffin is about the size of a golf ball. The 3oz muffin is about the size of a tennis ball. The 4oz muffin is around baseball-size and the 5oz muffin is as large as a softball. When confronted with the decision of the oat bran or the chocolate chip muffin, keep in mind that they will be very similar in both fat and calories. In fact, if they are the same size but the oat bran muffin feels heavier (it often does), it may even have *more* calories! Now, if you're thinking, "The oat bran muffin is healthier than all that chocolate," there may be some truth in that. But keep in mind that many commercial bran muffins have very little fiber. The brown color is more likely to come from the brown sugar and molasses rather than healthy fiber. So, you may want to eat the flavor you crave.

- **Pies** - Most pies contain 60-80 calories per ounce (except for pecan pies). The slices weigh more than an equal size of cake. A 9″ pie cut into eight slices (about 2¾″ slice) will contain anywhere from 270-300 calories (fruit and cream pies) to over

400 calories (pecan pie). Unfortunately, most restaurants cut the 9" pies into *six* slices (about 5" slice) so they range from 360-570 calories. If the restaurant makes a deeper 10" pie, you can count on 50% more calories!

Candy & Fudge

Stores that sell candy in bulk are popular in shopping malls, amusement parks, theatres, and airports. Since there is no nutrition information on the label, you may be consuming more calories than you realize. At the end of this chapter you'll find nutrition information for the most popular candies. Here are some general tips:

• **Buy just a little.** Let's face it. If you buy a big bag, you're more likely to eat the whole bag. So just select an ounce or two of your favorite candy. Since scales are often in pounds, keep in mind that 1oz is 0.06 pounds and 2oz is 0.13 pounds. Anything more than 4oz (or 0.25 oz) is just asking for trouble!

• **Consider sugar versus chocolate.** Candy, made mostly of sugar, has no fat and about 100 calories an ounce. On the other hand, chocolate and nuts are in the range of 150-160 calories and 9-10g fat per ounce. What's your "budget"?

Calorie-Meter (calories per oz):

160	Chocolate w/Nuts or Dark Chocolate, Chocolate Covered Almonds (8 pieces), or Hershey's Kisses® w/Almonds (6)
150	Milk Chocolate, Reese's Pieces® (35), M&M® (35), M&M® Peanut (12), Malted Milk Balls (10), Choc Nonpareils (7), Hershey's Kisses® (5), Hershey's® Minatures (3), or Reese's® Peanut Butter Cups (3 miniatures)
130	Peanut Brittle, Fudge (vanilla or chocolate w/ or w/o nuts), Pretzels (yogurt or chocolate covered), Boston Baked Beans (22), Raisinets® (22), or Candy Coated Almonds (8)
110	Chocolate Covered Thin Mints (4 sm), Tootsie Roll® (4 midgets) Caramel (3), or Caramels w/cream centers (2)
100	Cinnamon flavored (50 sm candies), Mints (34 soft dinner mints), SweeTarts (28), Candy Corn (17), Jaw Breakers (17-½" or two 1" balls), Gummy Bears (14), Gumballs (14-½" or two 1¼"), Jelly Beans (11 regular or 25 gourmet-sized), Gum Drop/Spice Drop (9), Smarties® (5), Bubble Gum (4), Hard Candies or Starlight Peppermints (4-5), Gummy Worms (4 reg or 3 sugar-coated), Licorice (3-6" sticks or 12 pieces)

Dried Fruit, Nuts & Seeds

Remember fruit has the same amount of calories whether it is dried or fresh. But since it's easier to pop large quantities of dried fruit into your mouth, we tend to eat more of that, consequently consuming more calories.

Nuts and seeds, while concentrated in healthy monounsaturated fat, are also concentrated sources of calories. A small handful (about 1oz or ¼ cup) contains 165-205 calories.

Pretzels

The original, plain, chewy pretzel (about the width of this book) has been sold at airports, amusement parks, and movie theatres for years. It had the same nutritional value of a plain bagel – around 350 calories and 1g fat. But the newer, more tender pretzels are more caloric.

• **Share your pretzel.** With the addition of butter, salt, sugar and/ or seasonings, most flavored pretzels are in the 400-500 calorie range. That's more than most of us can "afford" to eat for a snack.

• **Limit the dips.** Cheese dips and sweet caramel dips have more than 100 calories in a small dipping cup. If you must have a dip, try the marinara sauce or mustard dip at 30-40 calories.

Popcorn

Popcorn is often considered a healthy food due to its high fiber content (1g per cup). When air-popped, it's low calorie too (just 30 calories a cup). Unfortunately, movie theatres, malls, and convenience stores cook the popcorn in a lot of oil - and often a highly saturated fat. This increases the calories to about 55 calories a cup. And that's before the extra squirts of buttery topping! Here are some tips to keep your waistline and eat your popcorn, too:

• **Stick with the small.** While the small contains about 400 calories, the large size of popcorn has more than 1000 calories. And remember, the more you hold in your hand, the more you will eat.

• **Skip the "butter."** One squirt of butter-flavored oil has 130 calories! Since most people add four squirts on a large-size popcorn, this habit could add an extra 500 calories to this "snack"!

• **Select popcorn prepared with a healthier vegetable oil.** Most popcorn is still popped with coconut oil, a highly saturated (bad) fat. Some theatres are now using canola, a much healthier oil.

• **Estimate the size.** There are no standard sizes. Every theatre, airport, and sports concession stand offers a different size popcorn serving. How much popcorn is in your usual box, bag, or cup? Probably more than you think. Here are some tips to determine how many cups of popcorn are in your serving.

CUPS: If your popcorn was served in a cup, estimate how many fluid ounces it holds. Compare it to the cup sizes shown in the Beverages chapter or look for a size printed on the cup. The ounces may be labeled on the outside of the cup or on the bottom band (a code of "NO. 22P" is 22 oz). Then divide the number of ounces by 8 to see how many cups it will hold. For example, a 22 oz cup holds nearly three cups (22 ÷ 8 = 2¾ cups).

BOXES: The small, standard size found in many stores and airports measures 5½" X 8½" (a bit bigger than this book, but 2″ deep). This contains about 8 cups of popcorn when the cover is closed. If it is open and overflowing, count on at least 9 cups.

BAGS: Watch out, it's easy to overstuff bags. The measurements below are when the bag is filled, not overfilled. For visual assistance, the 12 cup bag (or a standard "medium" size) is a bit taller than the size of the front cover of this book (but 3.5" thick). The large might contain 20 cups and the tub at least 24 cups – that's around 1100-1320 calories!

Nutrition Information

	Calories	Fat (g)	Sat+Trans Fat (g)	Sodium (mg)	Carbohydrates (g)	Fiber (g)	Protein (g)
Fruits (per ½ cup):							
Fresh Fruit*	20-70	0	0	0	8-17	2	0
Fruit packed in or prepared w/sugar*	75-120	0	0	0	15-30	2	0

* For more detailed nutritional information on fruits, see the Breakfast chapter.

	Calories	Fat (g)	Sat+Trans Fat (g)	Sodium (mg)	Carbohydrates (g)	Fiber (g)	Protein (g)
Fruit Toppings:							
Fresh Whipped Cream, ¼ cup	104	11	7	10	1	0	0
Heavy Cream/Crème Fraiche, 2 Tbsp	104	11	7	10	1	0	0
Whipping Cream, canned, ¼ cup	40	3	2	20	2	0	0
canned (pressurized), ½ cup	75	7	4	40	3	0	0
Dried Fruits (1oz):							
Apple Rings, 4	70	0	0	25	17	3	0
Apricots, 8	65	0	0	2	16	2	0
Coconut, dried sweetened, ½ cup	95	7	6	5	9	1	0
Dates, 3½	80	0	0	1	19	2	0
Figs, 1½	70	0	0	3	18	4	0
Mixed Fruit	75	0	0	25	18	2	0
Peaches, 2	70	0	0	2	17	2	0
Pears, 1½	75	0	0	2	18	2	0
Pineapple Ring, 1	30	0	0	na	7	0	0
Prunes, 3	65	0	0	1	16	2	0
Raisins, 3 Tbsp	85	0	0	4	22	1	0
Nuts & Seeds (1oz):							
Cashews, dry roasted (18)	165	14	3	5	9	1	4
salted	165	14	3	90	9	1	4
Peanuts, dry roasted (40)	165	14	2	2	6	3	7
salted	165	14	2	150	6	3	7
honey roasted	170	13	2	180	8	3	7
Sunflower seeds or							
Pistachio Nuts, dry roasted (47)	165	14	2	3	8	3	6
salted	165	14	2	115	8	3	6
Almonds, dry or oil roasted, unsalted (24)	170	15	1	1	5	3	6
hickory smoked	165	15	1	120	5	3	6
Mixed Nuts, oil roasted & salted	175	16	3	100	6	2	7
Hazelnuts, dry roasted	190	19	2	1	6	2	7
roasted & salted	180	18	2	40	5	3	7
Pecans or Walnuts (15 halves)							
Macadamia Nuts, oil roasted	205	22	4	2	4	3	2
salted	205	22	4	75	4	3	2
Pretzels (1):							
Plain	375	5	2	950	72	3	8
w/o butter	330	1	0	900	72	3	8
Almond Pretzel	400	8	5	400	72	2	8
Cinnamon Sugar Pretzel	450	9	5	425	85	3	8
Iced Raisin Pretzel	510	4	2	480	110	4	8
Sesame Pretzel	410	12	4	860	64	7	10
Whole Wheat Pretzel	375	5	2	1100	72	7	8

	Calories	Fat (g)	Sat+Trans Fat (g)	Sodium (mg)	Carbohydrates (g)	Fiber (g)	Protein (g)
Frozen Desserts (per ½ cup):							
Ice or Sorbet	100	0	0	15	25	0	0
Nonfat Frozen Yogurt, soft serve	100	<1	0	50	19	0	3
Lowfat Frozen Yogurt, soft serve	120	4	3	65	17	0	3
Sherbet	130	2	1	25	27	0	1
Lowfat, No-Sugar-Added Ice Cream	150	3	2	140	30	1	3
Lowfat Ice Cream	180	4	2	120	32	1	3
Soft Serve	180	9	6	50	22	0	3
Regular Ice Cream or Concrete Mixers	250	14	9	120	27	<1	3
Ice Cream Toppings (2 Tbsp, unless noted):							
Fresh Strawberries	6	0	0	0	2	0	0
Fresh Blueberries	10	0	0	0	3	0	0
Fruit Cocktail, in own juice	15	0	0	10	4	0	0
Shredded Coconut	45	4	3	2	4	<1	0
Raisins or Strawberry Topping	60	0	0	0	15	<1	0
Grenadine, 1 Tbsp	60	0	0	0	15	0	0
Blueberry or Pineapple Topping	70	0	0	15	17	0	0
Whipped Topping, ½ cup (one big squirt)	75	7	4	40	3	0	0
No Sugar Added/ Fat-Free Hot Fudge	90	0	0	100	23	0	1
Marshmallow Creme	90	0	0	20	23	0	0
Chocolate Syrup	90	1	0	30	20	0	1
Caramel Topping	120	3	0	90	23	0	0
Hot Fudge Topping	120	5	3	35	19	0	1
Butterscotch Topping	130	1	0	110	29	0	0
Walnuts in Syrup	130	1	0	0	26	1	1
Candy & Nut Toppings (1oz, slightly rounded 2 Tbsp):							
Granola	60	3	1	5	9	1	1
Nuts, unsalted	100	9	1	0	3	1	3
Chocolate or Yogurt-covered Raisins	130	5	2	30	20	1	1
Butterfinger®, crumbled	130	5	3	60	23	0	1
Cookies, crumbled	135	5	2	95	23	0	2
Plain M&M® or Sprinkles ("Jimmies")	140	6	4	20	20	0	0
Reese's Pieces®	140	7	4	50	19	0	3
Heath® Bar, crumbled	140	9	5	105	15	0	1
Peanut M&M®	150	9	4	15	17	1	3
Cones (1):							
Cake	25	0	0	35	6	0	0
Sugar	60	<1	0	50	15	0	0
Large Waffle, commercial	120	2	0	55	23	0	0
Waffle Cone, fresh baked	150	2	0	5	33	0	0
Waffle Cone, chocolate covered	300	10	4	50	52	1	0
w/nuts	400	19	6	50	52	3	3

	Calories	Fat (g)	Sat+Trans Fat (g)	Sodium (mg)	Carbohydrates (g)	Fiber (g)	Protein (g)
Cakes:							
Angel Food, 1/12 tube or 2½" slice	160	<1	0	300	32	1	3
Carrot Cake w/frosting, 3" slice of 9" 2 layer	625	26	13	900	94	2	6
3" X 2" X 1" loaf slice w/frosting	360	15	8	530	54	1	3
Chiffon Cake, 1/12 of 10" tube pan	290	12	9	160	40	1	3
Chocolate w/frosting, 1/10 of 9" 2 layer	690	30	8	340	90	2	5
Devil's Food Cake, 1/12 of 9" 2 layer	530	19	5	250	70	2	4
Frosted Cake, 3" square X 2" high	375	18	5	340	55	2	3
unfrosted piece, same size	210	10	3	200	30	1	2
Fruitcake, ½" X 4" slice	210	7	1	175	40	3	2
Pineapple Upside Down, 3" square X 2"	360	14	3	350	55	1	3
Pound, 1" slice from rectangular pan	280	13	8	230	35	<1	2
Strawberry Shortcake, 2½" biscuit	430	24	12	240	45	1	3
Sponge Cake, 2½" slice	190	3	1	160	35	<1	2
Yellow, frosted, 1/12 of 9" cake	540	23	6	480	80	2	5
Cake Icing, chocolate, 2 Tbsp	140	5	1	50	23	1	0
Vanilla or Butter Cream Frosting, 2 Tbsp	150	6	1	20	25	0	0
Cheesecake (from 9″ tube pan):							
3oz, 1½" slice X 1½" high	330	23	14	310	25	1	5
6oz, 3" slice X 1½" high	660	46	28	620	50	1	10
9oz, 3" slice X 2½" high	990	69	42	930	75	2	14
Cobblers & Crisps:							
Fruit Cobbler, 1 cup	330	9	3	250	55	3	3
Fruit Crisp, 1 cup	260	8	3	120	45	2	2
Cookies:							
Peanut Butter, Chocolate Chip,							
Macadamia Nut, Chocolate Chunk, 1oz	135	8	4	100	16	1	1
2oz	270	15	8	200	34	2	2
3oz	405	23	12	300	50	3	3
Butter, Oatmeal Raisin, Sugar, 1oz	125	5	3	100	19	1	1
2oz	250	10	6	200	38	2	2
3oz	375	16	9	300	57	3	3
Doughnuts:							
Cake (compact)	360	22	10	330	44	1	3
Glazed, raised (fluffier)	250	14	6	330	31	1	3
raised and frosted (choc, van, straw)	270	15	7	340	31	1	3
filled w/jelly	290	14	7	340	36	1	3
filled w/crème	310	16	7	380	39	1	3

	Calories	Fat (g)	Sat+Trans Fat (g)	Sodium (mg)	Carbohydrates (g)	Fiber (g)	Protein (g)
Muffins:							
Mini (1oz)	110	5	1	110	13	<1	2
Tennis ball-sized (3oz), avg	330	15	3	330	39	2	6
banana nut, 3oz	315	13	3	190	47	2	7
bran, 3oz	320	12	2	375	45	6	6
chocolate chip, 3oz	330	17	5	170	56	2	6
cranberry nut, 3oz	330	13	3	150	45	3	6
lemon poppy seed, 3oz	330	17	5	450	45	2	6
Softball-sized (5oz), avg	550	25	5	550	65	3	10
Pudding (per ¾ cup):							
Bread Pudding,	280	10	6	250	40	1	6
Chocolate	250	13	7	180	32	2	6
Butterscotch	305	12	7	195	46	0	6
Vanilla	225	12	7	180	28	0	6
Rice	200	5	2	90	35	<1	6
Zabaglione (Italian frothy egg pudding)	110	6	1	25	8	0	6
Pies (from 9″ pan, unless noted):							
Apple, ⅛	270	13	3	240	34	2	2
⅙	360	17	4	320	45	3	3
Banana Cream Pie, ⅛	270	12	3	300	40	<1	3
⅙	360	16	4	400	45	1	4
Black Bottom Pie, ⅛ of 10"	380	16	7	na	45	1	2
⅙ of 10"	506	21	10	na	60	2	3
Blueberry Pie, ⅛	290	13	3	320	38	1	2
⅙	390	17	4	430	45	2	3
Brown Sugar Pie, ⅛ of 10"	590	25	5	na	68	1	1
⅙ of 10"	787	33	7	na	90	2	2
Cherry Pie, ⅛	350	17	4	410	40	1	2
⅙	465	23	5	540	56	2	3
Chocolate Cream Pie, ⅛	290	18	11	300	25	1	2
⅙	380	24	14	395	35	2	3
Coconut Cream Pie, ⅛	275	14	9	170	26	<1	2
⅙	365	19	12	220	40	1	3
Key Lime Pie, ⅙	460	20	9	na	57	1	3
Lemon Meringue Pie, ⅛	350	15	4	260	40	2	2
⅙	465	20	5	345	57	2	3
Pecan Pie, ⅛	430	24	6	230	40	2	3
⅙	570	32	8	310	55	2	4
Strawberry w/glaze + whip, ⅛	450	28	12	na	39	1	3

	Calories	Fat (g)	Sat+Trans Fat (g)	Sodium (mg)	Carbohydrates (g)	Fiber (g)	Protein (g)
Other Desserts (cont.):							
Baklava, 2" square X 2½" high	440	30	10	300	33	2	7
Biscotti, 7" long, chocolate or almond	130	6	3	45	16	2	2
Blintz, Cheese, 3" long	80	2	1	135	12	0	5
Fruit Filled, 3" long	125	5	2	95	17	<1	2
Brownie, 2½ oz, 2" square X 1" high	330	19	3	100	30	3	4
3½ oz, 2" X 3" X 1" high	475	28	4	150	45	4	5
Chocolate Croissant	370	23	8	260	40	1	4
Chocolate Mousse, 1 cup	380	32	16	60	15	0	6
Chocolate Pots de Crème, ²/₃ cup	270	21	12	30	23	0	4
Cinnamon roll (medium fast food)	225	10	2	230	31	2	3
large (mall-sized)	800	42	10	900	120	5	12
Cream Puff w/filling	300	18	5	380	28	<1	5
Crème Brûlée, ¾ cup	450	34	21	40	30	0	4
Crème Fraische or Heavy Cream, 2 Tbsp	104	11	7	10	1	0	0
Crepe, 1 w/o filling	135	7	2	40	15	0	2
w/chocolate filling, 1	280	16	6	40	33	1	2
w/fruit filling, 1	210	7	2	50	40	<1	2
Crepe Suzette, 1	160	6	2	75	16	<1	2
Custard, Baked or Stirred, ¾ cup	240	8	4	175	35	0	7
Flan, ¾ cup	225	6	4	225	37	0	6
Funnel Cake, 7" round w/sugar	1400	72	20	600	150	4	30
Gelatin, ½ cup	80	0	0	25	20	0	1
Marzipan or Almond Paste, 1oz (1½ Tbsp)	150	5	na	5	23	2	3
Pecan Roll, mall-sized	1100	50	20	1000	150	3	14
Scones, 2" wide wedge X 3" long	330	17	4	372	45	1	4
Snow Cone, 1 cup shaved ice w/syrup	120	0	0	10	25	0	0
Tiramisu, ¹/₈ of 9" pan (w/o cream)	220	14	8	40	12	0	5
Turnover, Fruit	330	15	4	305	38	2	5
Trifle: ¾ cup pudding+fruit+2 ladyfingers	450	15	14	400	70	4	6
Truffles, 1 Chocolate ball	80	7	3	5	4	0	1
1 Chocolate Nut ball	105	10	4	4	4	1	1
Popcorn (w/o butter):							
1 cup made /canola oil	55	4	1	100	6	1	1
1 cup made w/coconut oil	55	4	3	100	6	1	1
8 cups (small) w/coconut oil	440	32	24	800	48	8	6
12 cups (medium) w/coconut oil	660	48	36	1200	72	12	9
20 cup (large) w/coconut oil	1100	80	60	2000	120	20	14
24 cup (tub) w/coconut oil	1320	96	72	2400	144	24	17

	Calories	Fat (g)	Sat+Trans Fat (g)	Sodium (mg)	Carbohydrates (g)	Fiber (g)	Protein (g)

Butter-Flavored Oil:

	Calories	Fat (g)	Sat+Trans Fat (g)	Sodium (mg)	Carbohydrates (g)	Fiber (g)	Protein (g)
1 Tbsp (1 squirt)	130	14	4	0	0	0	0
4 Tbsp (4 squirts)	520	56	16	0	0	0	0

Candy:

	Calories	Fat (g)	Sat+Trans Fat (g)	Sodium (mg)	Carbohydrates (g)	Fiber (g)	Protein (g)
Bubble gum (4), Candy Corn (17), Cinnamon flavored (50 small candies) Gumballs (14-½" or 2-1¼"), Gum Drop/Spice Drop (9) Gummy Bears (14) Gummy Worms (4 reg or 3 sugar-coated) Hard Candies or Starlight Peppermints (4-5) Licorice (3-6" sticks or 12 pieces) Jelly Beans (11 regular or 25 gourmet-sized) Jaw Breakers (17-½" or two 1" balls) Mints (34 soft dinner mints) Smarties® (5) or SweeTarts (28)	100	0	0	10	25	0	0
Caramel (3) Caramels w/cream centers (2) Chocolate Covered Thin Mints (4 small) Tootsie Roll® (4 midgets)	110	2	0	50	24	0	1
Boston Baked Beans (22) Candy Coated Almonds (8) Fudge, vanilla or choc (w/ or w/o nuts) Pretzels (yogurt or chocolate covered) Peanut Brittle or Raisinets® (22)	130	5	2	na	20	1	1
Chocolate Nonpareils (7) Hershey's Kisses® (5) or Milk Chocolate Hershey's® Miniatures (3) Malted Milk Balls (10) Reese's® Peanut Butter Cups (3 miniatures) Reese's Pieces® (35) M&M® (35) or M&M® Peanut (12)	150	9	4	na	17	1	2
Chocolate Covered Almonds (8) Chocolate w/Nuts or Dark Chocolate Hershey's Kisses® w/Almonds (6)	160	10	5	na	15	1	4

PART 3

Favorite
Restaurants

A&W®

Tips:

- A combo meal includes regular Fries (310 calories and 12g fat) and regular Soda (250 calories).

- Many sandwiches are prepared with sauce - ask for without.

- Full nutrition information can be found at AWRestaurants.com.

Suggestions:

	Calories	Fat (g)	Sat+Trans Fat (g)	Sodium (mg)	Carbohydrates (g)	Fiber (g)	Protein (g)
Hamburger	380	19	7	860	33	3	21
Papa Single Burger	470	25	9	1000	38	4	23
Grilled Chicken Sandwich w/ dressing	400	15	3	820	31	4	35
Vanilla Cone, regular	200	5	3	115	32	0	6
A&W® Diet Root Beer Float, small	170	5	3	100	30	0	2
A&W® Diet Root Beer Freeze, small	260	8	5	170	39	0	7

Caveats:

- Stick with a single burger; the bigger ones are higher in fat:

Papa Burger®	690	39	15	1350	44	4	40
Original Bacon Double Cheeseburger	760	45	18	1570	45	4	44

- "Treats" should be consumed as treats - sparingly:

Polar Swirl®, avg all flavors	710	27	14	410	104	3	16
Milkshake, small, avg all flavors	700	30	18	200	96	1	11
A&W® Root Beer Freeze, small	370	8	5	170	68	0	7
Orange Freeze, small	450	8	5	170	108	na	7
A&W® Root Beer Float, small	330	5	3	100	70	0	2
Orange Float, small	320	5	3	115	74	8	4
Sundae, avg all flavors	330	9	5	180	53	0	8
Smoothies, avg all flavors	380	6	5	90	83	0	3
Reese's® PB Fudge Blendrr, sm 16oz	700	41	30	180	103	3	7
Slushee, sm 12oz, avg all flavors	300	0	0	40	75	0	0
A&W® Regular Root Beer, reg 20oz	270	0	0	50	72	0	0

Dr. Jo says

Beverages including juices, sodas, and coffee drinks are often not listed in this section of the book. Since they are similar from restaurant-to-restaurant, detailed nutrition information is in the Beverages Chapter.

Applebee's®

Tips:

- Try the Weight Watchers® or "under 500 calorie" entrées.

- Substitute. With any entrée, substitute steamed vegetables or fresh fruit in place of the mashed potatoes, fries, or onion rings. While the Seasonal Vegetables contain 35-50 calories, the Garlic Mashed Potatoes have 330 calories. Substitute grilled chicken or shrimp in place of fried chicken or shrimp.

- For more nutrition information, go to Applebees.com.

Suggestions:

	Calories	Fat (g)	Sat+Trans Fat (g)	Sodium (mg)	Carbohydrates (g)	Fiber (g)	Protein (g)
Under 500 calorie choices (includes sides):							
Asiago Peppercorn Steak	390	14	6	1520	25	5	44
Signature Sirloin w/Garlic Herb Shrimp	500	21	9	2440	31	6	51
Grilled Dijon Chicken & Portobellos	450	16	7	1820	30	6	55
Teriyaki Shrimp Pasta	440	8	2	3410	74	10	30
Teriyaki Chicken Pasta	450	8	2	2900	73	10	34
Grilled Shrimp & Island Rice	370	5	1	1990	56	5	29
Weight Watchers® options, as served:							
Chipotle Lime Chicken	490	12	2	4990	51	7	49
Cajun Lime Tilapia	350	5	2	1640	43	7	36
Spicy Pineapple Shrimp & Spinach	310	5	1	1690	48	5	22
Paradise Chicken Salad	340	4	1	2060	35	6	45
Steak & Potato Salad	380	12	4	1860	32	6	35
Veggie Burger	550	22	5	1560	60	7	29
Half Grilled Chicken Caesar Salad w/dressing	410	29	6	830	12	3	27
Chicken Noodle Soup, bowl	160	4	1	1100	17	1	13
Chicken Tortilla Soup	180	8	3	1540	18	2	9
Seasonal Vegetables (avg)	40	0	0	300	8	2	2
Fresh Fruit, side	90	0	0	0	24	3	<1

Caveats:

- Half portions are offered for all salads. The salads listed above are the lowest calorie ones. Full salads average about 1100 calories and 74g fat; half salads have about 630 calories, 44g fat.

- Most meals contain more than 1000 calories. Skillet Fajitas contain about 1400 calories; Cheeseburger Sliders have 1270.

- Skip the Side Salad. The Side Salad with dressing has as much fat and calories as the Garlic Mashed Potatoes.

- The small desserts are small in size, but not so small in calories. The Brownie Bite and the Shooters average close to 400 calories!

Arby's®

Tips:

- Roast Beef sandwiches are remarkably lower in calories than traditional burgers. Of course, much depends on the size and the toppings. Stick with the Jr. or Classic size.

- Most non-roast beef sandwiches contain mayo - so you may want to ask it to be left off.

- More nutrition information can be found at Arbys.com.

Suggestions:

	Calories	Fat (g)	Sat+Trans Fat (g)	Sodium (mg)	Carbohydrates (g)	Fiber (g)	Protein (g)
Jr. Roast Beef	210	8	3	520	24	1	12
Roast Beef Classic	360	14	6	950	37	2	22
Beef 'n Cheddar Classic	450	21	7	1240	43	2	22
Arby's Melt	390	16	6	1130	39	2	22
Ham & Swiss Melt	300	8	4	1070	37	2	18
Cravin' Chicken Sandwich, Roast	370	12	2	990	42	3	24
Chicken Bacon & Swiss, Roast	470	19	5	1310	43	2	32
French Dip & Swiss Toasted Sub au jus	450	17	8	2110	51	2	26
Roast Turkey & Swiss Wrap	500	24	7	1510	43	8	35
Roast Turkey & Swiss Sandwich	710	28	7	1780	78	5	39
Chopped Salads w/o dressing:							
Side Salad	70	5	3	100	4	1	4
Farmhouse Roast Chicken Salad	250	13	7	680	11	3	23
Balsamic Vinaigrette Dressing	130	12	2	470	5	0	0
Light Italian Dressing	20	5	1	790	3	0	0

Caveats:

- Market Fresh® Sandwiches are huge! Each sandwich contains 700-820 calories and 30-44g fat. The wraps are still high in fat, and have 500-630 calories. Best to share these.

- Combos come in small, medium, and large. If you must have a drink and fries, order the small combo consisting of a small drink (non-diet varieties contain about 180 calories) and small Curly Fries (450 calories and 24g fat).

- Think before you pop one of the Sides in your mouth. The Loaded Potato Bites® and Jalapeno Bites® have 60-70 calories (and 4g fat) per single piece. One Mozzarella Stick has 110 calories and 6g fat. Each Steakhouse Onion Ring has 90 calories and 5g fat. And, that's before you start dipping! While the Bronco Berry Sauce® adds another 90 calories (0g fat), the Ranch Dipping Sauce contains 160 calories and 16g fat.

Atlanta Bread®

Tips:

- Lower calorie bagels are: Wheat, Whole Grain, Cinnamon Raisin (see below). For the others add: Plain (30 calories), Apple Spice or Cinnamon Crisp (60), Poppy Seed or Everything (80).

- Sandwiches are served with potato chips and a pickle spear. For better health, ask for Fire Roasted Black Bean and Corn Salad (no nutrition information available).

- Basic sandwiches are prepared with mayo while most other sandwiches have added dressing and cheese. Leaving these off will save about 200 calories.

- Lower calorie sandwich breads include: French Roll, Baguette, or Rye, (170 calories/2 slices); French or Pumpernickel (220); Nine Grain (240); Sourdough, Ciabatta, or Honey Wheat (275).

- Salads come with bread. No nutrition info is available for the dressings, but expect about 60-80 calories/Tbsp. Many tablespoons are added so get the dressing on the side. Fat-Free Raspberry Vinaigrette is offered.

- For more nutrition information, go to AtlantaBread.com.

Suggestions:

	Calories	Fat (g)	Sat+Trans Fat (g)	Sodium (mg)	Carbohydrates (g)	Fiber (g)	Protein (g)
Wheat or Whole Grain Bagel	265	2	0	440	53	4	10
Cinnamon Raisin Bagel	270	1	0	420	55	3	10
Egg & Cheese Sandwich on bagel	440	17	6	790	52	2	20
Morning Classic with Ham	420	15	5	1440	39	2	37
Ham on Honey Wheat w/o mayo/cheese	410	5	2	1270	64	5	27
Turkey on Nine Grain w/o mayo/cheeese	370	6	2	1240	50	4	29
Chopstix Chicken Sandwich w/o dressing	240	10	2	530	22	4	18
Salsa Fresca Salmon Salad w/vinaigrette	560	29	5	590	40	6	38
French Onion Soup or Vegetable Soup	85	2	1	1420	14	2	3
Classic Chicken Noodle Soup	130	2	0	1050	15	1	11
Lowfat Apple or Pumpkin Muffin	235	2	<1	280	50	2	5

Caveats:

- Other soups average 260 calories...except for the Homestyle Chicken & Dumpling and Chicken Peppercorn at over 400!!

- The desserts (including Muffins, Danish, Croissants, Cookies, and Pies) average about 500 calories each. The Pecan Roll is the highest at 860 calories!

- Signature Sandwiches and Paninis contain an average of 670 calories and 36g fat. The highest is the Turkey Bacon Rustica at 960 calories and 56g fat.

Au Bon Pain®

Tips:

- Look for 90 calorie Whole Wheat Skinny bagels (most bagels have 300) and the Portions Menu (all under 200 calories).
- More nutrition information can be found at AuBonPain.com.

Suggestions:

	Calories	Fat (g)	Sat+Trans Fat (g)	Sodium (mg)	Carbohydrates (g)	Fiber (g)	Protein (g)
Oatmeal, large bowl (small = ½ of large)	340	6	1	15	63	9	13
Mini Cookies, average for one	85	5	3	55	10	<1	1
Breakfast: Egg on a Bagel®	430	12	4	580	58	2	22
Egg Whites & Cheddar on Skinny Bagel	250	11	6	550	23	6	20
Salmon & Wasabi on Onion Dill Bagel	430	12	5	1090	62	3	23
Sandwiches: Hummus/Olives on Tomato Bread	300	7	1	890	49	4	10
Grilled Chicken on Ciabatta w/o dressing	470	4	1	1660	67	4	39
Roasted Turkey on Baguette	490	5	2	1510	80	4	32
Chicken Salad Sandwich	490	11	2	1050	67	4	30
Roast Beef on Baguette	500	12	3	1370	65	3	33
Thai Peanut Chicken Wrap	560	17	5	880	68	8	34
Black Bean Burger	560	18	4	930	76	14	29
Mayan Chicken Hot Wrap	580	13	3	1190	93	5	25
Angus Steak Teriyaki Hot Wrap	630	15	3	1420	100	5	26
Mayan Chicken Harvest Rice Bowl w/br rice	550	11	3	910	87	3	27
Portion Menu (all have 200 calories or less):							
Hummus and Cucumber	130	8	0	460	10	3	3
Turkey, Asparagus, Chutney, Gorgonzola	140	5	3	550	10	1	15
Cheese, Fruit, and Crackers (avg)	195	11	6	340	19	<1	6
Apple, Blue Cheese, and Cranberries	200	10	4	270	27	3	4
Soups, 8oz cup or ½ large bowl:							
Veggies or Chicken Noodle	95	3	1	770	14	2	4
Lentil, White Beans or Black Eye Pea	130	2	0	820	22	7	7
Black Bean, Split Pea or Veg Chili	175	2	0	720	31	15	11
Salads: Asian or Thai Peanut Chicken	230	6	1	340	22	4	22
Fat-Free Raspberry Vinaigrette, 4Tbsp	50	0	0	190	12	0	0

Caveats:

- These items might have more calories than you would think:

Fruit Smoothie, medium (avg all flavors)	310	1	0	115	68	3	4
Lowfat Triple Berry Muffin	300	3	0	720	65	2	4
Fruit Yogurt w/granola, small	480	11	4	225	84	3	13

- Soups and salads are served with a 240 calorie Baguette. Most sandwiches above don't include mayo, pesto, and cheese.

- Here's the average calorie count for the sweets: Cupcakes (350); Bars, Danish, Strudels, and Cakes (450); Scones (500); Muffins (540); Croissants (240-540) and Pecan Rolls (810).

Auntie Anne's® Pretzels

Tips:

• All pretzels are brushed with butter. When you request "no butter," you'll save at least 30 calories and 4g fat, though the toppings may not stick as well.

• Reduce your sodium intake by asking for your pretzel without the salt topping. You'll reduce the sodium to less than 500mg.

• For more nutrition information, go to AuntieAnnes.com

Suggestions:

	Calories	Fat (g)	Sat+Trans Fat (g)	Sodium (mg)	Carbohydrates (g)	Fiber (g)	Protein (g)
Original Pretzel (or 6 Original Stix)	340	5	3	990	65	2	8
no butter, no salt	310	1	0	400	65	2	8
Jalapeno Pretzel	330	5	3	1060	63	2	6
Garlic Pretzel	350	5	3	990	65	2	8
Raisin Pretzel	360	5	3	390	69	2	8
Sour Cream & Onion Pretzel	360	5	3	1180	68	2	9
Almond Pretzel	390	6	4	400	74	2	6
Sesame Pretzel	400	10	4	990	67	3	10
Cinnamon Sugar Pretzel (or 6 Stix)	470	12	7	400	84	2	8
Pretzel Pocket, turkey & cheddar	470	10	5	1050	73	2	20
Pepperoni Pretzel, no butter	440	12	5	860	65	2	15
Pretzel Dog, no butter	320	16	6	740	33	1	11

Caveats:

• Think before you drink. Here are the counts for the smallest cup size (14-16oz). Expect 25-50% more for the next size up.

Sweetened Tea (all except raspberry)	130	0	0	30	34	0	0
Raspberry Sweetened Tea	150	0	0	5	36	0	0
ICEE® (all flavors)	140	0	0	10	38	0	0
Soda (avg)	150	0	0	20	40	0	0
HiC®	150	0	0	200	39	0	0
Dutch Ice (straw, blue rasp, kiwi banana)	160	0	0	40	40	0	0
w'melon, wild cherry, lemon, pina colada	210	0	0	25	50	0	0
Lemonade or Strawberry Lemonade	205	0	0	15	52	0	0
Lemonade Mixer (avg)	235	0	0	15	60	0	0
Dutch Smoothie (avg all except Mocha)	290	10	7	130	46	0	3
Mocha Dutch Smoothie	340	15	11	160	49	0	4
Dutch Latte, coffee	290	14	9	180	38	0	5
caramel and mocha	365	17	11	165	48	0	4
Dutch Shake, vanilla	510	27	18	300	57	0	9

• Want a meal? Choose the Turkey or Pepperoni Pretzel or Pretzel Dog (as shown above). The other meals contain 580-650 calories and 23-27g fat.

B.J.'s Restaurant & Brewhouse

Tips:

• Split an entree. Meals often contain 1000-2000 calories.

• Choose one of the suggested appetizers as your meal.

• For more nutrition information, go to BJsBrewhouse.com.

Suggestions:

	Calories	Fat (g)	Sat Fat (g)	Sodium (mg)	Carbohydrates (g)	Fiber (g)	Protein (g)
Breakfast Pizza, 1 slice	380	na	7	840	31	na	na
Minestrone Soup, small bowl	130	na	0	980	20	na	na
Thai Shrimp Lettuce Wraps	260	na	2	470	18	na	na
Thai Sauce	70	na	0	440	12	na	na
Chicken Pot Stickers	400	na	4	880	42	na	na
Soy Ginger Sauce	50	na	0	2340	9	na	na
Chicken Lettuce Wraps, full appetizer	530	na	4	2360	41	na	na
Hot Chinese Mustard	50	na	0	10	2	na	na
Sesame Soy Sauce	160	na	1	1510	20	na	na
Mini Beef or Chicken Tacos, 2 (avg)	255	na	3	500	22	na	na
Coleslaw	120	na	2	100	7	na	na
One large slice Pizza (avg):							
Cheese/Tomato, Vegetarian or Sweet Pig	310	na	4	810	38	na	na
BBQ Chicken or Buffalo Chicken	335	na	4	1120	41	na	na
Lunch Combo: ½ Spaghetti w/marinara	370	na	0	450	72	na	na
or ½ Spaghetti w/spicy tomato or meat sauce	440	na	4	560	72	na	na
with a House Salad w/lo-cal Italian, add:	180	na	1	840	19	na	na
Balsamic Glazed Chicken w/sides	740	na	12	2200	64	na	na
Fish/Grilled Shrimp Taco Combo w/sides	770	na	6	2400	77	na	na
Thai Salmon, entrée only	550	na	3	1410	33	na	na
Steamed Vegetables	120	na	1	270	10	na	na
Substitute Green Beans (instead of rice)	30	na	0	30	6	na	na

Caveats:

• Even the seemingly smaller lunch Combos are big on calories. The Mini Cheese Pizza *without toppings* has 600 calories. The leanest *half* sandwich option (California Chicken Sandwich) with fries has 810 calories. And, these are the leaner choices!

• Watch out for the extras. Sandwiches come with a side order of fries (415 calories). A side of rice or a baked potato adds on 520-630 calories. Want a small bowl of Tomato Bisque soup? Consider the calorie price tag of 450 calories before ordering. The plain Field of Greens Salad with dressing has 540 calories.

• Share dessert with many. Each "Mini" is over 500 calories. The Pizookies® average 1100 calorie and BJ's Brownie has 1280 calories.

Back Yard Burgers®

Tips:

- Burgers are big. The Junior Burger just might be enough to satisfy your burger craving.

- Mayo is standard for most burgers. Get yours plain. Or ask for a packet of Light Mayo.

- For more nutrition info, go to BackYardBurgers.com.

Suggestions:

Burgers and Sandwiches:	Calories	Fat (g)	Sat+Trans Fat (g)	Sodium (mg)	Carbohydrates (g)	Fiber (g)	Protein (g)
Grilled Chicken w/o mayo	350	5	<1	1280	47	3	31
Veggie Burger w/o mayo	400	8	2	1560	57	7	27
Hawaiian Chicken w/pineapple & sauce	450	11	2	1610	59	3	32
Blackened Chicken w/coleslaw	540	24	7	1810	53	4	32
Back Yard Burger®, junior w/mayo	530	27	10	1010	47	3	26
Salads w/o dressing:							
Side Salad	30	0	0	25	6	2	1
Garden Fresh Salad	100	2	0	160	20	4	4
Grilled Chicken Salad	220	4	0	950	23	4	27
Salad Dressing, 2 Tbsp:							
Ranch Dressing	150	15	2	310	2	0	0
Lite Ranch Dressing	80	6	1	310	6	0	0
Balsamic Vinaigrette	170	17	3	330	3	0	0

Caveats:

- Bigger burgers and fries might blow your calorie budget:

	Calories	Fat (g)	Sat+Trans Fat (g)	Sodium (mg)	Carbohydrates (g)	Fiber (g)	Protein (g)
Back Yard Burger®, 1/3# w/mayo	680	39	16	1040	47	3	36
w/cheddar cheese	790	48	22	1220	47	3	43
Bacon Cheddar Burger, 1/3#	850	54	24	1420	48	3	46
Back Yard Burger®, 2/3# w/mayo	620	26	4	1130	47	3	64
w/cheddar cheese	1290	88	42	1490	47	3	78
Seasoned Fries, regular-size	640	45	8	1160	58	6	6

- Share the cobbler. The Cobbler contains about 330 calories; add another 150 calories when topped with ice cream.

- That Lemonade is sweet! While the small Sodas contain about 250 calories, the Lemonade is listed in the nutrition information as containing 490 calories!

- Want a shake? Then, skip the burger! Shakes average 625 calories and 29g fat.

Baja Fresh®

Tips:

• Bare it. A Bare Burrito® is served in a bowl, rather than a tortilla. When you eliminate the tortilla, you've saved about 150 calories and 6g fat. A fried tortilla shell (served with the Tostada Salad) has 490 calories and 28g fat.

• Looking for meat? In most cases, dishes prepared with shrimp, chicken, or Mahi Mahi are the leanest options. Count on another 100 calories or so for carnitas, steak, and breaded fish.

• Think taco. A single taco contains just 210-250 calories each, while a burrito has about 800-1000+ calories each.

• Use salsa freely. Adding salsa to a salad adds just 15 calories. If you select one of the other dressings, it jumps 260-290 calories.

• Cut the cheese. The leanest burrito choice is the Burrito Mexicano (listed below). The calories aren't significantly lower, but because it's prepared without cheese, you save about 25g fat.

• For more nutrition information, go to BajaFresh.com

Suggestions:

	Calories	Fat (g)	Sat+Trans Fat (g)	Sodium (mg)	Carbohydrates (g)	Fiber (g)	Protein (g)
Original Baja Taco, chicken or shrimp (avg)	205	5	1	255	28	2	11
carnitas or steak	225	8	2	270	29	2	10
Americano Soft Taco, chicken or shrimp	230	10	5	565	21	2	15
carnitas or steak	255	13	6	640	21	2	14
Grilled Mahi Mahi Taco	230	9	2	300	26	4	12
Baja Ensalada® w/o dressing							
w/charbroiled shrimp	230	6	2	1110	18	6	28
w/charbroiled chicken	310	7	2	1210	18	7	46
Fat-Free Salsa Verde	15	0	0	370	3	1	0
Chicken Tortilla Soup w/chicken	320	14	4	2760	29	4	17
Bare Burrito®, veggie & cheese	580	10	4	1950	101	20	19
chicken	640	7	1	2330	97	20	45
carnitas or steak	690	15	5	2465	99	19	39
Burrito Mexicano (chicken, shrimp or Mahi)	780	13	4	2200	117	19	48

Caveats:

• Share the other items. Most are over 1000 calories (and more than double the fat) of the items above. These include: Taquitos (740-780 calories), Fajitas with flour tortillas (1120-1340 calories), Tostada Salads without dressing (1010-1230 calories), Quesadillas (1200-1430 calories), and Nachos (1890-2120 calories).

• Refrain from the chips. A small side of corn chips adds 210 calories and 9g fat; the larger side contains 740 calories!

Baskin Robbins®

Tips:

- Stick with the small scoop. One small 2.5oz scoop (not counting the cone) contains 150-210 calories. Fat grams vary from 8-13g. The larger 4oz scoop has 240-340 calories.

- Try the BRight Choices - Light Ice Cream and No-Sugar-Added varieties have 150 calories or less per small scoop.

- Select Strawberry. With Shakes, Ice Cream, Parfaits, and Soft Serve Sundaes, strawberry flavor is the lowest calorie choice.

- Act like a kid. The kid's soft serve is *half* the calories of the regular.

- For more nutrition information, go to BaskinRobbins.com.

Suggestions (per 2½ oz small scoop, add cone below):

	Calories	Fat (g)	Sat+Trans Fat (g)	Sodium (mg)	Carbohydrates (g)	Fiber (g)	Protein (g)
Ice or Sorbet	80	0	0	10	21	0	0
Fat-Free Vanilla Frozen Yogurt	90	0	0	65	20	0	4
Rainbow Sherbet	100	2	1	25	21	0	1
Very Berry Strawberry Ice Cream	140	7	4	45	18	0	2
Premium Churned Light Ice Cream (avg)	150	5	3	90	24	1	3
Reduced-Fat No-Sugar-Added Ice Cream:							
Pineapple Coconut	100	4	3	50	18	2	3
Caramel Turtle Truffle or Choc Overload	120	5	4	75	24	2	3
Key Lime Pie	130	5	3	70	23	2	3
Butter Almond Crunch	140	7	3	90	19	3	4
Vanilla Soft Serve, kid's	130	5	3	75	18	0	4
add Cake Cone	25	0	0	15	5	0	0
add Sugar Cone	45	1	0	35	9	0	1
Strawberry 'n Almonds Parfait, 8oz	300	11	6	140	43	2	9
Fruit Blast, sm (avg)	280	<1	0	10	70	2	1

Caveats:

- Avoid the waffle cone. While a single scoop on a sugar or cake cone contains only about 200-250 calories, a waffle cone with just one large scoop contains about 450-500 calories.

- Think before you drink. A small Fruit Blast Smoothie contains 420 calories while the small Shakes range from 560-750 calories.

- The specialty items can do you in. They range from:

  420-600 calories - small Fruit Creams, Ice Cream Float, or Soda; 8oz Parfait; or regular Soft Serve Sundaes

  600-1000 calories - small 31 Below™

  Over 1000 calories - Oreo® Layered Sundae, Reese's® Peanut Butter Sundae, Snickers® Sundae, or Classic Banana Split

Bertucci's® Italian Restaurant

Tips:

- Share a meal. Lunch pastas average 760 calories, while the dinner portions average well over 1100 calories. Even the Paninis and "Individual" Pizzas contain more than 1000 calories.

- Double the fiber. Multigrain pasta is available with any pasta dish, and whole wheat dough can be substituted for any torta.

- One slice of a large pizza has about 30-50 calories more than a slice of an individual pizza.

- For more nutrition information, go to Bertuccis.com.

Suggestions:

	Calories	Fat (g)	Sat+Trans Fat (g)	Sodium (mg)	Carbohydrates (g)	Fiber (g)	Protein (g)
Salads w/o dressing:							
Insalata or Chopped Salad	150	7	3	340	20	5	6
Insalata w/chicken	320	13	6	420	22	5	32
Venetian Spinach Salad	130	2	1	230	28	8	6
w/grilled chicken	300	9	5	330	29	8	31
Giardino Salad	150	5	3	270	22	6	7
w/grilled chicken	320	12	6	370	22	6	32
Dressing, 2 Tbsp: Lite Burgundy	20	0	0	280	2	0	0
Italian or Balsamic Vinaigrette	115	13	2	215	2	0	0
Soup, Minestrone, cup	100	3	2	640	14	2	6
Side Dishes: String Beans	150	11	7	320	10	5	3
Fresh Asparagus	180	15	10	260	7	2	7
Seafood Torta w/whole wheat dough	730	24	5	670	79	8	47
Pollo Parma Sandwich	630	19	6	590	81	4	33
Lunch (or roughly ½ dinner):							
Spaghetti Pomodoro	460	7	2	710	82	5	16
Rigatoni, Broccoli, Shrimp in wine sauce	530	16	8	620	68	4	30
Dinner: Lobster Ravioli	640	29	14	1730	64	3	28
Merluzzo di Mare	670	25	4	1350	25	3	80
Individual Pizza, one slice:							
Stella, Sofia or Nolio	240	9	3	450	31	2	8
Cheese or Margherita	250	11	4	345	30	1	9
Scallop di Mare	280	10	4	400	32	1	15

Caveats:

- There are 1740 calories and 85g fat in the "Taste of Bertucci's."

- Vegetables aren't always low-calorie. The Tuscan Vegetable Torta has 730 calories and 34g fat. Even a side of Roasted Tuscan Vegetables contains 320 calories and 27g fat!

- Don't dip. Most of the meals are already very high in fat. So, refrain from dipping that 140 calorie dinner roll in more oil.

Blimpie®

Tips:

- Slim it down. Nutrition info below is based on standard product formulations found on the menu. Leaving off the usual cheese, mayo, oil, and/or dressing will reduce both fat and calories.

- Keep it short. 6" Subs range from 350-635 calories.

- Take it up a notch. Order a wheat sub for an extra 3g fiber.

- For more nutrition information, go to Blimpie.com

Suggestions:	Calories	Fat (g)	Sat+Trans Fat (g)	Sodium (mg)	Carbohydrates (g)	Fiber (g)	Protein (g)
6" Subs: Blimpie Best®	450	17	6	1330	49	3	24
Cuban	410	11	5	1630	43	1	29
Chicken Teriyaki	450	12	5	1280	52	2	33
on wheat sub	450	14	6	1260	50	5	35
w/o cheese	370	6	2	1090	52	2	28
French Dip	410	11	5	1650	46	1	30
Tuna	470	21	3	770	43	2	24
Turkey, Ham, Roast Beef, or Club (avg)	420	14	5	1090	48	3	25
on wheat sub	420	15	5	1100	47	6	28
w/o cheese or sauce (avg)	310	5	1	1000	49	3	18
Turkey & Avocado	360	7	1	1340	51	4	21
Turkey & Cranberry	350	4	<1	1220	58	3	20
Veggie Max™ w/o cheese or sauce	390	8	1	950	55	5	23
Veggie & Provolone w/o sauce	330	9	4	940	49	3	14
Ciabatta: Mediterranean	450	8	3	1720	65	3	26
French Dip	430	11	5	1820	49	2	31
Salads: Garden Salad w/o dressing	30	0	0	15	6	3	2
Cole Slaw Salad, side	160	9	2	240	20	2	1
Chicken Caesar Salad w/o dressing	190	8	4	460	6	3	25
Potato Salad, side	230	12	3	490	28	3	3
Tuna Salad w/o dressing	270	19	3	370	6	3	18
Soups: Chicken Gumbo, Fr Onion, Garden Veg, Veg Beef,							
Minestrone, Yankee Pot Roast (avg)	80	2	<1	980	13	2	4

Caveats:

- Stay away from Super Stacked™ 12" Subs including Super Stacked™ Blimpie Best® (1100 calories), Super Stacked™ Trio (1030 calories), and Super Stacked™ B.L.T. (1270 calories).

- Most cookies and brownies contain between 180-230 calories and 7-13g fat (yes, even the Brownie and Peanut Butter Cookie). Not bad. The only exception is the (surprise!) Sugar Cookie which contains 320 calories and 16g fat.

Bob Evans®

Tips:

• Fit from the Farm® menu suggestions are 650 calories or less.

• Order your favorite egg meal with either Bob Evans Egg Lites or Egg Whites. Each contains 25-30 calories per egg (and no fat) versus 80 calories (5g fat) for the whole egg. Turkey sausage has about half the calories of the regular (70 vs. 130 per link).

• All appetizers are fried; select fresh fruit instead.

• For more nutrition information, go to BobEvans.com.

Fit from the Farm® Suggestions:	Calories	Fat (g)	Sat+Trans Fat (g)	Sodium (mg)	Carbohydrates (g)	Fiber (g)	Protein (g)
BE Fit Breakfast (cranberry sidecakes, fruit, no-cholesterol eggs, sugar-free syrup)	350	3	1	540	68	6	17
Blueberry-Banana French Toast	350	6	1	615	4	4	8
Strawberry-Blueberry French Toast	300	6	1	560	31	3	8
Fruit & Yogurt Crepe w/Quaker® Oatmeal	610	17	4	345	104	7	14
Veggie Omelet w/fruit, wheat toast, jelly	310	6	2	580	43	4	22
Fresh Fruit & Yogurt Plate	350	2	0	75	84	8	7
Apple-Cranberry Spinach Salad w/reduced-fat raspberry dressing	365	14	2	410	47	5	14
Plain baked potato, steamed broccoli and:							
Grilled Chicken Breast	415	8	2	630	57	9	40
Grilled Salmon Fillet	510	13	3	165	57	9	51
Potato Crusted Flounder	420	11	4	550	66	9	29
Chicken/Spinach/Tomato Pasta, savor-size	345	12	3	415	38	3	22
Chicken-N-Noodles	115	2	1	365	16	1	8

Other Suggestions:

	Calories	Fat (g)	Sat+Trans Fat (g)	Sodium (mg)	Carbohydrates (g)	Fiber (g)	Protein (g)
Fruit & Yogurt Parfait, mini	160	1	0	60	34	3	4
Farm-Grill Grilled Chicken Sandwich	400	7	2	1145	47	2	38
Wildfire Grilled Chicken Salad, dinner	390	13	5	965	37	6	32
Raspberry Reduced-Fat Dressing, dinner	200	10	2	170	27	0	0
Lite Ranch Dressing, dinner	190	18	3	700	4	0	2
Slow-Roasted Turkey, a la carte	115	4	1	725	3	0	15
Farm Favorite Grilled Chicken Sandwich	520	17	6	1385	48	2	45
Green Beans	30	1	0	415	5	2	2
Broccoli	35	0	0	35	7	3	3

Caveats:

• Garden vegetables are covered with an herb butter sauce - so each serving contains 150 calories and 12g fat (5g saturated).

• The No-Sugar-Added Apple Pie has 490 calories and 27g fat; the regular Apple Crumb Pie contains 510 calories and 23g fat.

Bojangle's®

Tips:

- Famous for Chicken and Biscuits, there's not much more on the menu. The best choices are the four sandwiches below.

- Breakfast is served all day.

- For more nutrition information, go to Bojangles.com.

Suggestions:

	Calories	Fat (g)	Sat Fat (g)	Sodium (mg)	Carbohydrates (g)	Fiber (g)	Protein (g)
Country Ham Biscuit Breakfast Sandwich	350	18	9	1440	33	0	15
Cajun Filet Sandwich w/o mayo	340	11	5	400	41	3	22
w/mayo	495	27	5	680	43	3	20
Grilled Chicken Sandwich w/o mayo	240	5	3	540	25	2	23
w/mayo	365	15	2	910	33	3	27
Grilled Chicken Salad w/o dressing	275	11	6	770	11	3	40

Caveats:

- The other breakfast biscuits are high in fat and calories:

Bacon, Egg & Cheese Biscuit	550	42	14	1250	27	1	17
Steak Biscuit	650	49	13	1130	37	1	14

- The smallest chicken meal is the One Breast Meal (breast, one "Fixin," and a biscuit) at 565-750 calories. This breakdown should convince you not to order the two or three piece dinners:

Breast, 1	280	17	na	560	12	<1	33
Biscuit, plain	240	12	3	660	29	2	4
Bo Berry™ Biscuit	220	10	3	410	29	1	3
Regular Soda	210	0	0	40	38	0	0
Sides: Green Beans	45	0	0	370	7	3	2
Potatoes w/o gravy	80	1	0	380	16	1	2
w/gravy	130	6	1	615	21	0	3
Bojangles' Cajun Pintos®	110	0	0	480	18	6	6
Marinated Cole Slaw	140	3	0	450	26	3	1
Bojangles' Dirty Rice®	165	6	2	760	24	1	5
Seasoned Fries, small	220	14	3	740	20	2	2
Bo-tato Rounds®, small	230	14	6	310	24	3	2

- Roasted Chicken Bites™ Combo might sound like a healthy choice (because the chicken is "roasted"), but it's not:

Combo w/bites, biscuit, fries, soda	990	39	14	2730	120	2	44
w/diet soda, biscuit, green beans instead							
	600	25	11	2335	49	3	44

Bonefish Grill®

Tips:

- No nutritional information is available on the web. Information below is from interviews with restaurant managers.
- A loaf of bread (and olive oil) is served with all meals.

Suggestions:

- Appetizers: Edamame is the leanest choice. The smaller portion of Ahi Tuna Sashimi (4.5oz) or the Sea Scallops (4 large) can also make a great entrée - complete the meal with some veggies. And, remove the bacon off the scallops.
- Salads: Citrus Herb Vinaigrette is an olive-oil based dressing - request this on the side.
- Hand Helds: If you have an appetite, Baja Fish Tacos are two large tacos prepared blackened (request without sour cream). The Fillet of Fish Burger is prepared with a 6oz fillet (4.5oz cooked). Request it without the sauce.
- Grilled Fish is cooked on an oak burning grill that is lightly brushed with oil - all varieties are moderate in calories. A house herb/spice mix is used for seasoning. Choose Mango Salsa for your topping (the other toppings are high in calories). Most fish portions are 8oz raw (6oz cooked). Some varieties are offered in a 6oz raw (4.5oz cooked) portion. The Ahi Tuna also comes in a 6-6.5oz dinner portion with a cup of Jasmine Rice and Steamed Vegetables.
- Sides: All entrées (except for pasta) are served with a seasonal vegetable, plus *one* other fresh side. Ask about the seasonal vegetable choice (Glazed Carrots are high in calories). For a slight upcharge you can opt for *two fresh* sides such as Jasmine Rice, Steamed Vegetable Medley, French Green Beans, Steamed Broccoli, or Steamed Asparagus. All steamed vegetables are steamed with butter, but you can request them without.

Caveats:

- Appetizers: Calamari and Coconut Shrimp are fried. The Mussels Josephine is prepared with a lot of lemon butter.
- Hand Helds: the Kobe Beef Burger is prepared with 8oz of high fat meat - and it's dressed with Cheddar cheese and special sauce. My guess is that it's 1500+ calories.
- Grilled Specialties: each are prepared with high-fat ingredients including buttery sauces and cheese.
- Desserts: all choices are large and best shared with 2-3 people.

Boston Market®

Tips:

• Remove the skin to save about 100 calories and 10g fat with the quarter chicken breast and 200 calories (and 19g fat) for the 3 piece dark order.

• Skip the cornbread. It's easy to pair one of the entrées and two sides (below) for under 500 calories. But that's without the cornbread served with all the meals.

• Go light. Though no information is available, light ranch dressing can also be requested.

• For more nutrition information, go to BostonMarket.com.

Suggestions:

	Calories	Fat (g)	Sat+Trans Fat (g)	Sodium (mg)	Carbohydrates (g)	Fiber (g)	Protein (g)
Roasted Turkey Breast, regular	180	3	1	620	0	0	38
Quarter White Rotisserie Chicken w/o skin	220	3	1	700	1	0	49
3 Piece Dark Skinless (thigh+2 drumsticks)	280	12	4	630	1	0	41
Beef Brisket, regular	230	13	4	570	0	0	28
Sides:							
Fresh Steamed Vegetables	60	2	0	40	8	3	2
Green Beans	60	4	2	180	7	3	2
Mediterranean Green Beans	120	9	3	220	10	4	3
Garlic Dill New Potatoes	140	3	1	120	24	3	3
Garlicky Lemon Spinach	140	10	6	440	9	5	6
Sweet Corn	170	4	1	95	37	2	6
Cornbread w/o butter	200	5	2	270	30	1	3
BBQ Chicken Slider, 1 (served in 3-pack)	210	5	1	520	35	0	10
Market Pair (pair any two):							
Chicken Noodle Soup	240	8	3	1360	23	2	21
Chicken Tortilla Soup w/o toppings	160	8	2	1640	13	2	10
Half Roasted Turkey Carver Sandwich	395	18	5	905	33	1	25
Half Pulled BBQ Chicken Sandwich	345	9	3	940	47	2	20
Half Caesar Salad w/dressing	330	21	5	800	16	1	19
Half Mediterranean Salad w/dressing	320	22	5	595	14	1	18
Half Southwest Salad w/dressing	370	23	5	620	25	3	18

Caveats:

• The sandwiches are big. All-White Rotisserie Chicken Salad sandwich contains 1050 calories (64g fat) and the Turkey BLT has 1030 calories and 57g fat.

• Skip dessert. The lowest calorie dessert is the Chocolate Chip Cookie with 370 calories and 19g fat. A Brownie has 470 calories. Both the Apple Pie and Chocolate Cake contain 580 calories.

Buca Di Beppo®

Tips:

- Don't eat it all! While lunch portions are considered just one serving, most dinner meals are served family-style and meant to be shared. Buca Small® serves three, while Buca Large® serves six. Nutrition information below is the average *per serving*.

- Share the luncheon portions, too. These are almost always larger than one serving of the family-style portions - sometimes as much as *four* times larger!!

- For more nutrition information, go to BucaDiBeppo.com.

Suggestions (*per serving* as noted above):

	Calories	Fat (g)	Sat Fat (g)	Sodium (mg)	Carbohydrates (g)	Fiber (g)	Protein (g)
Spaghetti Marinara	360	na	0	180	65	na	na
lunch portion	580	na	1	240	105	na	na
Spaghetti with Meat Sauce	390	na	2	706	63	na	na
lunch portion	650	na	3	1170	104	na	na
Ravioli Al Pomodoro	320	na	7	280	35	na	na
lunch portion	490	na	11	480	56	na	na
Baked Ravioli	320	na	7	290	36	na	na
lunch portion	485	na	11	440	53	na	na
Lasagna	350	na	7	1010	68	na	na
Baked Rigatoni	520	na	7	500	59	na	na
Veal or Chicken Parmigiana	250	na	2	600	20	na	na
Chicken Marsala or Roasted Salmon	395	na	6	655	11	na	na
Gnocchi Al Telefono	380	na	6	745	59	na	na
Pizza, per small, large, or luncheon serving							
Marghertia	250	na	3	310	34	na	na
Pizza Con Formaggio	185	na	0	320	35	na	na
Veggie	610	na	9	2025	64	na	na
Sides: Green Beans	90	na	1	470	9	na	na
Italian Broccoli Romano	90	na	1	490	6	na	na

Caveats:

- Count the Antipasti and Insalate. Most Antipasti, as well as Minestrone Soup, Mixed Green Salad, and Caesar Salad have an average of 150 calories *per serving* (3 servings in the small, 6 servings in the large). The Bruschetta, Spicy Calamari, and Mozzarella Caprese contain close to 300 calories *per serving*.

- Portions are huge - even when shared. While it may not be so shocking to discover that many meals have 2000-3000 calories in the entire "small" serving, there are 2840 calories in a small "side" of Fettucine Alfredo. A luncheon portion of Apple Gorgonzola Salad has 1140 calories and the kid's portion of Macaroni & Cheese has 1060 calories!

Buffalo Wild Wings®

Tips:

- Most meals are served with either French Fries or Tortilla Chips. And, as shown in the caveats below, most of the options are just as high in fat and calories. You can request a Veggie Boat with fat-free ranch dressing instead.

- For more nutrition information, go to BuffaloWildWings.com

Suggestions:

	Calories	Fat (g)	Sat+Trans Fat (g)	Sodium (mg)	Carbohydrates (g)	Fiber (g)	Protein (g)
Naked Tenders, each	43	2	0	570	6	0	2
Kid's Cheeseburger Slammer, 1 only	400	26	10	400	20	1	21
Naked Tenders Wrap	600	14	9	1980	68	6	54
Grilled Chicken Buffalitos	380	9	6	1240	44	4	40
Gardenburger, plain	450	5	2	1060	63	3	40
Grilled Chicken Sandwich, plain	470	7	3	750	50	3	51
Jerk Chicken Sandwich, plain	530	10	3	1140	56	3	51

Caveats:

- Most sides are high in fat and calories (choose the Veggie Boat):

Onion Rings, regular	460	26	5	960	52	4	4
French Fries	280	10	3	660	42	4	4
Potato Wedges, regular	280	14	4	1075	40	5	5
Buffalo Chips, regular (unsalted)	255	5	1	35	47	5	5
Tortilla Chips and salsa	250	15	8	590	23	1	2
Side Salad	210	15	5	385	14	4	6
Coleslaw	170	15	0	390	6	0	0

- Think before you dip. Here are the stats per 2 tablespoons:

Sweet BBQ	40	0	0	460	8	0	0
Hot BBQ	40	2	0	1200	2	0	0
Mild, Medium, Hot or Wild Sauce (avg)	45	5	0	1130	3	0	0
Spicy Garlic	50	4	0	1220	4	0	0
Teriyaki	70	0	0	1100	14	0	0
Honey BBQ	70	0	0	400	18	0	0
Honey Mustard	80	6	0	320	6	0	0
Asian Zing or Mango Habanera (avg)	85	0	0	520	21	0	0
Pepper Infusion®	90	9	2	780	2	1	0
Blue Cheese or Ranch (avg)	300	30	5	460	2	0	1
Southwestern Ranch	320	34	5	740	2	0	0

- Skip the salads. Entrée Salads range from 420-990 calories and 27-68 grams of fat. The Chicken Tenders Salad has more fat and calories than the 900 calorie Big Jack Daddy Burger™!

- Each Wing (boneless or not) contains about 80 calories and 6g fat. Rib plates range from 1480-2380 calories and 92-158g fat!

Burger King®

Tips:

• Craving a burger? Try the Burger King® WHOPPER JR® - just 260 calories when ordered without mayonnaise.

• Kid's meal options (also available for adults) include Apple Juice or fat-free milk, plus BK® Apple Fries or Apple Sauce.

• The BK Veggie® Burger is prepared with a Morningstar Farms® patty which contains milk, egg, wheat, and soy.

• If you want fries and a drink, request the "small combo" which includes 16oz soda (140 calories for non-diet choices) and small fries (340 calories and 17g fat).

• Go to BK.com for more nutrition information.

Suggestions:

	Calories	Fat (g)	Sat+Trans Fat (g)	Sodium (mg)	Carbohydrates (g)	Fiber (g)	Protein (g)
Quaker® Oatmeal Maple & Brown Sugar	270	4	2	290	55	5	5
Quaker® Oatmeal Original	140	4	1	100	23	3	5
CROISSAN'WICH® w/egg & cheese	320	16	7	680	26	0	11
w/ham	350	17	7	1110	27	0	18
BK® Egg & Cheese Muffin	290	14	5	175	24	1	11
Mott's® Harvest Plus Applesauce	50	0	0	0	13	1	0
BK® Fresh Apple Fries w/caramel sauce	70	<1	0	35	16	1	0
WHOPPER JR.® Sandwich	340	19	5	510	28	2	14
w/o mayo	260	10	4	440	28	2	13
BK VEGGIE® Burger w/o cheese	410	16	3	1030	44	7	22
w/o mayo	320	7	1	960	43	7	22
TENDERGRILL® Chicken Sandwich	470	18	4	1100	40	2	37
w/o mayo	360	7	2	1010	40	2	37
WHOPPER® Sandwich w/o mayo	510	23	10	980	51	3	29
CHICKEN TENDERS®, 4pc	190	11	2	310	10	1	10
TENDERGRILL® Chicken Garden Salad	290	12	6	1030	8	1	38
KEN'S® Fat-Free Ranch Dressing	60	0	0	740	15	2	0
KEN'S® Light Italian Dressing	120	11	2	440	5	0	0
BK® Chicken Fries, 6pc	250	15	3	820	16	1	14

Caveats:

• Mayonnaise is standard for nearly all sandwiches. Cutting out the mayo will save a whopping 80 calories on the small burgers and 160-210 calories on the larger sandwiches! And, each slice of cheese contains 45 calories and 4g fat.

• Think chicken and fish are healthy choices? Not when they are fried! TENDERCRISP® Chicken Sandwich contains 750 calories (45g fat); BK BIG FISH® SW has 590 calories, 31g fat.

California Pizza Kitchen®

Tips:

- This is the place to share. See the caveats below.

- Design your own meal. Pair a cup of soup (below) with just one Spring Roll. Or enjoy the Lettuce Wrap appetizer as a meal.

- Request fat-free vinaigrette, or dressing on the side, even if you order the half salads. Most half salads contain over 500 calories.

- Multigrain penne pasta and gluten-free pizza crusts are available.

- Get the vegetables. Salmon with vegetables contains 750 calories; when served with spaghettini it contains over 1200!

- Total fat info is not available at CPK.com. The info below uses a common scientific formula to estimate fat based on protein and carbohydrate values.

Suggestions:

	Calories	Estimated Fat (g)	Sat Fat (g)	Sodium (mg)	Carbohydrates (g)	Fiber (g)	Protein (g)
Cup of Soup: Artichoke + Broccoli	100	3	2	615	13	5	2
Dakota Smashed Pea/Barley	175	1	0	675	32	2	11
Small Cravings & Appetizers:							
Sesame Ginger Chicken Dumplings	465	13	1	1800	63	0	25
Lettuce Wraps w/chicken or shrimp (avg)	535	22	2	1455	55	6	31
Salads w/o dressing (half-size):							
Roasted Vegetable Salad w/shrimp	395	22	3	620	25	8	25
Caesar Salad w/shrimp	350	22	8	570	11	4	27
Miso Shrimp (or chicken) Salad	430	23	4	910	33	8	21
Fat-Free Vinaigrette, half size	105	0	0	220	26	0	0

Caveats:

- Most pasta, specialty dishes, and pizzas (even whole grain and thin crust) are over 1000 calories. Tacos and sandwiches average 965 calories. Here are some of the lowest calorie options:

Salmon w/wok-stirred vegetables	745	60	7	870	25	8	52
Margherita Thin Crust Pizza	995	42	20	2555	106	8	47
Veg. w/eggplant on whole grain crust pizza	1045	35	15	2135	134	17	48
Baja Fish Tacos w/o avocado	920	49	10	1410	86	8	3

- Think before you drink. Flavored Frozen Lemonade and Non-Fat Yogurt Smoothies average 210 calories while the Coladas are around 410 calories.

- Desserts range from 510-1388 calories. The Butter Cake or Red Velvet Cake a la Häagen-Dazs®, as well as all three Sundaes, are all over 1000 calories.

Captain D's Seafood Kitchen®

Tips:

- Salmon, tilapia, and shrimp dinners are served with rice, two sides, and a breadstick. Select wisely and the dinner is only 550 calories - otherwise, it could be close to 1000 calories.

- Watch the sauce. When offered your choice of sauce, choose Cocktail (25 calories) or Ginger Teriyaki at 60 calories - or none at all. Tartar Sauce, Sweet Chili Sauce, or Scampi Butter Sauce each contain 100 calories or more.

- For more nutrition information, go to CaptainDs.com.

Suggestions:

	Calories	Fat (g)	Sat+Trans Fat (g)	Sodium (mg)	Carbohydrates (g)	Fiber (g)	Protein (g)
Wild Alaskan Salmon	140	1	0	410	1	0	33
Seasoned Tilapia	130	3	2	520	1	0	24
Shrimp Skewers	50	0	0	390	0	0	11
Catfish, 1 piece	105	6	2	235	6	0	7
Sides: Baked Potato, plain	240	0	0	25	54	6	6
Roasted Red Potatoes	170	7	4	1200	25	3	3
Seasoned Rice	160	1	0	670	35	1	4
Corn on the Cob	190	2	0	10	37	4	5
Green Beans	60	2	0	400	10	3	1
Broccoli	40	1	0	30	5	2	2
Side Salad w/o dressing	15	0	0	10	2	2	1
Fat-Free Italian Dressing	10	0	0	440	2	0	0
Breadstick	150	6	3	150	21	1	3
Wild Alaskan Salmon Sandwich	520	18	2	980	48	2	42
Wild Alaskan Salmon Salad	180	1	0	430	8	3	35

Caveats:

- Request "no cracklins" (fried crumbs). Fried fish dinners are served with cracklins, two sides, and two hush puppies.

- The two piece fish dinner doesn't seem big, but the calories really add up:

Batter-dipped Fish, 2 pieces	360	24	14	910	16	2	18
Cracklins (served w/ all fried fish)	160	12	6	560	11	0	1
French Fries	310	15	18	450	38	4	3
Cole Slaw	170	12	2	310	13	2	1
Hushpuppies, 2	200	13	7	330	18	1	2
Tartar Sauce	100	10	2	75	1	0	0
TOTAL:	1300	86	49	2635	97	9	25

- Desserts range from 300 calories (Chocolate Cake) to 470 calories (Pecan Pie).

Carino's® Italian

Tips:

- Share a meal. Luncheon entrees average over 800 calories while dinner entrées average over 1000 calories - and that's before adding extras such as drinks, side dishes, and desserts.

- Luncheon portions aren't always smaller than dinner. Some lunch portions are 75% of the dinner, others are exactly the same.

- For more nutrition information, go to Carinos.com.

Suggestions:

	Calories	Fat (g)	Sat+Trans Fat (g)	Sodium (mg)	Carbohydrates (g)	Fiber (g)	Protein (g)
Minestrone Soup	160	8	2	1720	30	7	10
Classic Cheese Margherita	480	21	12	2070	75	7	35
Angel Hair w/artichokes, lunch	450	9	1	970	75	7	15
Angel Hair w/artichokes, dinner	660	14	1	1720	112	11	22
w/chicken or shrimp (avg)	740	15	1	1790	112	11	38
Create Your Own Pasta w/tomato or marinara	535	5	0	570	104	7	19
lunch portion	355	3	0	320	70	5	12
Create Your Own Pasta w/meat sauce	580	6	1	690	107	7	23
Chicken Parmigiana, lunch	640	18	6	1160	74	4	45
Lemon Rosemary Chicken meal	610	6	1	1460	67	8	64
Mini Chocolate Cake	140	4	2	100	23	1	2
Mini Cheesecake w/Amerena Cherries	230	13	8	160	25	0	3

Caveats:

- Even the mini appetizers are large. The minis (plus the regular Baked Stuffed Mushrooms) average 565 calories. The regular appetizers average over 1150 calories.

- Avoid the Italian Wedge Salad. Piled high with bacon, pecans, and dressing, it weighs in at 790 calories and 66g fat.

- Thinking Parmigiana? Pick the Chicken Parmigiana, instead of Eggplant. While similar in calories (around 660), eggplant soaks up more fat than chicken so the Eggplant Parmiagiana has nearly twice as much fat than the Chicken Parmigiana (31g and 18g respectively).

- The Paninis range from 820 calories (Smoked Turkey & Bacon) to 1332 (Italian Meatball). That's not counting the fries (for which no nutrition information was given).

- Desserts can be disastrous. While most regular desserts are 560-780 calories each, the Turtle Cheesecake has 1030 calories and the Mascarpone Bread Pudding contains 1680 calories! The mini Tiramisu has just 310 calories, but 25g fat!

Carl's Jr.®

Tips:

- These burgers are big - even the Turkey Burgers! Stick with a Grilled Chicken Sandwich to cut calories.
- Combo meals are served with small fries (310 calories and 15g fat) and drink (about 160 calories).
- For more nutrition information, go to CarlsJr.com.

Suggestions:

	Calories	Fat (g)	Sat+Trans Fat (g)	Sodium (mg)	Carbohydrates (g)	Fiber (g)	Protein (g)
Charbroiled BBQ Chicken™ Sandwich	390	7	2	990	50	3	30
Kid's Hamburger or Big Hamburger	490	18	8	1000	58	3	25
Teriyaki Turkey Burger	470	14	5	1120	55	3	32
Guacamole Turkey Burger	490	21	6	1120	43	3	33
Turkey Burger	490	23	5	960	45	3	29
Salads without dressing:							
Side Salad	120	5	2	250	13	2	4
Original Grilled Chicken Salad	270	9	3	800	23	4	25
Cranberry Apple Walnut Grilled Chicken	320	11	4	850	29	5	27
Salad Dressings:							
Lowfat Balsamic Vinaigrette	35	2	0	480	5	0	0
Raspberry Vinaigrette	160	12	2	150	12	0	0
Sourdough Breakfast Sandwich	450	21	8	1470	38	1	29

Caveats:

- Most breakfast options are big. The Breakfast Burger™ has 810 calories and 42g fat, while the Loaded Breakfast Burrito contains 780 calories and 48g fat.
- Not all salads are good for you. The Green Burrito® Taco Salad contains 880 calories and 53g fat.
- The Low Carb It® burgers are wrapped in lettuce, instead of a bun - and not low-calorie. For example, the Low Carb It® Six Dollar Burger® has 570 calories and 43g fat.
- The Charbroiled BBQ Chicken Sandwich (above) is a good choice. The other two Charbroiled Sandwiches are 580-640 calories and 29-36g fat.
- The Original Six Dollar Burger® will cost you 910 calories; get it with guacamole and bacon and you'll be out 1060 calories.
- If you have a sweet tooth, reach for one of the cookies or cakes. At 290-370 calories, these are lower in calories than the Hand-Scooped Ice Cream Shakes & Malts (at 690-780 calories and 34-39g fat).

Carrabba's Italian Grill®

Tips:

- No nutrition information is available at Carrabbas.com. Information below was obtained from interviews with restaurant managers.

- Avoid the Lemon Butter Sauce that's added to many dishes. Made with heavy cream, it's high in calories and saturated fat.

- Stick with the small. Fish and Chicken are offered in both small and regular sizes. Small-size portions weigh around 5-6oz raw, which will cook down to about 4-5oz. Regular-size meat portions are around 8oz raw (about 6oz cooked).

- Instead of Homemade Chips, request the Vegetable of the Day. It's prepared with butter or oil, but you can ask for less or none.

Suggestions:

- Antipasti - Order the smaller-sized Cozze in Bianco (steamed mussels) and request no lemon butter (it's added at the end). Shrimp Scampi can be requested to be served with "little" olive oil instead of lemon butter.

- Soup - both the Minestrone and Mama Mandola's Sicilian Chicken Soup are broth-based. They may make a filling enough meal since they are also chunky with ingredients.

- Cucina Casuale - Grilled Fish Ciabatta is a 4-5oz fish served open-faced on a grilled ciabatta. Or try the Insalata Johnny Rocco (without cheese) or Insalata Carrabba Caesar (without the bacon, egg, and cheese) with grilled chicken and lowfat sundried tomato vinaigrette.

- Marsala - Select the smaller portions of chicken or veal; request "very little Marsala wine sauce."

- Wood-Burning Grill - Choose the Spiedino Di Mare w/shrimp or scallops, Small Grilled Salmon (6oz), or Small Grilled Chicken (5oz). These dishes are served with soup or salad, plus a vegetable. Request two lower calorie vegetables instead.

Caveats:

- Boule bread is served with meals. I'm guessing around 400 calories worth. While low in fat, the fat and calories can increase significantly when dipped in the seasoned oil.

- Pasta servings are big (around 4 cups)! The optional Whole Grain Pasta has about the same calories as the white pasta.

- Mini-Desserts are offered, but may not be "guilt-free" as described on the menu. Estimate around 300 calories each.

Carvel®

Tips:

• Carvel® serves hand-dipped and soft-serve ice cream, not lower fat yogurt. The lowest calorie choices are listed below under "Suggestions."

• For more nutrition information, go to Carvel.com.

Suggestions:

	Calories	Fat (g)	Sat+Trans Fat (g)	Sodium (mg)	Carbohydrates (g)	Fiber (g)	Protein (g)
Lowfat Ice Cream, vanilla or chocolate (avg):							
in small cup	285	6	5	135	52	0	10
w/cake cone	310	6	5	140	55	0	10
w/sugar cone	330	6	5	145	62	0	10
Ice Cream, small cup:							
No-Sugar-Added Vanilla	260	7	5	190	51	0	11
Sherbet	290	3	2	115	67	0	2
Fruit Smoothies, small (avg all flavors)	315	0	0	35	78	2	0
Take Home Treats:							
Lil' Rounder®, avg all flavors	180	9	4	150	23	1	2
Flying Saucer w/lowfat van or choc, avg	190	5	3	135	35	0	5
Mini Sundae w/chocolate syrup	220	10	8	95	29	0	3
Slice of Carvel Ice Cream Cake	250	13	9	125	29	1	4

Caveats:

• Other ice cream desserts are high-calorie. Check these out:

Chocolate Ice Cream, small cup	410	21	13	220	48	2	10
Vanilla Ice Cream, small cup	450	26	17	210	47	0	6
Cake Cone w/vanilla or chocolate, avg	455	24	15	220	51	1	8
Sugar Cone w/vanilla or chocolate, avg	475	24	15	240	58	1	8
Waffle Cone w/vanilla or chocolate, avg	500	24	14	240	62	1	10

• Other specialty products are even higher (BTW these are all for the *small* size!). All flavors have been averaged:

Carvelatte® w/lowfat ice cream	465	7	6	210	93	0	10
Iceberg®	550	27	18	280	65	0	10
Classic Sundaes	615	33	34	275	70	2	8
Thick Shakes	635	30	19	295	83	1	12
Arctic Blender® w/lowfat ice cream	645	14	7	310	106	1	14
Carvelatte®	655	28	17	345	90	0	12
Cavelanche®	725	36	22	340	89	0	11
Dashers	785	29	20	410	94	4	11
Thick Shake Floats	785	37	24	360	99	1	14
Arctic Blender®	820	35	19	435	100	2	15
Banana Barge®	970	46	24	290	128	7	19

Casey's General Store

Tips:

- For more nutrition info, go to Caseys.com. Unfortunately, saturated and trans fat content is not available.

Suggestions:

Medium Pizza, 1 slice	Calories	Fat (g)	Sat+Trans Fat (g)	Sodium (mg)	Carbohydrates (g)	Fiber (g)	Protein (g)
Cheese, pineapple, Canadian bacon, ham, Hawaiian, or vegetable	370	11	na	660	49	2	16
Pepperoni	385	11	na	665	48	2	16
Beef	410	15	na	835	48	2	19
BBQ Beef	415	14	na	780	53	2	18
Breakfast Burrito	310	12	na	865	39	2	11
Marshmallow Rice Treats	170	2	na	115	23	0	2

Caveats:

- Think before you drink. Here are the stats:

	Calories	Fat (g)	Sat+Trans Fat (g)	Sodium (mg)	Carbohydrates (g)	Fiber (g)	Protein (g)
French Vanilla Cappucino, 12oz	250	8	na	300	40	0	3
Fat-Free French Vanilla Cappucino	210	0	na	290	48	1	3
French Vanilla Iced Coffee, 16oz	320	8	na	500	54	0	8
Hot Chocolate, 12oz	195	2	na	330	42	0	5
Mocha Iced Coffee, 16oz	320	8	na	520	54	0	8

- The other breakfast sandwiches range from 370-580 calories and 24-58g fat. The highest is the Sausage and Egg Biscuit.

- Other pizza slices range from 410-560 calories and 15-26g fat. Bacon Cheeseburger and Bacon Breakfast are the highest.

- Sandwiches range from 470-690 calories - with the Bacon Cheeseburger being the highest at 690 calories and 48g fat.

- Most bakery goods range from 50 calories (mini-cookie or doughnut hole) to 300 calories (regular cookie, unfrosted Apple Turnover, or Doughnut). Add another 100 calories if the turnover is frosted. The Blueberry Muffin, Brownie with icing, and Raspberry Cheese Flips have closer to 400 calories. The Sandwich Cookie has a whopping 790 calories!

Dr. Jo says

When looking at the fat content, remember there are 88g fat in a stick of butter!

Charley's® Grilled Subs

Tips:

• Ask for "no salt." Subs contain an average of 1500mg sodium. Many of the subs are salted - ask for yours without the sprinkle and save 390mg sodium.

• For more nutrition information, go to Charleys.com.

Suggestions:

	Calories	Fat (g)	Sat+Trans Fat (g)	Sodium (mg)	Carbohydrates (g)	Fiber (g)	Protein (g)
Breakfast Sandwiches:							
Egg & Cheese	470	17	6	950	54	2	29
Ham, Egg & Cheese	540	20	7	1440	55	2	39
Salads w/o dressing:							
Fresh Garden Salad	60	2	0	380	9	2	<1
Grilled Chicken Salad	200	7	2	530	10	2	25
Grilled Steak Salad	210	10	3	690	10	2	20
Buffalo Chicken Salad	210	8	2	1330	14	2	25
Chicken Teriyaki Salad	210	7	2	1140	12	2	22
Ranch or Italian Salad Dressing, 2Tbsp	140	16	3	250	1	0	0
Subs:							
Philly Veggie	450	15	8	1140	62	4	23
Turkey Cheddar Melt	470	12	6	1570	53	2	36
Philly Steak and Bleu	470	15	7	1400	56	3	32
Chicken California	500	16	7	1290	53	2	40
Philly Chicken	520	16	7	1290	58	3	42
Chicken Teriyaki	520	16	8	1280	58	3	43
Philly Ham & Swiss	520	16	8	1550	60	3	39
Philly Cheesesteak	520	19	8	1450	56	3	36
Mushroom Swiss Steak	520	19	8	1270	57	2	38
Chicken Buffalo	530	16	7	1700	59	4	42
Philly Steak Deluxe	530	19	8	1450	58	3	37
Chicken Cordon Blue	570	18	9	1210	54	2	53

Caveats:

• Skip the combo. Many subs are in the 500 calorie range, but when turned into a combo, the calories jump to 1210 calories. A regular combo includes fries (450 calories and 25g fat) and 21oz drink (about 260 calories).

• The Gourmet Fries won't look so lovely on your thighs. Count on 520-600 calories and 25-32g fat per order.

• The subs not mentioned above range from 560-640 calories and 20-32g fat. The highest calorie subs are the Bacon 3 Cheese and Sicilian Steak.

• Cut the cheese. Each sub includes 100-150 calories of cheese.

Checkers® and Rally's®

Tips:

- The restaurant's sign accurately describes the menu as, "Burgers, Fries, Colas." There are a few more offerings, but most are high-fat menu items.

- Want fries and a drink? Be sure to request the *small* combo consisting of small fries (230 calories and 13g fat) and small drink (170 calories).

- More nutrition information can be found at Checkers.com.

Suggestions:

	Calories	Fat (g)	Sat+Trans Fat (g)	Sodium (mg)	Carbohydrates (g)	Fiber (g)	Protein (g)
Grilled Chicken Breast Sandwich	360	9	2	710	38	3	32
Buffalo Chicken Sandwich	340	16	8	1340	34	2	16
Kid's Burger	280	12	6	570	28	2	15
Checkerburger®/Rallyburger®	390	22	8	680	32	3	16

Caveat:

- If you're craving wings, consider this: just *one* Big Boneless Wing (a breaded and fried chicken strip) contains around 300-350 calories. And the smallest order is three wings! The Classic Wings average 70-100 calories *per wing* (not per order).

Dr. Jo says

Ketchup contains just 15 calories per tablespoon (or 1 packet). Doesn't sound bad, does it? But how many level tablespoons can you eat with your meal. Two? Ten? All those calories add up!

Each tablespoon also contains 165mg sodium. Six packets will add another 1000mg sodium to your meal! Ouch!

Cheesecake Factory®

Tips:

• Look for specially-marked SkinnyLicious™ menu items inside the regular menu. Each contains less than 590 calories. Bread is not included in the nutrition information and is served on request only. Salad dressings contain 11-15 calories/tablespoon.

• No nutrition information is at TheCheesecakeFactory.com. Limited nutrition information can be obtained by calling customer service at 818-871-3281. Total fat is not available. Since this is generally many times the saturated fat, only those lowest in saturated fat are listed below.

SkinnyLicious™ Suggestions:

	Calories	Fat (g)	Sat Fat (g)	Sodium (mg)	Carbohydrates (g)	Fiber (g)	Protein (g)
Small Plates & Appetizers (all are <490 calories):							
Edamame	290	na	0	1250	27	na	na
Ahi Carpaccio or Tartare (avg)	250	na	2	990	12	na	na
Chicken Lettuce Wrap Tacos, Mexican	250	na	3	1015	14	na	na
Chicken Lettuce Wrap Tacos, Asian	470	na	4	870	50	na	na
Shrimp Summer Rolls	410	na	1	1495	61	na	na
Salmon Rolls	430	na	4	970	37	na	na
Chicken Pot Stickers	460	na	3	2470	44	na	na
Fresh Baked Flatbreads (all are <490 calories):							
Margherita	330	na	6	590	33	na	na
Roasted Pear and Blue Cheese	470	na	9	751	43	na	na
Salads (all are <590 calories):							
Tossed Green Salad	130	na	1	110	16	na	na
Spicy Chicken Salad	440	na	1	1105	42	na	na
Herb Crusted Salmon Salad	510	na	5	985	20	na	na
Pear & Endive Salad	520	na	5	1770	30	na	na
Mexican Tortilla Salad	560	na	5	1855	51	na	na
Asian Chicken Salad	570	na	2	2640	51	na	na
Seared Tuna Tataki Salad	580	na	4	1760	17	na	na
Specialties (all are <590 calories):							
Veggie Burger	530	na	3	1290	85	na	na
B.B.Q. Chicken	570	na	2	1090	33	na	na
Soft Taco, chicken or shrimp (avg)	570	na	4	1500	64	na	na
Fresh Vegetable Platter	580	na	3	1015	62	na	na
White Chicken Chili	585	na	5	1775	35	na	na
Tuscan Chicken	585	na	2	855	21	na	na

Caveat:

• Original Cheesecake contains 710 calories per slice (540 in the Low Carb) while the other cheesecake slices are much higher. Brownie Sundae Cheesecake has 1480 calories per slice.

Chevy's Fresh Mex®

Tips:

- Take half home, share a meal, or order a la carte (see caveats).

- Request Black Beans or Beans a la Charra, instead of Refried Beans to save nearly 100 calories and at least 10g fat. And pile on the naturally low-cal Pico de Gallo.

- For more nutrition information, go Chevys.com.

Suggestions (a la carte):	Calories	Fat (g)	Sat Fat (g)	Sodium (mg)	Carbohydrates (g)	Fiber (g)	Protein (g)
Homemade Tortilla Soup, bowl	420	18	4	1180	38	7	29
Salsa Chicken Enchilada, 1 enchilada	210	11	4	470	17	2	12
Soft Picadillo Beef Taco, 1 taco	280	14	4	500	27	2	11
Soft Salsa Chicken Taco, 1 taco	250	12	3	650	26	2	10
Mesquite Grilled Chicken Tacos, 2 (tacos only)	590	24	6	1280	49	3	41
Crispy Chicken Taco, 1	200	11	2	350	17	2	8
Pork Tamale, 1	250	10	4	690	30	2	10
Original Fajitas w/veggies, butter only (no accompaniments):							
Chicken	390	13	8	870	13	3	51
Chicken & Shrimp	410	17	7	1650	15	3	46
Chicken & Steak	450	22	9	860	13	3	48
Accompaniments: El Machino® Tortilla, 1	140	4	2	300	22	1	3
Black Beans	160	2	<1	720	27	9	10
Beans a la Charra	210	4	2	800	32	11	13
Fresh Mex® Rice	150	0	0	510	33	1	3
Guacamole	110	10	2	320	7	5	1
Side Salad w/fat-free salsa vinaigrette	190	5	1	480	35	5	5

Caveats:

- Upon being seated, a 450 calorie basket of chips and salsa arrives at your table. Before you dive in, remember that each *plain* chip contains about 25 calories.

- With a few exceptions, appetizers range from 1200-2500 calories. Sure, avocados contain healthy fats, but the entire Guac-My-Way order contains 730 calories and 52g fat.

- Salads are loaded in fat and calories. Sante Fe Chopped Salad contains 660 calories (39g fat); BBQ Chicken Salad has 880 calories (51g fat). The other salads range from 1220-1560 calories. Want dressing? Count on another 370-380 calories!

- Many entrées are over 1000 calories - even before factoring in the accompaniments. Most items are served with Fresh Mex® Rice, choice of beans, Sweet Corn Tamalito, guacamole, and sour cream (in total, these add at least 750 calories to the meal).

Chick-fil-A®

Tips:

• For breakfast choose multigrain oatmeal.

• Looking for a low-calorie option that's not soda? Check out the fresh squeezed diet lemonade.

• For more nutrition information, go to Chick-fil-A.com.

Suggestions:

	Calories	Fat (g)	Sat+Trans Fat (g)	Sodium (mg)	Carbohydrates (g)	Fiber (g)	Protein (g)
Fruit Cup, medium	50	0	0	0	13	1	0
Yogurt Parfait w/harvest nut granola	290	6	2	85	53	1	7
Multigrain Oatmeal	280	11	1	45	44	5	6
mixed fruit blend	45	0	0	10	12	1	0
roasted nut topping	80	8	1	10	3	1	2
cinnamon brown sugar	25	0	0	0	7	0	0
Chick-n-Minis™, 4 count	370	14	4	870	41	2	21
Chargrilled Chicken Sandwich	290	4	1	1030	36	3	29
Cool Wraps w/o dressing:							
Chargrilled Chicken Cool Wrap®	410	12	4	1290	50	9	33
Spicy Chicken Cool Wrap®	410	12	4	1350	48	8	34
Chicken Caesar Cool Wrap®	460	15	6	1510	47	8	40
Salads w/o dressing:							
Chargrilled Chicken Garden Salad	180	6	4	650	11	4	23
Chargrilled Chicken & Fruit Salad	220	6	4	640	22	4	22
Side Salad	70	5	3	110	5	2	5
Dressings, per packet:							
Fat-Free Honey Mustard Dressing	60	0	0	220	14	1	0
Reduced-Fat Berry Balsamic Vinaigrette	70	2	0	150	12	0	0
Light Italian Dressing	15	1	0	510	2	0	0
Hearty Breast of Chicken Soup, small	140	4	1	1110	19	2	7
Chick-fil-A® Diet Lemonade, small	15	0	0	10	4	0	0
Icedream®, small cup	290	7	5	200	50	0	8

Caveats:

• Milkshakes range from 550-770 calories. A better choice might be a small Icedream® cup at 290 calories and 7g fat.

• There's butter on some of the sandwiches. Order a Chick-fil-A® Chicken Sandwich with no butter on the bun and save 30 calories and 3g fat.

• Skip the dressing. All the Cool Wraps® are served with choice of dressing, but the wraps taste great without it. The dressings, not listed above, range from 140-160 calories and 14-17g fat per packet.

Chili's®

Tips:

• Try Chili's Guiltless Grills®. These modifications of Chili's favorites offer complete meals low in fat and calories, but high in fiber and flavor. These are identified as "GG" under the Suggestions below.

• Both the Fries and the Loaded Mashed Potatoes contain close to 400 calories. Instead, choose Steamed Veggies, Rice, or Corn on the Cob.

• For more nutrition information, go to Chilis.com.

Suggestions:

	Calories	Fat (g)	Sat Fat (g)	Sodium (mg)	Carbohydrates (g)	Fiber (g)	Protein (g)
Chili & Green Chile Soup, bowl	200	7	3	1250	21	3	16
GG Grilled Chicken SW w/veggies	610	13	5	1320	78	8	43
GG Santa Fe Chicken Wrap w/veggies	680	25	8	2210	80	8	37
GG Classic Sirloin, as served	370	9	4	3680	20	6	53
GG Salmon w/Garlic & Herbs, as served	480	17	5	1590	37	5	49
Caribb. Salad w/grilled chicken w/dressing	610	25	4	800	65	6	33
w/grilled shrimp instead	590	28	5	1030	65	6	19
Margarita Grilled Chicken, as served	600	13	3	1310	72	19	49
Chicken Fajitas & tortillas w/only salsa	590	17	6	1660	67	9	51
Beef Fajitas & tortillas w/only salsa	650	21	8	2580	70	9	42

Caveats:

• Most of Chili's® appetizers, meal, and desserts are over 1000 calories. Check these out (and remember that a stick of butter contains 88g fat):

Bottomless Tostada Chips w/salsa	1020	51	10	1210	125	12	11
Hot Spinach & Artichoke Dip w/chips	1610	103	43	1610	139	14	33
Skillet Queso w/chips	1710	101	37	3490	147	13	45
Quesadilla Explosion Salad w/dressing	1300	87	28	2050	75	8	62
Original Ribs as served	2170	123	44	6510	137	20	133
Oldtimer® Burger (w/mustard/onion) w/fries	1310	65	20	3230	128	10	51
Jalapeno Smokehouse Burger w/ranch, fries	2210	144	46	6600	136	11	92
Big Mouth® Bites w/ranch, fries	2120	133	38	4810	163	7	66
BBQ Pulled Pork Sandwich w/fries	1670	85	16	4240	172	13	54
Bacon Ranch Chicken Quesadilla	1480	103	39	2900	69	4	73
Cajun Pasta w/grilled chicken	500	76	36	4130	124	6	79
Beef Fajitas, tortillas, rice, beans, and condiments	1170	48	20	4260	125	18	63
Brownie Sundae	1290	61	30	930	195	8	14

Chipotle Mexican Grill

Tips:

- What's the best way to build a meal at Chipotle? Start with corn tortillas or shells for the leanest meal. As far as the other choices, it doesn't matter whether you choose a base of a burrito, soft flour taco, or salad - you'll end up with about the same number of calories.

- After selecting a base, add one of four meats or a vegetarian option. Chicken and steak are just slightly lower in total fat and saturated but the calories are all similar.

- The meal includes choice of two carbs - Cilantro-Lime Rice, plus either Black Beans or Pinto Beans. Each choice is almost identical in calories and fat. So to cut calories, select just one. Hint: beans contain healthy soluble fiber.

- Add salsa for a total of 615-790 calories (when both rice and beans are selected). Cheese and sour cream are additional.

- For more nutrition information, go to Chipotle.com.

Suggestions:

	Calories	Fat (g)	Sat+Trans Fat (g)	Sodium (mg)	Carbohydrates (g)	Fiber (g)	Protein (g)
Choice of: Soft Corn Tortillas (tacos), 3	180	2	0	75	39	1	6
Crispy Taco Shells, 3	180	6	2	30	27	3	1
Flour Tortillas (tacos). 3	270	8	3	600	39	1	6
Romaine Lettuce & Vinaigrette (salad)	270	25	4	705	14	2	1
Flour Tortilla (burrito), 1	290	9	3	670	44	2	7
Choice of: Barbacoa	170	7	3	510	2	0	24
Vegetables + Guacamole (vegetarian)	170	14	2	360	12	7	3
Chicken	190	7	2	370	1	0	32
Steak	190	7	2	320	2	0	30
Carnitas	190	8	3	540	1	0	27
Choice of: Cilantro-Lime Rice	130	3	<1	150	23	0	2
Black Beans	120	1	0	250	23	11	7
Pinto Beans	120	1	0	330	22	10	7
Choice of: Green Tomatillo Salsa	15	0	0	230	3	1	1
Tomato Salsa	20	0	0	470	4	<1	1
Red Tomatillo Salsa	40	1	0	510	8	4	2
Corn Salsa	80	2	0	410	15	3	3

Caveats:

- Adding the usual cheese (100 calories and 9g fat) and sour cream (120 calories and 10g fat) would bring the meal to a grand total of 835-1010 calories...and as much as 63g fat!

- Chips add another 570 calories and 27g fat.

Chuck E. Cheese®

Tips:

• Let the kids focus on the play, not the food.

• Go dipless. Take advantage of the Veggie Platter (carrot sticks and celery sticks). The calories are negligible. Nearly all the calories come from the dressing.

• For more nutrition info, go to ChuckECheese.com.

Suggestions:

	Calories	Fat (g)	Sat+Trans Fat (g)	Sodium (mg)	Carbohydrates (g)	Fiber (g)	Protein (g)
Individual Cheese Pizza	540	19	8	1260	69	3	21
Large Pizza slice, avg:							
Cheese or Veggie Combo	170	6	3	400	24	1	8
BBQ Chicken or Super Combo	210	8	3	480	26	1	7
All Meat Combo	240	11	4	570	24	1	10
Medium Pizza slice, avg:							
Cheese or Veggie Combo	160	6	2	365	22	1	6
BBQ Chicken or Super Combo	185	7	3	460	23	1	7
All Meat Combo	215	11	4	610	21	1	9
Small Pizza Slice, avg:							
Cheese or Veggie Combo	135	5	2	310	20	1	5
BBQ Chicken or Super Combo	155	6	3	390	20	1	6
Cinnamon Stick, 1 stick	70	2	1	90	11	0	1
Side Fruit Garnish	65	0	0	0	9	1	0
Side Mandarin Oranges	60	0	0	0	15	1	0

Caveats:

• Little things add up. Calculate these nibblers into your total:

Breadstick, 1	175	9	2	410	18	1	6
Mozzarella Stick, 1 stick	90	6	2	210	6	0	4
Buffalo Wing, 1 wing	75	5	1	330	4	1	4
Celery Stick w/Bleu Cheese, 1 stick	70	7	1	150	2	<1	1
Carrot Sticks & Lite Ranch, side order	180	15	2	450	12	2	2

• Veggie Platter has over 1000 calories and 88g fat. So, snatch up the veggies and leave most of the bleu cheese dressing behind.

• Hot Dog and French Fries shouldn't be called a kid's meal. Excluding the drink the meal adds up to 730 calories, 38g fat.

• The Oven-Baked Sandwiches average 730 calories and 31g fat each. Skip the mayonnaise and balsamic vinaigrette to reduce both fat and calories.

• Count dessert. Each cake slice contains about 300 calories and 15g fat. One slice of Apple Dessert Pizza has 190 calories and 5g fat.

Church's Chicken®

Tips:

- Main courses consist of only fried chicken, fried chicken sandwiches, and wings. Below are the leanest choices of what's offered.
- For more nutrition information, go to Churchs.com

Suggestions:

	Calories	Fat (g)	Sat+Trans Fat (g)	Sodium (mg)	Carbohydrates (g)	Fiber (g)	Protein (g)
Original or Spicy Chicken Sandwich	360	18	6	660	35	3	14
Southern Style Sandwich	450	16	4	1210	50	2	23
Original Breast	200	11	5	440	3	1	22
Original Leg	110	6	8	280	3	0	10
Mashed Potatoes & Gravy	110	2	<1	780	21	2	3
Corn	140	3	0	15	24	9	4
Collard Greens	35	0	0	240	7	3	3
Green Beans	35	0	0	360	7	2	2

Caveats:

- Every chicken piece is fried. Original pieces are lower in calories and fat than the Spicy:

Original Breast	200	21	5	440	3	1	22
Leg	110	6	8	280	3	0	10
Thigh	330	23	9	680	8	1	21
Wing	300	18	8	540	7	3	27
Spicy Breast	320	20	9	760	12	2	21
Leg	180	11	5	470	8	1	12
Thigh	480	35	14	1040	20	2	22
Wing	430	27	11	1020	17	2	29

- Meals come with choice of sides and biscuits. The leaner ones are listed in the Suggestions. Here are the rest:

Honey Butter Biscuit	240	12	6	540	28	1	3
Cole Slaw	155	10	2	170	15	2	1
Okra	300	19	7	500	31	4	3
Sweet Corn Nuggets, 8	250	12	2	530	30	2	3
French Fries, regular	280	12	4	800	40	3	3
Jalapeno Cheese Bombers, 4	160	8	2	680	20	0	8
Cajun Rice, regular	130	7	3	260	16	0	1
Macaroni & Cheese	190	7	4	640	24	2	8

- All sandwiches are prepared with fried chicken; those not mentioned above range from 500-740 calories and 26-38g fat.

- Dip lightly. Ketchup has just 15 calories a packet, the others are higher: Hot Sauce (20), BBQ Sauce and Tartar Sauce (25), Creamy Jalapeno (80), Honey Mustard (90), and Ranch (100).

Cici's Pizza

Tips:

- Pizzas on the "All-You-Can-Eat" buffet are mostly 12" pizzas and range from 110-180 calories per slice. The "To-Go" Pizzas are 15" pizzas and range from 160-240 calories per slice.

- Pizzas lowest in fat and calories include Cheese, Classic Chicken, Ham, Ole, Veggie, and Alfredo (no, that's not a typo). Those on the high-calorie end include Bar-B-Que, Cheeseburger, Macaroni & Cheese, Pepperoni, and Sausage.

- For more nutrition information, go to Cicispizza.com

Suggestions (per slice):

	Calories	Fat (g)	Sat+Trans Fat (g)	Sodium (mg)	Carbohydrates (g)	Fiber (g)	Protein (g)
Buffet Slices:							
Thin Crust Italiano	80	4	1	230	9	0	4
Regular Crust Pizza, avg	140	4	2	340	19	<1	5
Deep Dish Pizza, avg	180	6	3	340	19	<1	7
To-Go 15" Pizza Slices:							
Higher Calorie Pizza (see list above)	225	8	4	730	29	<1	10
Other varieties	180	7	3	500	23	<1	8
Deep Dish Pizza	200	7	4	390	22	<1	8
Other Choices:							
Pasta with red sauce	240	1	0	300	48	3	8
Chicken Noodle Soup, 1 cup	120	3	0	1040	16	0	6

Caveats:

- Count the extras:

	Calories	Fat (g)	Sat+Trans Fat (g)	Sodium (mg)	Carbohydrates (g)	Fiber (g)	Protein (g)
Garlic Bread Stick, 1	100	5	2	120	10	0	4
Mild Wings, 4	320	26	6	980	1	0	22
BBQ Wings, 4	270	18	5	730	6	<1	22
Hot Wings, 4	280	21	5	1130	2	0	22
Fudge Brownie, 1 slice	140	6	1	125	23	<1	1
Cinnamon Roll, 1 roll	140	5	1	100	20	0	2
Bavarian Dessert, 1 slice	170	3	1	210	32	<1	3
Apple Dessert, 1 slice	240	6	1	290	43	<1	5

Dr. Jo says

As with all buffets, it's not just *what* you eat, but also *how much* you eat.

Cinnabon®

Tips:

• Get a Minibon rather than a Classic, or better yet, share a four-pack of the Bites with three other people. Just one of these "bite-sized goodies" still has over 100 calories.

• For more nutrition information, go to Cinnabon.com.

Suggestions (per 1 piece):

	Calories	Fat (g)	Sat Fat (g)	Sodium (mg)	Carbohydrates (g)	Fiber (g)	Protein (g)
Minibon® Roll	350	14	7	330	51	1	5
Cinnabon® Classic Bite (in packs of 4-6)	105	4	2	90	15	<1	2
Caramel Pecanborn Bite (in packs of 4-6)	135	7	2	110	17	1	2
Cinnabon Stix® (from a 5-10 count pack)	80	4	2	90	9	0	1

Caveats:

• Don't eat a Classic all by yourself:

Cinnabon® Classic	880	36	17	830	127	2	13
Caramel Pecanbon®	1080	50	20	960	147	3	14

• Most beverages are high in calories. Here's how the 16oz (often the smallest size) stacks up:

Classic Lemonade	190	0	0	5	50	0	0
Orange Juice	220	2	0	0	50	1	4
Raspberry Lemonade	230	0	0	10	58	0	0
Chocolate Mocha Chillattas®	370	14	8	200	61	3	8
Hot Cocoa w/Ghiradelli sauce and whip	370	15	9	160	50	3	14
Chocolate Reduced Fat Milk	380	9	6	330	61	3	15
MochaLatta Chill®	420	17	10	290	63	1	10
Tropical Blast® Chillattas	500	8	4	105	107	1	1
Strawberry Chillattas®	510	8	4	260	111	2	1
Strawberry Banana Chillattas®	520	8	4	75	113	0	1

• Think before you take home a box. Pre-packed versions are even higher in calories than the in-store ones. The Minibon® has 30 additional calories and the Cinnbon® has 60 calories extra. In addition, do you really need the temptation of a box of these high-calorie treats in your kitchen?

• Don't dip. A frosting cup contains 180 calories and 11g fat.

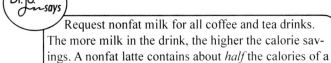

Request nonfat milk for all coffee and tea drinks. The more milk in the drink, the higher the calorie savings. A nonfat latte contains about *half* the calories of a latte prepared with whole milk!

Cold Stone Creamery®

Tips:

- Customized Creations™ mix ice cream, yogurt, or sorbet with a variety of goodies. Stick with the smallest "Kid's" or "Like It" in a cup or sugar cone. Kid's (for anyone) has half the calories of the Like It.

- For more nutrition info, go to ColdStoneCreamery.com

Suggestions (avg per "Like It"):

	Calories	Fat (g)	Sat+Trans Fat (g)	Sodium (mg)	Carbohydrates (g)	Fiber (g)	Protein (g)
Frozen Sorbet Base:							
Lemon, Raspberry or Watermelon Sorbet	160	0	0	15	41	0	0
Straw Mango or Pink Lemonade Sorbet	230	0	0	20	57	0	0
Frozen Yogurt Base:							
Most Flavors, except those listed below	180	0	0	150	40	0	5
Cake Batter™, Chocolate Malt, Cinn Bun,							
Cookies & Creamery, or Key Lime	210	2	0	200	46	0	5
Choc Hazelnut, Cookie Batter, Peanut Butter	240	5	1	215	43	0	6
Ice Cream Base:							
Sinless Sans Fat™ Sweet Cream	170	0	0	160	35	1	8
Sinless Cake Batter Ice Cream	210	1	<1	250	43	1	7
Pumpkin Ice Cream	290	15	10	105	33	1	4
Other flavors (except those in caveats)	330	19	13	100	36	0	5
Mix-Ins:							
Blueberries or Blackberries	10	0	0	0	2	1	0
Banana, P/apple, Strawberry, Raspberry	20	0	0	0	5	<1	0
Nuts	70	6	<1	30	2	1	2
Black Cherries or Raisins	75	0	0	5	19	<1	0
Sinless Smoothies:							
Berry Trinity™	110	1	0	25	28	6	2
Straw Bonanza™ or Berry Lemony™	145	1	0	25	38	3	1

Caveats:

- Cookie Batter, Peanut Butter, Choc Peanut Butter, and Oreo® Creme ice cream contain 360-440 calories per "Like It" size.

- Add no more than one non-fruit mix-in. Most add 25-95 calories. Brownies, chocolate, peanut butter, cookie dough, and candy with nuts and chocolate add 100-225 calories.

- Waffle cones or bowls contain 160 calories and 4g fat while the dipped waffle cone has about 310 calories and 15g fat.

- Avoid larger sized Creations™. Like It size contains 5oz ice cream; Love It and Gotta Have It have 8 and 12oz, respectively.

- Sinless Shakes are still sinful (500-670 calories/small), though half the calories of regular shakes.

Corner Bakery Cafe

Tips:

• Order egg dishes prepared with egg whites - and save 80-160 calories.

• Go Topless. Oatmeal is topped with a 150 calorie "sweet crisp" unless requested otherwise. Get dried fruit and nuts instead.

• Do the combo. Combine half portions of any two: soup, salad, sandwiches, paninis, and pasta (find all the options at 100under600.com). Best choices are listed below.

• For detailed nutrition info, go to CornerBakeryCafe.com

Suggestions:

	Calories	Fat (g)	Sat+Trans Fat (g)	Sodium (mg)	Carbohydrates (g)	Fiber (g)	Protein (g)
All American Scrambler w/bacon & egg whites	190	11	4	800	2	0	19
Harvest Toast w/o butter	160	1	<1	280	31	3	7
Fruit Medley (instead of potatoes)	70	0	0	10	13	<1	<1
Ham & Swiss Panini w/egg whites	460	14	6	1540	47	2	33
Seasonal Fruit Medley	70	0	0	10	16	2	<1
Oatmeal w/o toppings or sweet crisp	140	2	<1	230	21	1	10
toasted walnuts & cranberries	75	5	<1	0	7	1	1
toasted almonds & currents	70	3	<1	0	9	1	1
Swiss Oatmeal w/o sweet crisp	360	3	1	130	78	5	11

Combo Suggestions (pick 2 half portions, unless already combined):

	Calories	Fat (g)	Sat+Trans Fat (g)	Sodium (mg)	Carbohydrates (g)	Fiber (g)	Protein (g)
½ Penne w/Marinara w/mixed green salad	450	14	3	535	62	5	14
Mom's Chicken Noodle soup, cup	140	4	2	1080	19	1	8
Three Lentil Vegetable soup, cup	140	3	0	930	24	9	8
Tomato Basil soup w/croutons, cup	200	7	0	1500	30	3	8
DC Chicken Salad on Steakhouse Rye, ½	275	8	1	900	39	2	13
Turkey on Pretzel Bread, ½	335	8	3	1410	43	2	22
Uptown Turkey on Harvest Bread, ½	320	10	3	910	37	5	20
Tuna Salad on Harvest Bread, ½	310	11	2	635	35	4	17
Mom's Roasted Chicken or Turkey on Harvest Bread							
w/out mayo or cheese, ½ (avg)	235	2	<1	650	34	3	19
California Grille Panini, ½	310	14	6	650	34	4	13
Green Chile & Chicken Panini, ½	375	15	6	890	37	2	22
Mixed Greens Salad, ½	220	17	2	460	13	3	3
Asian Wonton Salad, ½	270	8	<1	960	33	6	20
Trio Salad w/edamame, chicken salad & fruit	400	19	2	1080	39	7	18

Caveat:

• Full-size Sandwiches, Paninis, Pasta, Soups & Salads are served with extras (chips, roll...) so could easily end up over 1000 calories. Baby Carrots are available, instead of chips.

Cosi®

Tips:

- Sandwiches and melts are served with chips or baby carrots; salads are served with your choice of flatbread (see below).

- "Light" options are prepared with fat-free or reduced-fat vinaigrette - though the Cobb Light Salad still has 34g fat!

- T.B.M. is Cosi's® abbreviation for tomato, basil, & mozzarella.

- For more nutrition information, go to GetCosi.com

Suggestions:

	Calories	Fat (g)	Sat+Trans Fat (g)	Sodium (mg)	Carbohydrates (g)	Fiber (g)	Protein (g)
Breakfast: Oatmeal, plain	220	3	0	100	45	4	5
Roasted Veggie & Egg White Wrap	265	12	4	685	22	11	26
Most Squagels® (see caveat)	350	3	<1	240*	66	3	14
Lighter Side Menu Options:							
Tandori Chicken Sandwich Light	375	3	1	890	50	2	35
Hummus & Veggies Sandwich	400	7	0	530	72	7	13
T.B.M. Sandwich Light	440	16	9	325	49	2	29
Grilled Chicken T.B.M. Chicken SW Light	530	17	7	435	49	3	46
Bombay Chicken Salad Light w/dressing	165	2	0	735	19	4	19
Signature Salad Light w/dressing	380	19	1	505	47	6	10
Sandwiches: Fire Roasted Veggie SW	330	9	4	265	51	4	12
Turkey Light Sandwich	390	5	1	525	63	2	26
Cosi Club Sandwich w/lowfat mayo	465	14	4	965	49	3	31
Tuscan Pesto Chicken Sandwich	510	18	6	455	49	5	39
Chicken Tinga Sandwich	555	21	7	1215	60	7	37
Shanghai Chicken Salad w/dressing	315	13	2	850	27	5	26
Rustic Flatbread	215	1	0	40	43	2	8
Whole Grain Cosi Bread	235	2	0	70	46	3	9
Shareable Flatbreads:							
Smoky BBQ Chicken Flatbread Pizza	890	21	11	1400	123	4	49
Margarita Flatbread Pizza	740	27	10	410	91	5	38

* "Everything" Squagels® contain 1150mg sodium

Caveats:

- Original Flatbread pizzas contain 710-920 calories and 22-41g fat. Interestingly, Thin Flatbread Pizzas have 210 calories less, but still have the same amount of fat.

- Squagels® (bagels) over 400 calories include: Cinnamon Raisin, Asiago, Cranberry Orange, Jalapeno Cheddar, and Choc Chip.

- Cosi Break Bar®, while prepared with healthful ingredients, contains 360 calories and 18g fat; Yogurt Parfaits are over 330 calories. Scones and Muffins range from 360-510 calories. Cinnamon Apple Pie has 960 calories and 41g fat. The other desserts range from 570-700 calories.

Cracker Barrel®

Tips:

- No nutrition information is available at their website (Cracker Barrel.com). Information below is from a review of the menu and interviews with restaurant managers.

- Special order! Although it's not mentioned on the menu, feel free to order menu items ala carte (perhaps just one pancake), order foods not listed on the menu (such as sliced tomato, fresh fruit cup, or cottage cheese), or a half order of select items (such as bacon or sausage).

- Know your no-extra-charge substitutes. Egg Beaters® (or egg whites) are available instead of whole eggs for all egg dishes. In addition, there's Sugar-Free Syrup, Low Sugar Fruit Spread, Promise® Spread, and Turkey Sausage (instead of the regular).

- Be a kid. Anyone can order off the kid's menu. Choices include Two Pancakes, Grilled Chicken Tenderloin (3 strips with 1 side), and One Egg with a half order of bacon (2 strips).

- Choose the grilled. Fried menu items tend to have twice as many calories as their grilled counterparts.

- Select the Country Dinner Plate rather than the Fancy Fixin's®. The meat portion is generally smaller and it's served with two sides rather than three.

Suggestions:

- Sugar-Free Stewart's bottled Root Beer is available.

- Breakfast: Egg Beaters®, Sourdough Toast, and Sliced Tomatoes; Oatmeal with skim milk, Pecans, Raisins, or Bananas; Kid's One Egg with half-order Bacon or Turkey Sausage, or Kid's Two Pancakes (ask for no butter on top) and Sugar-Free Syrup.

- Lunch & Dinner: Country Dinner Plate with Ham, Pork Chop, Grilled Chicken Tenderloin, Grilled Catfish, or Rainbown Trout; Kid's 3 piece Grilled Chicken Tenderloin dinner with one side; or Kid's Country Vegetable Plate (choice of two sides).

Caveat:

- Limit the bread and butter. Unlimited bread (cornbread and biscuits) are served with meals. Neither are lowfat, and probably contribute about 150 calories each. The Apple Bran and Wild Maine Blueberry Muffins served at breakfast are even bigger - ask for a fresh fruit cup instead.

Culver's®

Tips:

- While Culver's® is known for its high-fat ButterBurgers® and Concrete Mixers, it is possible to eat responsibly.
- Stick with the Single Burger. Combos come with regular fries (385 calories, 17g fat) and drink (300 calories).
- For more nutrition information, go to Culvers.com.

Suggestions:

	Calories	Fat (g)	Sat+Trans Fat (g)	Sodium (mg)	Carbohydrates (g)	Fiber (g)	Protein (g)
ButterBurger® "The Original" Single	350	15	6	670	36	1	19
w/cheese	420	21	9	990	38	1	22
Flame Roasted Chicken Sandwich	310	8	2	980	36	0	27
Beef Pot Roast Sandwich	360	16	9	950	33	1	24
Garden Fresco Salad w/o dressing	230	10	4	380	19	4	16
Side Salad (reg or Caesar) w/o dressing	55	2	1	140	6	2	3
Classic Caesar w/chicken, w/o dressing	340	16	6	1450	14	3	34
Reduced-Calorie Raspberry Vinaigrette	45	0	0	180	11	0	0
Tomato Basil Ravioletti Soup	110	3	1	650	18	1	4
Soups: Chix Noodle, Veg Beef & Barley, Minestrone, Tomato Florentine (avg)	110	2	1	1340	17	2	6
Mini Scoop Vanilla Cake Cone	200	10	6	60	22	0	3
Mini Scoop Chocolate Cake Cone	190	8	5	80	25	1	4
Lemon Ice, 1 scoop	80	0	0	0	21	0	0

Caveats:

- Wisconsin Cheese Curds are the highest fat and calorie side offered at 670 calories and 38g fat.
- The dinners are huge. While the Pot Roast and Chopped Steak Dinners contain 750 and 850 respectively (still very high in fat), the other dinners range from 1265-2220 calories.
- Avoid the Green Beans. Prepared with butter, it contains 10g saturated fat - more than a ButterBurger® Single.
- Count on about 600 calories for a single scoop Sundae, about 1000 calories for a double, and 1200 for a triple.
- Each scoop of Ice Cream contains around 300 calories. Add another 25 calories for a cake cone, 90 calories for a waffle cone, and 240 calories for the chocolate-dipped waffle cone.
- Keep it short. A short Shake or Malt contains about 610-740 calories, a short Root Beer Float has around 470 calories, and a short Concrete Mixer adds up to 680-850 calories (and 40+g fat).

D'Angelo®

Tips:

• Stick with small. Small *Cold* Subs range from 290-940 calories (Small *Toasted* Subs range from 550-920 calories). Large subs are twice as big as the small; the medium-size is in between.

• Multigrain Subs and Honey Whole Wheat Wraps have similar nutrients as white or plain - but with an extra gram of fiber.

• For more nutrition information, go to DAngelos.com.

Suggestions, condiments additional:

	Calories	Fat (g)	Sat+Trans Fat (g)	Sodium (mg)	Carbohydrates (g)	Fiber (g)	Protein (g)
Veggie Quesadilla	280	13	1	810	33	3	12
Ham Sub, small	310	4	1	1190	48	2	20
Roast Beef Sub, small	330	5	2	970	45	2	26
Turkey Sub, small	340	3	1	510	43	2	31
Chicken Stir Fry Quesadilla	350	14	2	1050	32	2	25
Number 9 Quesadilla	370	19	4	850	31	2	22
Grilled Chicken Sub, small	380	7	2	880	47	3	31
Ham Wrap	390	10	2	1320	53	4	20
Capicola & Cheese, small	390	13	4	1470	45	2	27
Turkey Wrap	410	10	2	640	49	3	31
Roast Beef Wrap	410	12	4	1100	50	3	26
Ham & Cheese Sub, small	420	12	1	1830	48	2	27
Grilled Chicken Wrap	440	13	3	1010	50	3	30
Classic Veggie, small	450	17	3	1100	55	4	22
Steak, small	490	18	7	1120	44	2	37
Chicken Stir Fry, small	510	14	2	1360	52	3	41
Chicken Honey Dijon, small	540	16	7	1240	54	3	44
Greek Salad w/dressing	510	23	7	1470	58	7	21

Caveats:

• Count the condiments. Cheese and mayonnaise adds another 100 calories each. Olive Oil Blend has about 240 calories per tablespoon.

• Other than the one listed above, the other Salads with dressing contain 630-940 calories and 31-56g fat.

• Got a sweet tooth? Keep in mind that the Cookies and Bars average 520 calories.

Dairy Queen®

Tips:

- Skip the Combo. Regular Fries contain 310 calories while the medium drink has 220 calories. If you're craving fries and a regular drink, think about ordering a kid's meal instead.

- Want ice cream? Stick with a small cone - even a dipped cone, rather than a milkshake or Blizzard® Treat. The freezer case also has several bars at 50-80 calories each (some are sugar-free).

- For more nutrition information, go to DairyQueen.com.

Suggestions:

	Calories	Fat (g)	Sat-Trans Fat (g)	Sodium (mg)	Carbohydrates (g)	Fiber (g)	Protein (g)
Deluxe Hamburger	350	14	7	680	34	1	17
Grilled Chicken Sandwich	370	16	3	810	32	1	24
Grilled Chicken Salad	280	11	5	840	4	1	31
Grilled Chicken Wrap	200	13	4	450	9	1	12
Iron Grilled Cheese Sandwich	290	13	8	1020	30	1	13
Kid's Hamburger and fries	540	22	8	1080	61	3	19
Vanilla Orange Bar	60	0	0	40	18	6	2
Fudge Bar	50	0	0	70	13	6	4
DQ® Cone, vanilla or chocolate, kids	170	5	3	70	27	0	4
small	230	7	5	100	36	0	6
Dipped Cone, all flavors, kids (avg)	220	9	7	75	30	0	4
Fruit Flavored Sundae, small (avg)	240	7	5	100	40	0	6
Chocolate Sundae, small	280	8	5	115	48	0	6

Caveats:

- Mini Blizzard® Treats range from 290-450 calories and 8-19g fat. Those in the lower calorie range include Banana Split, Strawberry CheeseQuake®, and Hawaiian (290-330 calories and 8-12g fat). On the highest end are the Peanut Butter Parfait, Oreo® Brownie Earthquake® Treat, and Pecan Mudslide® Treat. But, the mini size is still way lower than the small size Blizzard® Treats (which range from 440-750 calories).

- Drinks can really add up. A small Artic Rush® contains no fat, but 230 calories. Small Milkshakes range from 500-660 calories (and 20-35g fat) while a small Malt is even higher (570-710 calories, 20-35g fat). As you might expect, fruit flavored ones are on the lower end, chocolate and caramel are in the middle range, while peanut butter Shakes and Malts are the highest. Small MooLattes® contain 460-530 calories and 15-18g fat.

Del Taco®

Tips:

• Taco Del Carbons are small, flavorful tacos prepared with California chili sauce, onion and fresh cilantro - great for a snack. Or pair two together for a meal.

• For more nutrition information, go to DelTaco.com.

Suggestions:

	Calories	Fat (g)	Sat Fat (g)	Sodium (mg)	Carbohydrates (g)	Fiber (g)	Protein (g)
Breakfast Del Carbon Taco	140	4	1	170	18	2	7
Breakfast Burrito	280	13	6	570	28	1	13
Egg & Cheese Burrito	400	17	6	770	22	1	18
Chicken Taco Del Carbon	150	4	0	300	19	2	10
Steak Taco Del Carbon	210	8	2	400	18	2	9
Soft Taco	150	6	3	330	15	2	8
Pollo Asado Taco	170	7	0	380	21	3	10
Half Pound Burrito, red or green	440	9	4	2080	54	12	18
Half Pound Bean & Cheese Burrito Deluxe	490	12	6	2090	56	12	19
Veggie Works Burrito	620	14	6	2200	83	9	18
Spicy Chicken Burrito	610	13	4	2450	82	7	27
Kid's Burrito, red or green	320	8	1	1320	44	7	14
Kid's Quesadilla, 2 pack	280	13	7	540	28	3	12
Guacamole, side	25	2	0	65	1	1	0

Caveats:

• Combo meals are served with small fries (260 calories and 15g fat) and small drink (250 calories).

• Don't pick the salad. The Deluxe Taco Salad™ has 845 calories and 47g fat (17g saturated fat).

• Steer clear of the Macho menu items. They often have twice as many calories as their "regular" counterpart. Check it out:

Macho Taco®	300	17	7	630	16	2	20
Taco	130	7	3	180	9	1	7
Chips & Salsa, Macho	400	25	4	450	42	3	5
Chips & Salsa, regular	200	12	2	220	21	2	2
Macho Beef Burrito™	1010	44	19	2140	82	6	61
Del Beef Burrito™	470	19	8	1060	24	2	29
Macho Nachos®	1000	56	4	530	28	1	5
Nachos	370	22	4	530	28	1	5
Macho Fries	515	30	4	630	56	6	6
Small Fries	260	15	2	310	28	3	3

• Desserts have 180-235 calories each - one Churro, one Chocolate Chip Cookie, or one Caramel Cheesecake Bite (again, just one...not one order!)

Denny's®

Tips:

- Make special requests. Order Egg Whites or Substitutes (instead of eggs) and Sliced Tomatoes (instead of hashbrowns).

- Build Your Own Grand Slam®. Request egg substitutes, bacon, and Hearty Wheat Pancakes (no butter) with sugar-free syrup - all for about 450 calories.

- Select Fit Fare® (lighter) menu items.

- Kids and Senior options are smaller and contain fewer calories (anyone can order these).

- For more nutrition information, go to Dennys.com.

Suggestions (as described on menu):

	Calories	Fat (g)	Sat+Trans Fat (g)	Sodium (mg)	Carbohydrates (g)	Fiber (g)	Protein (g)
Seasonal Fruit	70	0	0	7	18	3	1
Build Your Own Grand Slam® choices:							
Egg Whites, 2	50	0	0	180	1	0	11
Turkey Bacon Strips, 2	90	5	3	360	1	0	10
Bacon Strips, 2	70	5	2	230	1	0	5
Hearty Wheat Pancakes, 2	310	2	0	950	64	8	10
Buttermilk Pancakes, 2	320	4	1	1170	67	2	8
Fit Slam®	390	12	4	850	46	5	27
Fit Fare® Omelette w/bacon, fruit	390	18	8	870	25	4	34
Hearty Oatmeal Breakfast w/bacon, fruit	530	11	5	600	93	9	19
Veggie Burger w/Fit Fare® veggies	540	13	5	1340	76	11	31
Chicken Avocado SW w/Fit Fare® veggies	520	16	5	2040	48	6	46
Cranberry Apple Salad w/vinaigrette, half	310	10	2	590	21	2	36
Grilled Chicken Deluxe Salad only	340	13	6	530	13	4	44
Lowfat Balsamic Vinaigrette, 1oz	35	1	0	140	7	0	0
Fit Fare® BBQ Chicken w/broccoli, corn	630	13	4	1230	56	2	78
Fit Fare ® Tilapia Ranchero w/potatoes	450	19	6	930	40	3	53
Senior Grilled Shrimp Skewer only	280	6	2	650	36	2	18
Senior Fit Fare® Grilled Chicken w/sides	540	16	7	810	52	8	48
Broccoli	25	0	0	20	4	2	2
Green Beans, average	35	<1	0	250	6	2	1
Smoked Cheddar Mashed Potatoes	120	5	3	390	49	1	4

Caveat:

- Most meals are high in calories. The All-American Slam® with hashbrowns and toast adds up to 1280 calories and 93g fat (that's more than a stick of butter)! Classic Cheeseburger & Fries contains 1250 calories and 67g fat. And, though it may sound lean, the Hickory Grilled Chicken Sandwich (without fries) has 900 calories and 47g fat.

Domino's Pizza®

Tips:

- Surprise! The Philly Steak Pizza is lower in calories and fat than the plain cheese.

- Thin crust pizza slices are lower in both carbohydrates and calories (than hand tossed), but may not be any lower in fat.

- Multiple the info for the large slices X 0.7 to estimate the nutrition info for the medium slices.

- For more nutrition information, go to Dominos.com

Suggestions, per large slice:

	Calories	Fat (g)	Sat+Trans Fat (g)	Sodium (mg)	Carbohydrates (g)	Fiber (g)	Protein (g)
Philly Steak, hand tossed	270	9	4	565	34	2	11
thin crust	210	10	4	385	19	1	8
Veggies, hand tossed	270	10	4	570	34	2	10
thin crust	210	11	4	390	19	1	7
Ham & Pineapple, hand tossed	280	10	4	665	36	2	11
thin crust	220	10	4	485	21	1	8
Grilled Chicken & Veggies, hand tossed	280	10	4	620	34	2	13
thin crust	220	10	4	440	19	1	10
Cheese, hand tossed	290	11	6	640	35	2	12
thin crust	230	12	5	460	20	1	9
Pacific Veggie, hand tossed	320	14	7	640	34	2	13
thin crust	230	13	6	450	20	2	10
Deluxe Feast®, hand tossed	320	14	6	730	36	2	13
thin crust	250	15	6	550	21	2	10
Honolulu Hawaiian, hand tossed	350	16	7	790	36	2	15
thin crust	260	15	6	600	22	2	12

Caveats:

- Baked Sandwiches range from 680 (Mediterranean Veggie) to 870 calories (Chicken Bacon Ranch).

- The Marinara and Hot Dipping sauces are low in calories (25-50 per cup), but the rest have 200-310 calories. Resist your temptation to dip.

- Pasta in the dish contains 540-670 calories...without the bread bowl. Best choice is the Pasta Primavera.

- Pick your extras wisely. There are 1000-1100 calories in an order of Buffalo Wings. And the sticks (Breadsticks, Cheesy Bread and Cinna Stix®) have 110-120 calories *each*. The Chocolate Lava Cake contains 350 calories.

Dunkin'Donuts®

Tips:

- Flatbread Sandwiches are available all day.

- Select a "yeast" or "raised" doughnut, rather than a denser "cake" doughnut. The plain cake doughnuts and cake sticks contain about 100 calories more (mostly from fat) than "raised" doughnuts of similar size and variety.

- Request nonfat milk and sweetener in your coffee drinks.

- For more nutrition information, go to DunkinDonuts.com.

Suggestions:

	Calories	Fat (g)	Sat+Trans Fat (g)	Sodium (mg)	Carbohydrates (g)	Fiber (g)	Protein (g)
Egg White Veggie or Turkey Wake Up Wrap w/cheese	150	6	3	370	14	1	10
Ham, Egg & Cheese Wake Up Wrap	200	11	5	600	14	1	11
White Turkey Sausage Flatbread	280	8	3	770	32	3	19
Egg White Veggie Flatbread	280	10	4	690	32	3	16
Ham & Cheese Flatbread	310	11	5	880	35	1	19
Turkey Cheddar & Bacon Flatbread	410	20	7	1140	36	1	22
Egg & Cheese on English Muffin	320	15	5	820	34	1	14
w/ham	360	16	6	1080	34	1	20
w/bacon	370	18	6	1030	34	1	18
Egg & Cheese on Bagel	480	15	5	1130	66	5	20
w/ham	510	16	6	1390	66	5	26
w/bacon	530	19	7	1340	66	5	24
Turkey/Bacon Club or Turkey/Cheese SW	445	13	4	1650	52	3	35
Bagel (Plain, Wheat, Sour Cream & Onion							
Cinn Raisin, Blueberry, Garlic, or Onion)	325	3	<1	600	64	5	12
Sugar Raised Doughnut	230	14	6	330	22	1	3
Glazed Doughnut	260	14	6	330	31	1	3
Frosted Raised Doughnuts (choc, strawberry,							
maple, marble, Bavarian Kreme...), avg	270	15	7	350	31	1	3
Jelly Filled Doughnut	290	14	7	340	36	1	6

Caveats:

- Bagel or doughnut? One bagel with cream cheese has more calories than one doughnut - but are you eating just one?

- Biscuit and croissant breakfast sandwiches have about as many calories as the bagel sandwiches, but contain twice as much fat (mostly saturated fat).

- The Reduced Fat Blueberry Muffin still contains 430 calories and 11g fat, though much less saturated fat than a doughnut.

- Coolata® drinks range from 200-850 calories!

Einstein Bros.® Bagels

Tips:

- Take advantage of Bagel Thins - with nearly half the calories of a typical bagel for breakfast and other sandwiches. These are offered in plain, honey wheat, and everything varieties.

- For more nutrition information, go to EinsteinsBros.com.

Suggestions:

	Calories	Fat (g)	Sat+Trans Fat (g)	Sodium (mg)	Carbohydrates (g)	Fiber (g)	Protein (g)
Honey Whole Wheat Bagel Thin	140	2	0	120	28	4	6
Light Whipped Plain Cream Cheese, 1.25oz	80	6	4	200	4	0	3
Bacon & Cheese on Bagel Thin Panini	370	17	9	740	32	3	22
Turkey Sausage w/Salsa on Bagel Thin	240	6	2	560	31	4	20
Asparagus, Mushroom, Swiss on Bagel Thin	270	11	4	420	30	5	16
Fruit Salad	140	0	0	25	36	3	2
Fruit & Yogurt Parfait	170	1	0	115	34	3	7
BLT with Avocado Bagel Thin Sandwich	390	24	5	620	35	7	12
Turkey or Tuna on Bagel Thin Sandwich	280	7	2	800	34	3	24
Turkey or Ham Deli Sandwich	480	16	6	1700	60	6	31
Turkey Tornado Wrap	300	14	4	710	30	4	15
Turkey Chili Bowl	400	8	0	1430	28	8	24
Half Bros Bistro Salad w/chicken	450	36	6	450	18	3	19
Half Chicken Chipotle Salad w/chicken	320	20	4	900	19	3	16
Chipotle Vinaigrette, per tablespoon	50	4	1	200	2	0	0
Cafe Latte, regular w/nonfat milk	100	0	0	160	15	0	11
Iced Latte, medium w/nonfat milk	60	0	0	100	9	0	7
Cappuccino, regular w/nonfat milk	70	0	0	115	11	0	8

Caveats:

- Bagels and Ciabatta bread, no matter which flavor, are the caloric equivalence of three or four slices of bread:

Good Grains Bagel, 1	280	3	0	440	58	3	10
Ciabatta Bread, 1	220	1	0	610	43	2	0

- The smears, even the reduced-fat varieties, add up:

Regular Plain Cream Cheese	120	12	8	115	2	0	2
Reduced-Fat, avg all flavors	110	9	6	135	7	0	2

- Specialty drinks can be quite high in calories:

Chai Tea Latte, medium w/whole milk	240	9	5	135	66	0	9
Caramel Macchiato, large w/whole milk	400	13	8	170	60	2	13
Cafe Mocha, frozen 18 fl oz	650	19	7	230	109	2	10

- Salads, even the half salads listed above, are very high in fat. For example, Bros Bistro Salad (without chicken) has 810 calories and 68g fat. On top of that, all salads are served with a bagel (240-310 calories). Yikes! Most of the fat is in the dressing; Chipotle Vinaigrette is *slightly* lower.

El Pollo Loco®

Tips:

- Plenty of options whether you're reducing calories, fat, or carbs.
- Remove the skin off the chicken breast to save 40 calories and 6g fat.
- For more nutrition information, go to ElPolloLoco.com.

Suggestions:

	Calories	Fat (g)	Sat+Trans Fat (g)	Sodium (mg)	Carbohydrates (g)	Fiber (g)	Protein (g)
Small Garden Salad w/o dressing, strips	35	2	1	170	4	1	2
Chicken Caesar Salad w/o dressing	230	7	2	520	18	3	25
Sirloin Steak Tostada Salad w/o dressing or shell	480	15	7	1270	55	6	29
Chicken Tostada Salad w/o dressing, shell	470	13	7	1190	52	6	34
Light Creamy Cilantro dressing	70	5	1	400	6	0	1
Light Italian dressing	20	1	0	770	2	0	0
Regular Chicken Tortilla Soup w/o strips	140	6	2	1040	8	2	15
Sirloin Steak Chili, small	160	3	1	810	20	7	12
large serving	430	8	2	2150	60	18	31
Taco al Carbon only	160	6	1	290	17	1	10
Chicken Breast, skinless	180	4	1	560	0	0	35
BRC Burrito	450	12	5	1050	69	5	15
The Original Pollo Bowl®s	680	11	2	1870	106	12	40
Sirloin Bowl	700	12	3	1980	110	12	35
Pinto Beans	200	4	<1	370	29	8	11
Fresh Vegetables w/margarine	60	3	0	65	8	3	2
w/o margarine	35	0	0	35	8	3	2
BBQ Black Beans	200	3	<1	520	36	4	7
Corn Cobbette	110	3	1	40	19	2	2
House Salsa, 1.5oz	10	0	0	160	2	0	0
Pico del Gallo, 1.5oz	15	1	0	170	2	0	0

Caveats:

- Avoid fried tortillas. Consider these estimated counts:

Fried Tortilla Salad Bowl	430	30	5	300	34	1	7
Tortilla Chips, 1.3oz	170	8	1	250	23	2	2
Tortilla Strips on Soup	70	3	1	na	2	1	0
Tortilla Strips on Garden Salad	35	2	1	na	4	1	0

- The three highest calorie items on the menu include the Ultimate Pollo Bowl® at 1040 calories and 34g fat, Chicken Tostado Salad in a fried tortilla bowl (before you add the dressing) at 900 calories and 43g fat, and Twice Grilled Burrito® with 800 calories and 40g fat.

Fazoli's®

Tips:

- If you're looking for a small entrée, choose a Flatbread Pizza (500 calories or less), one of the Mini Bakes (400 calories or less), or a kid's meal (220-300 calories and 1-13g fat).

- All of the salads are offered with either grilled chicken or crispy (fried) chicken - choose the grilled.

- For more nutrition information, go to Fazolis.com.

Suggestions:

	Calories	Fat (g)	Sat+Trans Fat (g)	Sodium (mg)	Carbohydrates (g)	Fiber (g)	Protein (g)
Bakes, 400 Calories or less:							
Chicken Penne & Peppers	340	12	5	920	37	5	21
Three Cheese Baked Ravioli	340	19	11	940	26	2	17
Chicken Mushroom Alfredo	400	17	9	1070	37	2	23
Flatbread Pizza, 500 Calories or less:							
Chicken Broccoli Florentine	500	19	9	1440	53	3	27
Tuscan Chicken	480	17	7	1570	55	4	26
Cheese Pizza, one slice	290	12	6	730	32	2	14
other varieties (avg)	320	14	6	820	33	2	15
Choice of Pasta w/marinara sauce:	560	3	0	970	111	9	19
w/sliced grilled chicken, add	100	3	0	570	1	0	18
w/broccoli, add	25	0	0	10	5	3	3
w/broccoli & fire-roasted tomatoes, add	35	0	0	85	5	2	1
Choice of Pasta w/meat sauce	680	12	4	1640	113	10	28
Baked Spaghetti	640	22	13	1340	80	7	29
Cherry Almond Chicken Salad w/dressing	490	26	6	1160	38	5	28
Side Chopped Salad w/o dressing	60	4	2	130	5	2	4
Salad Dressings, 3 Tbsp:							
Fat-Free Italian	25	0	0	390	6	0	0
Red Wine Vinaigrette	110	10	2	410	3	0	0
Italian Citrus	110	9	2	590	7	0	0

Caveats:

- Though the breadsticks are *unlimited*, you may want to limit how many you take or order it *dry*:

Garlic Breadstick, 1	150	7	2	290	20	1	3
Dry Breadstick, 1	100	2	0	160	20	0	3

- All of the other pasta dishes, not mentioned above, contain 670-1150 calories and 25-51g fat (and 11+g saturated fat).

- Baked Submarino's® are big, ranging from 660-1070 calories and 31-65g fat. Save calories - omit the mayo and dressing.

- Sweet Treats add another 510-700 calories each. A regular-size Italian Ice contains 170 calories.

Firehouse Subs®

Tips:

- Go wheat. Wheat Sub Rolls have an extra 4g fiber.

- Stick with the medium. The medium subs average 765 calories, while the large subs average 1230 calories. Tuna is the highest!

- Leave off the mayo and/or cheese. As shown below, cutting both save about 300 calories. Subs contain about 200 calories of mayo and 100 calories in the cheese - mostly all fat!

- For more nutrition information, go to FirehouseSubs.com.

Suggestions:

	Calories	Fat (g)	Sat+Trans Fat (g)	Sodium (mg)	Carbohydrates (g)	Fiber (g)	Protein (g)
Chicken or Turkey Salad w/o dressing	360	17	7	1220	18	5	38
Fat Free Ranch dressing, packet	40	0	0	550	11	1	0
Fat Free Raspberry Vinaigrette, packet	45	0	0	110	12	0	0
Balsamic Vinaigrette	160	17	3	400	2	0	0
Medium Subs on wheat:							
Turkey	660	34	8	1940	59	6	37
w/o mayo or cheese	370	4	1	1470	56	6	29
Engineer	680	35	9	2000	62	6	39
w/o mayo or cheese	380	5	1	1720	58	6	31
Pastrami	680	37	10	2200	57	6	33
w/o mayo or cheese	390	7	3	1730	54	6	25
Chicken	680	38	9	1840	55	5	37
w/o mayo or cheese	380	7	2	1370	53	5	29
Engine Company	690	36	10	1840	57	6	36
w/o mayo or cheese	390	5	1	1450	55	6	30
Hook & Ladder	690	36	10	1750	65	6	35
w/o mayo or cheese	400	5	1	1360	62	6	29
Roast Beef	700	36	9	1910	55	6	39
w/o mayo or cheese	410	6	2	1430	52	6	31
Steamer	710	43	11	2450	51	4	33
w/o mayo or cheese	410	12	4	1980	49	2	25
Veggie	710	45	13	1610	60	6	25
w/o mayo or cheese	420	15	6	1140	58	6	17
Corned Beef	720	42	11	2380	55	6	35
w/o mayo or cheese	430	12	4	1910	52	6	27
Ham	730	37	9	1720	71	6	37
w/o mayo or cheese	430	6	2	1250	68	6	29

Caveat:

- Don't forget about the extras. Sodas contain about 260-300 calories, a Cookie adds another 310 calories or so, and brownies contain 490 calories.

Five Guys® Burgers & Fries

Tips:

- Five Guys® offers a simple menu - mostly burgers and fries.

- Don't be shy. Even big guys should feel comfortable ordering the Little Hamburger - it's like the competitor's quarter pound burgers.

- Add lower calorie toppings. These include lettuce, tomatoes, green peppers, mushrooms, onions, jalapenos, mustard, hot sauce, relish, and pickles.

- For more nutrition information, go to FiveGuys.com.

Suggestions:

	Calories	Fat (g)	Sat+Trans Fat (g)	Sodium (mg)	Carbohydrates (g)	Fiber (g)	Protein (g)
Little Hamburger, plain	480	26	12	380	39	2	23

Caveats:

- Don't forget to consider the toppings:

Cheese, 1 slice	70	6	4	310	<1	0	4
Bacon, 2 slices	80	7	3	260	0	0	4
Mayonnaise, 1 Tbsp	100	11	2	75	3	2	0
BBQ Sauce, 1 Tbsp	60	0	0	400	16	0	0

- The bigger burgers are...well, big:

Hamburger	700	43	20	430	39	2	39
Cheeseburger	840	55	27	1050	40	2	47
Bacon Burger	780	50	23	690	39	2	43
Bacon Cheeseburger	920	62	30	1310	40	2	51

- The Veggie Sandwich consists of just veggies and a bun. The flavor increases with cheese, but so do the calories:

Veggie Sandwich (veggies on a bun)	440	15	6	1040	60	2	16
w/1 slice cheese	510	21	10	1350	60	2	20

- Share the fries. Sold separately, even the regular order of fries is huge:

Fries, regular order	620	30	6	90	78	6	10
Fries, large order	1470	71	14	210	184	14	24

- There are a few other options, though none are low in calories:

Grilled Cheese Sandwich	470	26	9	715	41	3	11
Hot Dog	545	35	16	1130	40	2	18
Bacon Cheese Dog	695	48	22	1700	41	2	26

Freshëns®

Tips:

- Truvia®, a zero calorie sweetener, is used in all the proprietary smoothie and yogurt base mixes.

- Want toppings on your yogurt? Fruit or sprinkles add just 10 calories while cereal contains just 15 calories. The other toppings have 35-70 calories each.

- For more nutrition information, go to Freshens.com.

Suggestions:

	Calories	Fat (g)	Sat+Trans Fat (g)	Sodium (mg)	Carbohydrates (g)	Fiber (g)	Protein (g)
Breakfast Crepes: Egg White Florentine	270	8	5	710	24	2	22
Savory Crepes: Greek Salad	370	9	4	660	52	5	15
Pesto Chicken	440	13	5	1030	48	5	32
Honey Mustard Chicken	470	14	6	1160	52	3	31
Havana Chicken	470	15	6	1400	46	3	35
Fajita Chicken	500	13	7	1310	58	6	32
Harvest Salad	520	12	4	1060	73	6	30
Low-Cal Smoothies, avg all flavors	80	0	0	55	50	1	0
Fat-Free Yogurt, 7oz cup:							
Tart	240	<1	0	150	48	0	10
Vanilla	240	0	0	150	48	0	7
Fat-Free Vanilla Yogurt w/cake cone	200	0	0	120	40	0	5

Caveats:

- Blended Fruit Classic Smoothies and Rainforest Energy Smoothies contain fruit, along with fruit juice blend, sherbet, or fat-free yogurt. They contain between 250-350 calories and 0-7g fat.

- High Protein Smoothies are much higher in calories. The Strawberry 'n Cream has 370 calories and 1g fat, while the Peanut Butter Protein™ contains 540 calories and 12g fat.

- Indulgent Shakes contain 490-610 calories and 4-7g fat.

- Fro-Yo Blasts have between 430-680 calories. Not surprisingly, the Reese's Pieces® & Peanut Butter Fro-Yo Blast is the highest.

- Dessert Crepes contain an average of 560 calories and 18g fat. Sure, you can order a *half*, but the calories aren't really cut in half - count on about 320 calories and 11g fat.

Friendly's®

Tips:

- Friendly's® offers a limited number of meals that are "Under 550 Calories."

- For more nutrition information, go to Friendlys.com.

Suggestions:

	Calories	Fat (g)	Sat Fat (g)	Sodium (mg)	Carbohydrates (g)	Fiber (g)	Protein (g)
Half Turkey Club Supermelt & Salad							
w/fat-free Italian dressing	420	17	6	1730	40	3	25
Caprese Chicken Sandwich & Salad							
w/fat-free Italian dressing	550	13	3	1970	66	5	42
Chicken Ginger Stir-Fry	530	10	1	1930	73	4	35
Sweet & Spicy Grilled Shrimp	490	9	0	1660	80	4	22
Side Salad w/lite balsamic vinaigrette	150	9	1	720	15	2	2
w/light Italian dressing	80	1	0	820	15	2	2
Soup, cup:							
Chicken Noodle Soup	280	9	3	1970	31	2	20
Broccoli Cheddar Soup	190	13	7	780	14	1	7
Strawberry or Nonfat Vanilla Yogurt							
Sundae, 2 scoops	250	3	2	130	48	1	7

Caveats:

- Read carefully. Nutrition info at Friendlys.com is per menu item; you may need to add up several items to find your total. For example, a "single scoop" cone contains 2 scoops - for a total of 270-410 calories on a sugar cone.

- Serving sizes are huge. Therefore, meals may have more calories than you would think:

Buttermilk Pancakes w/syrup only	930	17	8	2140	175	5	14
Caramel Cinnamon Swirl French Toast	2090	57	28	1610	374	4	23
Super Sizzin Bacon w/3 eggs, bacon, home fries,							
grilled sourdough bread, orange slice	1010	54	15	1740	89	6	42
Ultimate Grilled Cheese Burgermelt	1500	97	38	2090	101	9	54
Strawberry Lowfat Smoothie	520	4	2	290	105	2	17
Fribble Shake, avg all flavors	660	20	12	380	104	0	16
Double Thick Milkshake, vanilla	770	32	21	270	106	0	15
Grilled Chicken Pesto Supermelt w/fries	1360	82	26	2060	98	6	59
Asian Chicken Salad w/dressing	760	34	5	2160	77	6	36
Grilled Chicken Deluxe Wrap w/fries	1000	45	9	1810	108	8	43
Hunka Chunka Peanut Butter Fudge®							
Lava Cake Sundae	1700	104	33	1060	157	14	36

Fuddrucker's®

Tips:

• Not all menu items are available at all restaurants.

• Request the smaller bun and save 57 calories. Also, ask for the bun to be "grilled dry" (instead of brushing with butter first).

• Information below does not include toppings from the "bar."

• Limited nutrition information (no fat, fiber, or protein) is available at FuddruckersNebraska.com.

Suggestions:

	Calories	Fat (g)	Sat Fat (g)	Sodium (mg)	Carbohydrates (g)	Fiber (g)	Protein (g)
Veggie Burger w/wheat bun	435	na	2	1190	67	na	na
Buffalo Burger w/wheat bun	555	na	8	995	48	na	na
Ostrich Burger w/wheat bun	555	na	3	1035	48	na	na
Original 1/3# Burger w/bun	560	na	9	475	40	na	na
Grilled Chicken Sandwich	625	na	5	1125	55	na	na
Salmon Filet w/wheat bun	715	na	5	1215	64	na	na
Napa Valley Salad w/grilled chicken	455	na	5	800	24	na	na
Market Toss Salad w/grilled chicken	510	na	9	930	15	na	na

Caveats:

• Watch the toppings. Lettuce, tomato, onion, and salsa have negligible calories. But count on another 100 calories for a (level) tablespoon mayonnaise or a slice of cheese. Want bacon and cheese? That adds about 175 calories more on a smaller sandwich.

• Fruit instead of fries? A regular order of French Fries contains 300 calories while a fruit cup has just 60 calories.

• The bigger Hamburgers (and the Turkey Burger) are quite high in calories:

Turkey Burger w/wheat bun	790	na	10	1090	45	na	na
Original 1/2# Burger w/bun	780	na	13	645	53	na	na
Original 2/3# Burger w/bun	922	na	17	685	53	na	na
Original 1# Burger w/bun	1565	na	27	1292	106	na	na

• Got a sweet tooth? Cookies average 180 calories while the Crispy Squares have 445 and the Brownie contains about 500 calories. Even the Kid's Shakes average 465 calories (over 800 calories for the regular-size). Ice Cream Treats average over 600 calories - except for the Ice Cream Brownie Blast at 1365 calories!

Gatti's Pizza®

Tips:

• Go for Original or Thin pizza. Interestingly, a slice of Thin has as much fat as a slice of Original - but fewer carbs and calories.

• Medium slices (⅛ pizza), while not listed below, contain about 20 calories more than the large slices ($1/12$ pizza) of the same variety and have an extra gram of fat.

• Count your slices. Adding meat to your pizza won't add nearly as many calories as when you add another slice or two of pizza to your plate.

• For more nutrition information, go to MrGattis.com.

Suggestions:

	Calories	Fat (g)	Sat+Trans Fat (g)	Sodium (mg)	Carbohydrates (g)	Fiber (g)	Protein (g)
Original Crust, large slice:							
Cheese or Canadian Bacon	170	5	2	345	24	<1	8
BBQ Chicken	180	7	3	120	19	0	10
Pepperoni, Bacon, or Burger	190	6	3	405	24	0	9
Sausage or Spicy Sausage	205	7	3	465	25	0	9
Meat Market or Sampler	210	8	0	530	25	<1	10
Thin Crust, large slice:							
Cheese or Canadian Bacon	115	5	3	255	11	1	8
BBQ Chicken	125	7	4	124	12	0	9
Pepperoni, Bacon, or Burger	130	6	3	320	12	1	8
Sausage or Spicy Sausage	150	7	3	370	12	1	8
Meat Market or Sampler	150	8	3	435	13	1	8
1 cup Spaghetti w/½ cup marinara	290	1	0	630	35	2	6
w/½ cup meat sauce	340	5	1	520	37	3	9

Caveats:

• Skip the Cheeseburger. Compare these slices to the ones above:

Bacon Double Cheeseburger, Original	240	9	4	575	27	1	13
Bacon Double Cheeseburger, Thin	185	9	4	480	15	1	11

• Pass up the Perfect Pan Pizza. Thicker pizza slices have about *twice* as much fat as the other crusts - and way more calories. Check out these large slices of Perfect Pan pizza:

Cheese or Canadian Bacon	225	10	4	380	25	1	10
BBQ Chicken	235	12	5	155	20	0	12
Pepperoni, Bacon, or Burger	240	10	4	440	26	1	11
Sausage, Meat Market, or Sampler	260	12	5	535	27	1	11

• Watch the extra nibbles. Garlic Sticks contain 110 calories and 5g fat each, while Cheese Sticks have 140 calories (7g fat). A serving of Dessert Pizza (⅛) has an average of 260 calories.

Godfather's®

Tips:

• Think thin. While the fat content is about the same, Thin Crust is lower in calories than Golden. Original is highest in calories.

• Cheese, Hawaiian, and Veggie are the leanest pizza toppings. Next, is Pepperoni and Super Hawaiian. Super Taco and Super Combo are the fattiest.

• For more nutrition information, go to Godfathers.com.

Suggestions:	Calories	Fat (g)	Sat Fat (g)	Sodium (mg)	Carbohydrates (g)	Fiber (g)	Protein (g)
Cheese, Hawaiian, or Veggie (avg per slice):							
Mini, Original	160	4	2	270	21	1	7
Small, Golden	210	7	3	390	26	1	10
Small, Original	240	7	3	450	32	2	11
Medium, Thin	180	8	3	280	16	1	8
Medium, Golden	230	8	3	420	27	1	10
Medium, Original	270	7	3	520	35	2	12
Large, Thin	220	10	4	330	19	1	10
Large, Golden	260	9	4	480	29	1	11
Large, Original	300	9	4	580	37	2	14
Pepperoni or Super Hawaiian (avg per slice):							
Mini, Original	165	5	2	290	21	1	8
Small, Golden	240	10	4	430	26	1	11
Small, Original	265	9	4	480	32	2	12
Medium, Thin	215	11	4	340	17	1	10
Medium, Golden	250	10	4	475	27	1	11
Medium, Original	290	10	5	555	35	2	14
Large, Thin	240	12	5	390	19	1	11
Large, Golden	285	12	4	535	29	1	13
Large, Original	330	12	5	625	37	2	16
Gluten-Free: Cheese (per slice)	140	5	2	380	18	1	5
Beef, Pepperoni, or Sausage (avg)	170	7	3	460	18	1	7
Fruit Dessert or Streusel, alum. pan, 1/6	155	3	<1	160	29	1	3
Medium on Golden crust, 1/8	220	5	1	220	39	1	4
Breadstick, 1	110	2	0	160	20	1	3
Breadstick w/cheese, 1	140	4	2	220	20	1	5

Caveats:

• Pizzas with toppings other than those listed above have about 50% more calories and fat as the "Cheese." So if a Cheese slice contains 200 calories, the other varieties are about 300 calories.

• Calzones are colossal. They average 1500 calories and 43g fat.

• Monkey Bread is monstrous - averaging 760 calories, 24g fat.

Golden Corral®

Tips:

• "Make Peace with Your Plate" as discussed in the *General Tips* chapter. Using the peace sign as your guide, fill one-quarter of your plate with a lean protein (3oz is the size of a deck of cards). Fill half of the remaining area with healthy starches, and the other half with fruits and vegetables.

• Pick and choose. You don't have to give up all your favorites, just don't select all the higher calorie items on the same visit.

• For more nutrition information, go to GoldenCorral.com.

Salad Buffet Suggestions:	Calories	Fat (g)	Sat+Trans Fat (g)	Sodium (mg)	Carbohydrates (g)	Fiber (g)	Protein (g)
Lettuce, Spinach, Spring Mix, 1 cup	10	0	0	10	2	1	<1
Fresh Veggies such as Tomatoes, Cucumbers, Broccoli, Carrots, Cauliflower, 1 spoon	5	0	0	5	1	0	0
Fresh Fruit, 1 spoon	35	0	0	5	9	2	<1
Asian Salad, 1 cup	80	5	1	110	8	1	1
Marinated Vegetable Salad, ½ cup	30	2	0	90	3	1	1

Hot Buffet Suggestions:

	Calories	Fat (g)	Sat+Trans Fat (g)	Sodium (mg)	Carbohydrates (g)	Fiber (g)	Protein (g)
Chicken Breast, 1	100	3	0	390	2	0	17
Baked New Orleans Style Fish, 1 piece	100	5	3	220	0	0	13
Fajita Chicken, 3oz	110	4	0	500	2	1	16
Pot Roast, Salmon, Machaca Chicken, 3oz	110	5	2	415	3	1	38
Breaded Bay Scallops, 10	140	6	1	260	13	0	8
Sirloin, London Broil, Beef Tips, Fajita Beef, 3oz	150	6	3	340	1	0	22
Chipotle Chicken Breast, Jalapeno Tilapia, 1	175	8	2	405	11	0	17
Turkey, 3oz	180	8	3	125	0	0	23
Hickory Bourbon Chicken Breast, 1	190	4	0	590	22	0	17
Steamed Vegetables, ½ cup	35	1	0	85	5	2	2
Vegetable Medley, Sitr Fry Veggies, ½ cup	80	5	2	150	5	2	1
Corn on Cob, 1 or Peas, ½ cup	70	1	0	90	12	2	3
Beans such as Lima, Black Eyed Peas, ½ c	110	2	0	400	18	4	6
Red Potatoes, ½ cup	80	2	0	80	13	1	2

Caveat:

• Desserts range from 70-420 calories. For 100 calories, grab a small cookie, an unfrosted Rice Krispy Treat, or a half cup of sherbet, frozen yogurt, or soft serve (without toppings). Bars and cobblers are around 200 calories, while a piece of cake or pie is generally in the higher range of 300-400 calories.

Great American Cookies®

Tips:

• For more nutrition information, go to GreatAmericanCookies.com.

Suggestions:

	Calories	Fat (g)	Sat+Trans Fat (g)	Sodium (mg)	Carbohydrates (g)	Fiber (g)	Protein (g)
Chewy Chocolate Supreme, 1.5oz	180	7	2	80	27	2	2
Sugar Cookie, 1.5oz	200	9	4	310	29	<1	2
Other Smaller Cookies, 1.5-1.8oz (avg)	240	12	5	215	31	1	3

Caveat:

• The other sweets are much bigger - and higher in calories:

	Calories	Fat (g)	Sat+Trans Fat (g)	Sodium (mg)	Carbohydrates (g)	Fiber (g)	Protein (g)
Brownies, 4oz	465	24	11	290	61	3	5
Original M&M® Big Bite Doozie	340	17	9	190	46	1	3
Double Doozie, Original	690	34	17	520	94	3	6
Cookie Cake by the Slice	580	27	13	630	83	2	5

Great Harvest Bread Co.®

Tips:

• For more nutrition information, go to GreatHarvest.com.

Suggestions per 2oz slice, unless noted:

	Calories	Fat (g)	Sat+Trans Fat (g)	Sodium (mg)	Carbohydrates (g)	Fiber (g)	Protein (g)
Low Carb Breads, avg	110	4	na	180	13	3	6
Most Breads made w/100% whole wheat	135	2	na	300	24	3	5
Pecan Swirl Bread	190	8	na	220	26	4	4
Batter Bread: Zucchini	130	4	na	105	23	2	3
flavors other than zucchini	180	8	na	125	25	1	3
Muffins: Blackberry Bran, 1	260	2	na	520	58	8	8
Oat Berry Muffin, 1	360	12	na	460	66	8	10
Cookie: Chocolate Bliss, 1	290	15	na	80	41	3	4
Coffee Cake: Apple Strussel or Blueberry	165	7	na	125	25	1	2
Biscotti: Vanilla Almond	200	7	na	135	29	2	6

Caveat:

• Other breads are bigger and have more calories:

	Calories	Fat (g)	Sat+Trans Fat (g)	Sodium (mg)	Carbohydrates (g)	Fiber (g)	Protein (g)
Focaccia, 4oz (avg)	280	4	na	730	54	2	7
Brownies	370	22	na	55	41	3	6
Other Cookies not listed above, avg	470	23	na	275	59	4	8
Other Muffins not listed above, avg	575	30	na	170	67	4	10
Scones, 1	635	28	na	815	88	3	27
Kahuna Bar	1620	70	na	580	230	14	22

Hardee's®

Tips:

• Most menu items are really big. Below are the leanest choices - though many are still very high in fat and saturated fat.

• Small combo meals include small fries (320 calories and 14g fat) and small drink (160 calories).

• For more nutrition information, go to Hardees.com.

Suggestions:

	Calories	Fat (g)	Sat Fat (g)	Sodium (mg)	Carbohydrates (g)	Fiber (g)	Protein (g)
Frisco Breakfast Sandwich®	430	19	7	1510	41	2	23
Cinnamon 'N' Raisin™ Biscuit	300	15	3	680	40	1	3
Pancakes, 3 w/out syrup, butter	300	5	1	830	55	2	8
Charbroiled BBQ Chicken Sandwich	380	6	1	1220	58	4	26
Regular Roast Beef Sandwich	300	14	5	850	28	2	18
Hot Ham 'N' Cheese™ Sandwich	280	12	4	1140	29	1	19
Small Hamburger	310	15	4	500	32	1	14
Original Turkey Burger	480	17	4	930	47	4	31

Caveats:

• Hardee's® is home of the ⅔LB Monster ThickBurger® - weighing in at a hefty 1290 calories and 92g of fat (more fat than a stick of butter). Even the "Little" ThickBurger® has 570 calories and 39g fat. Omitting the mayo will help a little.

• If you want ice cream, order the Single Scoop Ice Cream Cone (285 calories, 13g fat) rather than the Hand-Scooped Ice Cream Shake or Malt (705-780 calories and 33-35g fat).

• Sandwiches ordered "Low Carb" will get the burger bun replaced with a lettuce wrap. This is still a high-calorie, high-fat option.

Dr. Jo says

It's true that a level teaspoon of sugar has just 16 calories and a tablespoon of half & half creamer has just 20 calories. But all those additions can add up over time. Just one coffee creamer and two packets of sugar can add 52 calories to a cup of coffee. And, how many cups of coffee do you drink everyday?

Hometown Buffet®/Old Country/Ryan's

Tips:

• "Make Peace with Your Plate." As discussed in the *General Tips* chapter, fill a quarter of your plate with lean protein. Split the rest of the plate with healthy starches and fruits & vegetables.

• Stick to just one treat. Craving a fried entrée? Then skip dessert. You can eat all your favorites while eating out healthy - just not at the same visit.

• For more nutrition information, go to HometownBuffet.com.

Suggestions:

	Calories	Fat (g)	Sat+Trans Fat (g)	Sodium (mg)	Carbohydrates (g)	Fiber (g)	Protein (g)
Leaner Protein:							
Peel & Eat Shrimp, 1 shrimp	5	0	0	40	0	0	1
Diced Egg, 1 spoon	20	2	<1	20	0	0	2
Diced Chicken Breast, 1 tong	45	1	0	160	0	0	9
Cheese (except feta), 1 spoon	25	2	1	75	1	0	3
Kidney or Garbanzo Beans, 1 spoon	10	0	0	40	2	1	<1
Baked Fish or Oven Roasted Chicken, pc	100	5	1	280	1	0	14
Rotisserie Chicken, breast or thigh+drumstick	300	17	5	700	1	0	35
Grilled Pork Steak or Loin, 1 piece	145	9	3	450	1	0	14
Healthier Starch:							
Rice, Rice Pilaf or Mashed Potatoes, 1 spoon	75	0	0	210	16	<1	1
Corn on Cob, 1 piece	80	3	<1	20	13	2	2
Red Potatoes, Risotto, Dirty Rice, Corn, 1 spoon	95	4	<1	230	16	1	2
Wheat Bread, 1 slice	70	1	0	130	12	1	3
Fruits & Veggies (1 spoon, unless noted):							
Lettuce, Spinach, Spring Mix, 1 cup	5	0	0	10	2	1	<1
Raw Veggies (e.g. tomatoes, cucumbers, broccoli, carrots, peppers, cauliflower)	5	0	0	5	1	0	0
Simple Veggies (e.g. Gr Beans, Broccoli/Caul)	25	0	0	30-340	5	2	1
Seasoned Veggies (e.g. Grilled Veggies)	50	3	<1	200	4	1	1
Fresh Fruit, 1 spoon	35	0	0	5	9	2	<1

Caveats:

• While a slice of bread has about 70 calories (1g fat) and a dinner roll has 130 (5g fat), the other bread choices (biscuits, bagels, and muffins) range from 180-320 calories and 8-13g fat.

• Size matters when it comes to dessert. Count on 100-200 calories per cookie (larger ones have more). One spoon of cobbler/crisp has about 150 calories. A piece of cake, cupcake, slice of pie, brownie, or bar ranges from 150-350 calories.

Houlihan's®

Tips:

- Not all restaurants have all menu items or sell them the same way. Instead of an entrée, consider making a meal by ordering a couple of suggested appetizers, soups, and small plate items.

- Skinny Alcoholic Drinks, under 125 calories, are offered.

- Combo meals at lunch are served with a choice of sides. Instead of fries (270 calories, 12g fat), select the orzo or green beans.

- For more nutrition information, go to Houlihans.com.

Suggestions:

	Calories	Fat (g)	Sat Fat (g)	Sodium (mg)	Carbohydrates (g)	Fiber (g)	Protein (g)
Appetizer: Lettuce Wraps	540	17	4	1870	71	4	25
Chicken Noodle or Tortilla Soup, avg	165	7	3	1755	13	2	13
Salads: Spinach Salad	265	19	2	110	20	4	4
Grilled Asparagus Salad	255	21	4	290	9	3	7
Small Plates: Gazpacho Shrimp Shooter	50	3	0	110	1	0	5
Chicken Skewers/Kabobs	250	10	3	220	5	1	32
Pot Roast Slider, single	230	10	4	450	20	1	13
Pulled Smoked Pork Slider, single	280	12	5	460	23	1	18
Veggie Mini Burger Slider, single	305	14	4	720	35	4	10
Mini Chicago Dog Slider	225	13	5	715	20	1	8
Vietnamese Spring Spring Eggrolls	205	1	0	310	30	1	13
ADD three dipping sauces	100	9	1	430	10	0	5
Fancy Spaghetti Small Plate	400	17	5	640	44	3	16
Grilled 4oz Atlantic Salmon	330	22	8	490	10	2	24
Seared Sea Scallops	315	20	6	610	11	2	20
Sandwiches: Farmhouse Club	540	25	9	2120	41	2	38
Taos Turkey Wrap	470	21	6	1890	39	4	33
Sides: French Green Beans	115	8	1	290	9	4	2
Mediterranean Orzo	155	7	1	705	20	1	4
Mashed Potatoes	335	23	15	610	26	4	3
Dinners w/panzanella bread salad & grilled asparagus:							
Grilled Shrimp	555	26	4	1240	32	5	48
Atlantic Salmon, Simply Prepared	550	29	6	760	25	3	44
5oz Petite Sirloin dinner	520	31	12	600	25	3	35
Other Dinners:							
Grilled Rosemary Chicken Breast							
w/orzo and french green beans	580	27	7	1200	29	5	50
Seared Scallops w/asparagus risotto	590	32	8	1510	31	3	44

Caveat:

- Many of the suggested menu items listed above, while reasonable in calories, are still high in fat - so pair accordingly.

IHOP®

Tips:

- Select substitutes to save calories: egg substitutes for omelettes (save 300 calories, 28g fat), sugar-free syrup instead of regular (save 170 calories per ¼ cup), and sliced tomatoes instead of hash browns (save 300 calories, 10g fat).
- For more nutrition information, go to IHOP.com.

SIMPLE & FIT (S&F) Suggestions:

	Calories	Fat (g)	Sat+Trans Fat (g)	Sodium (mg)	Carbohydrates (g)	Fiber (g)	Protein (g)
Spinach, Mushroom, Tomato Omelette w/fruit	330	12	5	690	31	5	29
S&F Veggie Omelet w/fresh fruit	320	10	1	420	40	8	21
S&F Turkey Bacon Omelette w/fresh fruit	420	20	9	720	25	2	38
S&F 2 Egg Breakfast w/egg subs, fresh fruit, turkey bacon, whole wheat toast	350	8	2	710	48	7	25
S&F Oatmeal	290	5	2	25	58	4	7
S&F Whole Wheat French Toast Combo	490	15	4	930	56	5	33
Seasonal Fresh Fruit Crepes	580	24	6	430	82	7	12
S&F Blueberry Harvest Grain 'N Nut® Combo	560	23	4	1040	64	8	25
Buttermilk Pancakes, 3	490	18	9	1610	69	4	13
S&F Two X Two X Two	400	12	3	1450	48	3	25
S&F Fresh Fruit & Yogurt Bowl	320	3	<1	45	73	7	7
S&F Fruit Bowl	130	0	0	0	33	4	1
S&F Simply Chicken Sandwich w/fresh fruit	500	10	4	840	65	4	40
S&F House Salad	50	2	0	140	9	3	2
Add Reduced-Fat Italian Dressing	15	1	0	105	1	0	0
S&F Grilled Tilapia Dinner	490	23	4	1270	27	8	49
S&F Grilled Balsamic-Glazed Chicken Dinner	440	22	4	940	25	8	39

Caveat:

- Think before you build. Most breakfast meals are over 1300 calories (before butter & syrup). Consider these breakdown stats:

Plain Omelette w/cheddar cheese only	680	52	23	770	12	2	42
Add Bacon Strips, 2	80	6	2	300	<1	0	6
Add Pork Sausage Links, 2	180	16	6	290	1	0	6
Original Buttermilk Pancakes, 3	490	18	9	1610	69	4	13
Harvest Grain 'N Nut® Pancakes, 3	700	39	10	1380	71	8	18
CINN-A-STACK™ Pancakes, 3	690	23	9	1700	106	4	14
Original French Toast w/butter	920	50	16	1100	88	8	31
CINN-A-STACK™ French Toast	1120	54	16	1190	126	8	32
Plain Belgian Waffle	360	15	9	520	47	2	8
Add Blueberry Compote w/topping	170	3	2	80	37	2	<1
Syrup, avg all flavors, ¼ cup	210	0	0	30	54	0	0
Seasoned Hash Browns	320	20	4	590	31	3	3

In-N-Out Burger®

Tips:

- Expect a simple menu of burgers, fries, shakes, and soda.

- Request your burger to be prepared with mustard and ketchup instead of "spread" to save 80 calories and 9g fat.

- For more nutrition information, go to In-N-Out.com.

Suggestions:

	Calories	Fat (g)	Sat+Trans Fat (g)	Sodium (mg)	Carbohydrates (g)	Fiber (g)	Protein (g)
Hamburger w/onion, ask for mustard & ketchup instead of "spread"	310	10	4	730	41	3	16
Cheeseburger w/onion, ask for mustard & ketchup instead of "spread"	400	18	10	1080	41	3	22

Caveats:

- If you get the Combo meal, you've added another:

	Calories	Fat (g)	Sat+Trans Fat (g)	Sodium (mg)	Carbohydrates (g)	Fiber (g)	Protein (g)
French Fries	395	18	5	245	54	2	7
Soda (avg of non-diet flavors)	205	0	0	45	55	0	0

- Order a milkshake, and your drink is even more caloric:

	Calories	Fat (g)	Sat+Trans Fat (g)	Sodium (mg)	Carbohydrates (g)	Fiber (g)	Protein (g)
Milkshake (avg of all flavors)	585	29	20	300	73	0	9

- Bigger isn't better:

	Calories	Fat (g)	Sat+Trans Fat (g)	Sodium (mg)	Carbohydrates (g)	Fiber (g)	Protein (g)
Double-Double® w/onion	670	41	19	1440	39	3	37

Dr. Jo says

Take your pick. Whether dining out at a full-service restaurant or a buffet, decide what your "pleasers" are today. If you want the creamy entrée, skip dessert. Want fried fish? Then order steamed vegetables instead of fries. Craving dessert? Drink water instead of soda. You can eat all your favorite higher-calorie foods, just not all at the same meal.

Jack in the Box®

Tips:

- Skip the mayo and cheese. There are 45 calories of mayo on the regular Hamburger (and 280 calories worth on the Sirloin Swiss & Grilled Onion Burger). One slice of cheese adds 40 calories - and some of the bigger burgers have more than one slice.

- Skip the combo. A small soda has 230 calories while the small fries contains about 300 calories and 14g fat.

- For more nutrition information go to JackInTheBox.com.

Suggestions:

	Calories	Fat (g)	Sat+Trans Fat (g)	Sodium (mg)	Carbohydrates (g)	Fiber (g)	Protein (g)
Breakfast Jack	290	11	5	780	30	1	16
Chiquita® Apple Bites w/caramel	70	0	0	55	17	2	0
Chicken Fajita Pita w/salsa	320	11	5	870	33	4	24
Chicken Teriyaki Bowl	580	5	1	1460	106	4	26
SW Grilled Chicken Salad w/o corn sticks	350	15	6	1010	29	7	34
Grilled Chicken Salad w/o croutons	250	10	4	660	15	5	28
lowfat Balsamic dressing	35	2	0	480	5	0	0
croutons	70	5	2	230	13	0	2
Grilled Chicken Strips w/Teriyaki dip sauce	310	8	2	1600	16	0	44
Hamburger Deluxe	340	16	6	540	33	2	15
Fruit Smoothie, avg all flavors, 16oz	290	0	0	75	71	1	2

Caveats:

- Even the smaller-sized snacks add up:

Egg Roll, 1	150	7	2	320	15	2	5
Beef Taco, 1	190	11	3	320	17	2	6
Stuffed Jalapenos, 3 piece	220	12	5	730	21	1	6
Mozzarella Sticks, 3 piece	280	16	6	580	22	2	12
Seasoned Curly Fries, small	290	16	2	610	30	3	3
French Fries, small	330	15	2	610	45	3	4
Onion Rings	450	28	2	620	45	3	6
Bacon Cheese Potato Wedges	680	42	10	1270	58	5	18

- Keep to the smaller sandwiches. Check out these shocking stats:

Jumbo Jack	500	27	11	790	45	2	19
Ultimate Cheeseburger	830	57	28	1430	44	2	36
Steak & Egg Burrito w/salsa	820	50	16	1620	56	5	37
Hearty Breakfast Bowl	850	65	19	1390	41	4	27
Sirloin Cheeseburger	900	60	21	1870	52	3	40

- The smallest size Vanilla Shake contains about 700 calories and 38g fat. The other flavors can have over 100 calories more. Skip the whipped topping and cherry to save 75 calories.

Jamba Juice®

Tips:

• More than juice and fruit smoothies - the menu has expanded to include a variety of foods including Fruit & Yogurt Parfaits and Oatmeal.

• Wraps, sandwiches and salads are available at some locations. Save calories (mostly fat) by using less sauce or dressing.

• For more nutrition information, go to JambaJuice.com.

Suggestions:

	Calories	Fat (g)	Sat+Trans Fat (g)	Sodium (mg)	Carbohydrates (g)	Fiber (g)	Protein (g)
Juice (12oz):							
Carrot Juice	100	<1	0	170	22	0	3
Orange Juice	170	0	0	45	14	0	3
Smoothies (16oz unless noted):							
Light Smoothies, avg all flavors	150	<1	0	180	30	2	6
Fruit & Veggie Smoothies, orange carrot	180	<1	0	90	43	3	3
Apple n'Greens or Berry upBEET™ (avg)	225	1	0	130	50	7	4
All Fruit Smoothies, avg all flavors	230	<1	0	20	56	4	1
Probiotic Smoothies, avg all flavors	240	0	0	150	49	2	10
Classic Smoothies: Blackberry Bliss™	230	1	0	25	55	4	1
Strawberry, Caribbean, Pomegranate, Peach,							
Razzmatazz® or Banana Berry™, (avg)	260	1	0	50	61	3	2
Pre-Boosted Smoothies: Protein Berry	280	0	0	115	52	3	17
Coldbuster® or Energizer™ (avg)	260	2	0	20	62	4	2
Acai Super Antioxidant Pre-Boosted	260	4	0	45	53	3	4
Steel Cut Oatmeal: plain w/brown sugar	220	4	1	20	44	5	8
Banana, Apple or Blueberry Oatmeal (avg)	290	4	1	25	53	6	8
Berry Cherry Pecan Oatmeal	340	9	2	55	62	7	9
Fruit/Yogurt Parfait, Berry or Mango,12oz	310	5	1	85	62	7	9
Spinach n'Cheese Breakfast Wrap	240	8	6	530	30	3	15
MediterraneanYUM® Flatbread, 1	320	8	4	770	49	3	13
Smokehouse Chicken Flatbread, 1	390	10	4	690	53	5	19

Caveats:

• Fruit Tea Infusions contain about 150 calories per 16oz.

• Most of the "shots" have few calories, but one Matcha Energy shot adds another 65-70 calories and 13-14g carbs.

• Stick with the Sixteen (ounces, that is). The Power size is about twice as large - with the Original size in between the two.

• Move away from the Moo. Creamy Treats start at 300 calories; the smaller cups of the Peanut Butter Moo'd® and the Chocolate Moo'd® contains 470 and 430 calories respectively.

Jason's Deli®

Tips:

- There's a full salad bar with some organics and a wide variety of veggies, fruits, meats, and several lowfat and fat-free dressings.

- To reduce the calories of your build-your-own sandwich, choose a half sandwich or half the meat (Slim Sandwich). Instead of chips, request fresh fruit, steamed vegetables, or one of the soups below (for an additional charge).

- Jason's Just Right Kid's entrée menu has plenty of options within the range of 220-500 calories (just avoid the kid's baked potato at 800 calories).

- For more nutrition information, go to JasonsDeli.com

Suggestions:

	Calories	Fat (g)	Sat+Trans Fat (g)	Sodium (mg)	Carbohydrates (g)	Fiber (g)	Protein (g)
Chicken Noodle Soup, bowl	150	5	1	900	16	1	10
Vegetarian Vegetable Soup, bowl	160	7	0	1030	24	4	4
Club Lite	475	14	5	1530	49	7	44
Spinach Veggie Wrap	360	16	8	620	40	6	16
Mediterranean Wrap	320	11	2	940	47	6	14
Turkey Reuben	510	13	6	3050	53	6	44
Savory Chicken Salad Wrap	355	14	3	535	45	5	16
Turkey Wrap	360	14	4	1060	40	5	22
Amy's Turkey-O	590	22	7	1430	68	7	31
"Lighter" Nutty Mixed Up Salad w/o dressing	170	6	3	170	29	3	4
w/chicken	240	6	3	430	30	3	17
Lowfat Raspberry Vinaigrette, 4 Tbsp	90	5	0	170	10	0	0
Whole Sandwich: Turkey or Ham (slim portion)							
on Whole Wheat Bread (avg)	290	5	1	890	45	6	22
"Lighter" Chicken Pasta Primo or Portobello							
Garden Pasta w/mushrooms, no bread (avg)	420	20	7	1390	44	4	19

Caveats:

- Many of the options are big, even some of the "Lighter" ones:

	Calories	Fat (g)	Sat+Trans Fat (g)	Sodium (mg)	Carbohydrates (g)	Fiber (g)	Protein (g)
Plain Jane® Potato (butter, cheese...)	2320	150	61	1750	192	13	56
"Lighter Plain" Jane Potato	1130	55	23	690	135	9	29
Turkey Muffaletta, half	1490	103	14	5100	77	3	53
Pastrami Melt	1230	94	42	1630	44	1	50
The New York Yankee, no dressing	1190	69	32	2270	47	2	92

- Most of the other sandwiches (not listed above) average 700-1000 calories. Entrée salads with dressing have even more!

- The offer of free ice cream is tempting. A very small cone has about 200 calories (5g fat). Other desserts contain 300-625 calories.

Jersey Mike's® Subs

Tips:

- Go mini. These smaller-size sandwiches range from 425-645 calories (w/o mayo or oil) while the regular-size sandwiches contain between 540-940 calories. Wraps have about the same number of calories (and *more* carbs) as the regular-size subs (the regular wraps have 20 calories more while the reduced-carb wraps have 20 calories fewer).

- Dress it down. Nutrition information below does not include vinegar, oil, or mayo. The calories in vinegar are insignificant, but adding oil and mayo to a "mini" adds 255 calories.

- Fill up with soup. Most are under 150 calories per cup (black bean, vegetable, clam chowder, tomato bisque, and chicken noodle). A bowl contains 50% more.

- More nutrition information can be found at JerseyMikes.com.

"Mini" Suggestions on wheat (w/o oil or mayo):

	Calories	Fat (g)	Sat+Trans Fat (g)	Sodium (mg)	Carbohydrates (g)	Fiber (g)	Protein (g)
#2 Jersey Shore Favorite	425	12	5	990	55	4	22
#3 American Classic	435	13	6	1320	54	4	25
#5 Super Sub	455	13	6	1260	56	4	27
#4 Provolone, Prosciuttini & Cappacuolo	425	12	5	930	55	4	22
#7 Turkey Breast & Provolone	425	11	5	1100	53	4	27
#11 Ham & Salami	435	14	6	1100	54	4	21
#14 Veggie	515	21	11	720	55	5	25

"Regular" Suggestions on wheat (w/o oil or mayo):

	Calories	Fat (g)	Sat+Trans Fat (g)	Sodium (mg)	Carbohydrates (g)	Fiber (g)	Protein (g)
#17 Steak Philly	620	24	11	1700	64	4	41
#18 Chicken Parmesan	650	22	7	1590	77	5	37
#19 BBQ Beef	710	15	5	1520	83	4	59
#20 Pastrami & Swiss	580	18	9	2660	60	3	45

Caveats:

- Some sandwiches (on wheat) sound leaner than they actually are:

	Calories	Fat (g)	Sat+Trans Fat (g)	Sodium (mg)	Carbohydrates (g)	Fiber (g)	Protein (g)
#10 Tuna, mini	645	37	7	980	56	5	22
#17 Chicken Philly, regular	630	25	13	1730	65	4	39
#18 Grilled Chicken, regular	670	33	5	1290	60	4	34
#43 Chipotle Chicken, regular	910	56	19	2200	68	4	40

- Rethink the "Sub in a Tub." Any sub can be served as a salad. But, the 185 carb calories you'll save from omitting the bread will be easily replaced with fat calories from the salad dressing!

- While Cookies range from 170-210 calories, a Chocolate Brownie contains 440 calories.

Jimmy John's® Gourmet Sandwiches

Tips:

• Select a Sub, rather than a Club. Clubs offer larger bread and double the meat and cheese - and an extra 200 calories.

• Ditch the mayo (or at least ask for less). Subs and Clubs contain almost 200 calories and 8g fat of the stuff.

• Don't be fooled by the Plain Slims®. For a dollar less, they remove the veggies and sauce from the regular subs. Instead, order the Sub and remove the sauce - that way you can fill up with all the veggies (including lettuce, cucumbers, peppers...)

• Combos include a small drink (250 calories for a regular soda) and chips (150 calories and 8g fat). Thinny chips are slightly lower in calories. And, unsweetened tea is available.

• A nutrition calculator can be found at JimmyJohns.com.

Suggestions:

	Calories	Fat (g)	Sat Fat (g)	Sodium (mg)	Carbohydrates (g)	Fiber (g)	Protein (g)
#1 Pepe (ham & cheese) w/o mayo	420	10	5	1090	50	1	28
#2 Big John® (roast beef) w/o mayo	340	3	1	840	49	1	26
#4 Turkey Tom®	510	22	3	1090	50	1	24
w/out mayo	320	1	0	920	50	1	24
#12 Beach Club w/o mayo	535	10	5	1345	71	2	36
Any Sub with 7-Grain Bread instead, ADD	100	5	0	90	18	5	4
Thinny Chips	130	5	1	105	19	2	2

Caveats:

• Most sandwiches, as described on the menu, average 590 calories for the Subs and 790 for the Clubs. Check these out:

	Calories	Fat (g)	Sat Fat (g)	Sodium (mg)	Carbohydrates (g)	Fiber (g)	Protein (g)
#6 Vegetarian Sub	580	30	8	870	52	2	19
Slim 3 Tuna Salad	720	31	4	1750	68	1	35
#17 Ultimate Porker™ on 7-Grain Wheat	760	39	9	1750	67	6	37
# 9 Italian Night Club®	950	51	12	2170	70	1	44
The J. J. Gargantuan®	990	54	13	2890	65	0	29

• Thick Sliced 7-Grain can be substituted on any Sub or Club. Though higher in fiber, it contains 100 calories more than a Sub.

• Don't Unwich®. An Unwich® contains the same ingredients as a Sub or Club, but with a lettuce wrap instead of bread. With all the mayo, vinaigrette and/or cheese, they still contain 22-54g fat.

• Want a cookie? Though the Raisin Oatmeal Cookie sounds like a better choice than the Chocolate Chunk, each have 420 calories. The Raisin Oatmeal contains a couple fewer grams of fat and three additional grams of fiber.

Joe's Crab Shack

Tips:

• Substitute and save calories. Many of the meals are served with Cheesy New Potatoes (250 calories and 15g fat) or Fries (370 calories and 19g fat). Request Broccoli (80 calories and 6g fat) or Ear of Corn (60 calories and 1g fat) instead.

• Drop the butter. Most entrées are finished with melted butter (120 calories a tablespoon) - ask for your meal without. Just one cup of Dipping Butter contains 400 calories and 44g fat.

• Limit the seasonings. While most added flavors add minimal calories, they are loaded in sodium. Enjoy your crab plain or with Garlic Herb (just 15mg sodium). Spicy Boil adds 950mg sodium; Fire-Grilled and Joe's Famous BBQ flavors contain more than 7700mg sodium (about three days worth)!

• Share a Steam Pot. The "Steampots for One" start at 1180 calories (including corn and potatoes).

• For more nutrition information, go to JoesCrabShack.com

Suggestions:

	Calories	Fat (g)	Sat+Trans Fat (g)	Sodium (mg)	Carbohydrates (g)	Fiber (g)	Protein (g)
Bucket of Shrimp, 12	190	3	0	2400	9	1	31
Grilled Malibu Shrimp w/rice & veggies	540	19	4	2400	55	5	39
Maui Mahi w/seasonal veggies, potatoes	680	28	11	3400	49	8	56
Bucket King Crab, potatoes, corn w/o butter	430	3	0	1410	68	7	33
Snow Crab or Dungeness Crab	475	4	0	835	69	7	43
Crab Daddy Feast	510	4	0	1410	69	7	49
Lobster Daddy Feast	580	4	1	1420	69	7	66
Share a Steampot for One (½ order each)							
Samuel Adams or Old Bay® Steampot, ½	595	37	17	1240	36	4	29
Joe's Classic Steampot, ½	605	38	17	1555	35	4	31

Caveats:

• Salads sound slimming yet the Crab Cake Chipotle Caesar has more fat than ¾ of a stick of butter (970 calories and 72g fat). Even a simple Caesar Salad with dressing contains 450 calories and 37g fat. The other entrée salads with protein added range from 530-860 calories and 38-61g fat.

• Joe doesn't skimp on portions. The lowest calorie sandwich is the Grilled Chicken Club Sandwich at 790 calories (this doesn't count the 370 calorie fries)! Most meals contain an excess of 1000 calories - the Skillet Paella has 1990 calories and 84g fat. The Bean Town Bake Steampot has 1470 calories. And, the desserts range from 980-1530 calories!

KFC®

Tips:

- KFC® offers bone-in grilled chicken pieces (see below) and several choices of vegetables to make a complete meal.

- Plated meals include chicken, two sides (see below), and a biscuit (180 calories and 8g fat).

- Full nutrition information is available at KFC.com.

Suggestions:

	Calories	Fat (g)	Sat+Trans Fat (g)	Sodium (mg)	Carbohydrates (g)	Fiber (g)	Protein (g)
Grilled Chicken, breast	220	7	2	730	0	0	40
thigh	170	10	3	530	0	0	19
drumstick	90	4	1	290	0	0	13
whole wing	80	5	2	250	1	0	10
Green Beans, individual	25	0	0	260	4	2	1
Mashed Potatoes w/gravy, individual	120	4	1	530	19	1	2
w/o gravy	90	3	<1	320	15	1	2
Corn on the Cob, 3"	70	5	<1	0	16	2	2
5½" cob	140	10	1	5	33	4	5
Sweet Kernel Corn, individual	100	<1	0	0	21	2	3
BBQ Baked Beans, individual	210	2	0	780	41	8	8
Honey BBQ KFC Snacker®	210	3	1	470	32	2	13
Honey BBQ Sandwich	320	4	1	770	47	3	24
Roasted Chicken Caesar Salad, plain	220	7	4	740	6	3	33
Fat-Free Hidden Valley® Ranch, 1 packet	35	0	0	410	8	0	1
Marzetti Light Italian Dressing, 1 packet	15	<1	0	510	2	0	0
Snack-Size Bowl	260	13	4	760	26	1	12

Caveats:

- Fried chicken pieces may contain more than *twice* as many calories and grams of fat as grilled chicken. And, as you can see, the crispier it is, the more calories (and fat) each piece has:

Original Chicken, breast	360	21	5	1080	11	0	34
drumstick	120	7	2	310	3	0	11
thigh	250	17	5	730	7	0	17
Extra Crispy, breast	510	33	7	1010	16	0	39
drumstick	150	10	2	360	5	0	12
thigh	340	24	5	780	10	0	20
Spicy Crispy, breast	420	25	5	1250	12	1	38
drumstick	160	10	2	440	5	0	11
thigh	360	27	6	1010	13	1	17

- No grilled pieces? Then, remove the skin and breading.

Original Chicken, breast	360	21	5	1080	11	0	34
w/o skin or breading	160	4	1	580	2	0	31

Krispy Kreme®

Tips:

• While known for doughnuts, there are some healthier options including oatmeal with many different toppings like fresh fruit and nuts.

• Choose the Whole Grain Bagel with reduced-fat cream cheese. While about the same calories as a doughnut, you'll get far more fiber and about half as much saturated fat.

• For more nutrition information, go to KrispyKreme.com.

Suggestions:

	Calories	Fat (g)	Sat+Trans Fat (g)	Sodium (mg)	Carbohydrates (g)	Fiber (g)	Protein (g)
Lowfat Fruit Yogurt (avg all flavors)	150	2	1	85	29	0	5
Quaker® Organic Instant Oatmeal	100	2	0	0	19	3	4
Pecan Cranberry Mix	100	6	<1	35	11	1	1
½ banana	60	0	0	0	15	2	1
Dried Fruit Blend	80	0	0	0	20	2	0
Apple Cinnamon Medley	70	0	0	5	17	1	1
Wholegrain/Whole Wheat Bagel	290	5	<1	500	54	9	11
Reduced Fat Plain cream cheese, 1oz	60	5	3	130	2	0	2
Reduced Fat Triple Berry Muffin	300	6	2	400	57	2	5
Doughnut hole, 1 (avg)	50	3	1	50	6	0	0
Mini Original Glazed	90	5	3	40	10	0	1
Mini Chocolate Iced Glazed	110	5	3	45	16	0	1
Mini Chocolate Iced w/sprinkles	130	5	3	45	20	0	1
Original Glazed or Sugar doughnut (avg)	190	11	5	90	21	0	2
Traditional Cake doughnut	190	12	6	260	19	0	2
Glazed Cinnamon	200	11	5	90	25	<1	2
Apple Fritter	210	14	7	110	18	1	3
Glazed Crueller	220	12	5	260	27	<1	2
Powdered Cake	220	11	5	240	27	0	2
Maple Iced Glazed	230	11	5	90	32	<1	2

Caveats:

• Think before you drink. A 16oz bottle of Naked® Juice contains 220-440 calories. The small (12oz) Chillers have 620-670 calories and 28-29g fat (all saturated). That's more saturated fat than most people should have for the entire day! Artic Avalanches® are almost as bad. A small 12oz contains 510-750 calories. Stick with a simple cone (300 calories) instead.

• The doughnuts not mentioned above contain 240-400 calories and 12-21g fat. There are 670 calories (38g fat) in the Cinnamon Roll (the Cinnamon Roll Lite contains 330 calories and 19g fat). The Pecan Roll has 840 calories and 51g fat (20g saturated)!

Krystal®

Tips:

- Krystal® serves a limited menu of tiny burgers (called Krystals), fried chicken sandwiches (Krystal Chik) and pieces (Chik'N Bites), fried chicken salad, hot dogs (Pup), and chili. Most are high in fat so the key to moderating calories is to limit the portion.

- Combo meals include medium fries (310 calories and 13g fat) and medium drink (160 calories).

- For more nutrition information, go to Krystal.com.

Suggestions:

	Calories	Fat (g)	Sat+Trans Fat (g)	Sodium (mg)	Carbohydrates (g)	Fiber (g)	Protein (g)
Krystal Sunriser	200	11	4	620	16	1	11
Egg on Toast	230	9	3	580	26	1	12
Grits w/margarine	160	2	0	570	33	1	4
Pancakes, 4	280	8	2	500	44	1	7
Syrup, 1	120	0	0	25	31	0	0
Krystal, 1	130	6	3	330	20	1	6
Cheese Krystal, 1	160	8	4	470	20	1	7
Plain Pup, 1	150	8	4	450	15	2	6
Chik'N Bites, small	200	7	2	690	20	1	15
Large Chili	300	11	6	200	33	10	17
Side Salad	70	5	3	95	4	2	4
Lite Italian Dressing, packet	45	4	1	530	3	0	0
Honey Dijon Dressing, packet	120	7	1	390	15	0	0
Kid's Meal: 1 Krystal, sm fries, sm drink	430	13	7	370	79	4	8

Caveats:

- The smallest combo (4 Krystals with fries and soft drink) add up to nearly 1000 calories:

	Calories	Fat (g)	Sat+Trans Fat (g)	Sodium (mg)	Carbohydrates (g)	Fiber (g)	Protein (g)
Krystals, 4	520	24	12	1320	80	4	24
French Fries, medium	310	13	7	65	46	5	4
Soda, medium	160	0	0	10	44	0	0
TOTAL:	990	37	19	1395	170	9	28

- Most of the menu items are high in fat, sugar or calories:

	Calories	Fat (g)	Sat+Trans Fat (g)	Sodium (mg)	Carbohydrates (g)	Fiber (g)	Protein (g)
Breakfeast	780	51	17	1240	45	1	27
Fruit-Flavored Freeze	230	0	0	10	58	0	0
BA Burger	550	35	11	770	46	3	17
BA Double Bacon Cheese	850	59	24	1580	48	3	32
Milkquake, avg all flavors	875	49	36	260	95	1	17
Oreo® Chocolate Sandwich Cookie	100	5	1	105	16	1	1
Apple Turnover	220	8	5	330	34	2	2
Lemon Icebox Pie	320	9	4	230	56	2	6

Lee's Famous Recipe Chicken®

Tips:

• Opt for Oven Roasted Chicken pieces or strips. Breading and frying adds to both the fat and calories of the fried chicken pieces. Famous Recipe Chicken has 50-60% more calories than the Roasted Chicken while the Crispy Plus has more than *double* the calories of the Roasted! Also, the Famous Breast Strips have double the calories of the Oven Roasted Strips.

• For more nutrition info, go to LeesFamousRecipe.com.

Suggestions:

	Calories	Fat (g)	Sat Fat (g)	Sodium (mg)	Carbohydrates (g)	Fiber (g)	Protein (g)
Oven Roasted Chicken:							
Breast w/o wing (1 piece option)	270	11	3	100	<1	0	41
Drumstick and Thigh (2 piece option)	340	20	6	240	<1	0	37
Breast and Wing (2 piece option)	430	22	6	210	<1	0	56
Chicken-on-a-Stick Strips, 3	200	4	1	250	<1	0	35
Sides:							
Green Beans	30	<1	0	425	3	1	3
Mashed Potatoes w/gravy	125	5	1	390	18	1	2
Corn on the Cob	155	3	1	10	25	7	5
Baked Beans	310	1	<1	740	47	7	7
BBQ Chicken Sandwich	325	5	1	810	34	1	37
White Chicken Chili	140	4	0	620	12	5	15

Caveats:

• Avoid the standard. Select Oven Roasted Chicken and ask for a leaner substitution for the coleslaw. Check out the difference these requests make in a standard two piece meal:

Famous Recipe Breast and Wing	540	27	8	1480	15	0	53
Mashed Potatoes w/gravy	125	5	1	390	18	1	2
Coleslaw	190	10	2	290	22	3	1
Biscuit	195	10	3	605	22	1	4
TOTAL:	1050	52	14	2765	77	5	60
Oven Roasted Breast and Wing	430	22	6	210	<1	0	56
Mashed Potatoes w/gravy	125	5	1	390	18	1	2
Green Beans	50	3	1	620	4	2	1
Biscuit	195	10	3	605	22	1	4
TOTAL:	800	40	11	1495	44	4	63

• It all adds up. A Biscuit (195 calories and 10g fat) is served with both snacks and meals. And, that's without the butter. A small soda contains 250 calories, while the large has 400.

Little Caesars®

Tips:

• A slice or two of regular crust pizza can fit into a healthy lifestyle, especially when paired with a veggie or fruit salad from home.

• For more nutrition information, go to LittleCaesars.com.

Suggestions:

	Calories	Fat (g)	Sat+Trans Fat (g)	Sodium (mg)	Carbohydrates (g)	Fiber (g)	Protein (g)
Pizza Slices, 1:							
Just Cheese	250	9	4	440	32	1	12
Veggie	270	10	5	560	33	2	13
Hula Hawaiian™	280	9	5	640	35	2	15
Pepperoni	280	11	5	560	32	2	14

Caveats:

• The extras really add up:

	Calories	Fat (g)	Sat+Trans Fat (g)	Sodium (mg)	Carbohydrates (g)	Fiber (g)	Protein (g)
Crazy Bread, 1 piece	100	3	<1	150	15	1	3
Italian Cheese Bread, 1 piece	130	6	3	240	13	1	6
Pepperoni Cheese Bread, 1 piece	150	8	3	280	13	1	6
Crazy Sauce®, 1 container	45	0	0	260	10	1	2
Caesar Wings®: 1 oven roasted wing	50	4	1	150	0	0	4
mild or hot, 1 wing (avg)	50	4	1	300	0	0	4
barbecue, 1 wing	70	4	1	220	3	0	4

• Don't dip. Each of the containers has 100-170 calories and 10-18g fat.

• Avoid the Deep Dish, including Baby Pan! Pan!®. Each Just Cheese slice (or pan) contains 320-360 calories and 13-18g fat. The meat varieties are even higher.

Dr. Jo. says

Cheese has a healthy reputation because it's rich in calcium and protein. But, let's face the facts...cheese has as much calories and fat (ounce-for-ounce) as fried chicken. So, keep cheese as a garnish, not an entrée. To save calories you might want to leave the cheese off your burger or salad, and request your pizza to be prepared "light" on the cheese.

Lone Star Steakhouse™

Tips:

• Limited nutrition information was available by asking at LoneStarSteakhouse.com. Some information was obtained from interviewing restaurant managers.

• For sides, request Fresh Green Beans, Steamed Spinach, and Broccoli "without added butter." Prepared this way, they should be under 100 calories per serving.

• Sandwiches are served with Fries, but you can request steamed vegetables instead.

Suggestions (a la carte):

	Calories	Fat (g)	Sat Fat (g)	Sodium (mg)	Carbohydrates (g)	Fiber (g)	Protein (g)
Sweet Bourbon Salmon	310	18	5	540	0	0	36
lunch	240	11	2	680	0	0	34
Mesquite-Grilled Shrimp on rice	230	8	1	3665	17	1	21
lunch portion	190	7	1	2365	17	1	12
Mesquite-Grilled Chicken	170	4	<1	1335	0	0	33
6oz Bacon-Wrapped Sirloin	245	7	3	1935	1	0	43
6oz Filet	330	18	7	230	2	0	42
Plain Baked Potato	225	0	0	35	50	5	6
Plain Sweet Potato	330	0	0	135	76	12	7

Caveats:

• The "Starters" are as big as Texas. Most of these appetizers are well over 1000 calories, including 2640 calories in the Amarillo Cheese Fries. The lowest calorie dish is the Spinach & Artichoke Dip at 880 calories and 62g fat (picture yourself eating ¾ stick of butter because it's the same as the amount in this dish).

• Be prepared. Bread (either a Bavarian Loaf or Yeast Rolls), along with honey cinnamon butter, is served before all meals.

• Get everything "on the side" since butters, toppings, and dressings are very high in fat and calories.

• The Salads are described as "big," and they are. While lettuce is low-calorie, each of the salads have a number of other high-fat ingredients including cheese, fried chicken, croutons, tortilla strips, and dressing. For example, the Grilled Chicken Caesar dressing (as prepared) contains 820 calories and 67g fat.

• Skip the "Add-Ons." Each of these toppings add about 100 calories (or more).

Long John Silver's®

Tips:

- Freshside Grille® Smart Choices are available. The fish entrées, served with long grain rice and steamed vegetables, range from 280-330 calories.

- Get the corn unbuttered and save about 60 calories and 7g fat.

- For more nutrition information, go to LJSilvers.com.

Suggestions:

	Calories	Fat (g)	Sat Fat (g)	Sodium (mg)	Carbohydrates (g)	Fiber (g)	Protein (g)
Freshside Grille® entrées w/rice & veggies:							
Salmon	280	7	2	1010	27	3	27
Tilapia	250	5	2	820	27	3	25
Shrimp Scampi	330	15	4	1230	29	3	20
Corn Cobbette w/o butter oil	90	3	<1	0	14	3	3

Caveats:

- "Battered" Fish and Chicken are fried - and high in calories and fat (especially unhealthy trans fats).

- Sandwiches and tacos have 360-470 calories - but are high-fat:

Alaskan Pollock Sandwich	470	23	10	1180	49	3	18
Baja Fish Taco	360	23	8	810	30	3	9
Zesty Chicken Strip Sandwich	380	19	7	880	39	3	14

- Baskets consist of two pieces of chicken or fish (or an order of popcorn shrimp), plus fries and a medium drink. Add it up - a fish basket contains 1230 calories:

Battered Fish, 1 piece	260	16	9	790	17	0	12
Chicken Strips, 1 piece	140	8	5	480	9	0	8
Battered Shrimp, 3 pieces	130	9	5	480	8	0	5
Popcorn Shrimp, snack box	270	16	9	570	23	1	9
Fries, basket portion	310	14	7	460	45	3	3
Soda, medium	400	0	0	100	112	0	0

- Don't forget to count the extras:

Breadstick, 1	170	4	1	290	29	1	6
Breaded Mozzarella Sticks, 3 pieces	150	9	4	350	13	1	5
Broccoli or Jalapeno Cheese Bites, 5 pcs	235	13	9	640	24	2	5
Chocolate or Pineapple Cream Pie (avg)	290	17	11	240	32	0	3

- Skip the "Crumblies®." These fried crumbs, spread on the bottom of each of the platters, add on 170 calories and 12g fat.

- Platters are large! A fish platter contains 2 pieces of fried fish, 8 fried shrimp, cole slaw, fries, hushpuppies, Crumblies®, and a medium drink for a grand total of about 1800 calories!

LongHorn Steak House®

Tips:

• Entrées are served with choice of side or salad - pick a veggie from the suggested list or ask for the fat-free dressing.

• For more nutrition info, go to LongHornSteakHouse.com.

Suggestions:

	Calories	Fat (g)	Sat+Trans Fat (g)	Sodium (mg)	Carbohydrates (g)	Fiber (g)	Protein (g)
Salads w/dressing:							
Grilled Salmon Salad	490	24	10	600	28	na	40
Grilled Chicken Salad	470	21	9	750	26	na	46
Mixed Greens Side Salad	110	5	2	200	12	na	4
Dressing, 1½ oz (3 Tbsp):							
Fat-Free Ranch	45	0	0	560	11	na	0
Balsamic or Ranch dressing	195	20	3	340	2	na	0
Entrées: Renegade Top Sirloin, 6oz	380	23	7	520	0	na	43
LongHorn Salmon, 7oz, lunch or dinner	290	13	3	300	3	na	40
Grilled Rainbow Trout, lunch or dinner	280	15	3	460	0	na	37
Redrock Grilled Shrimp, dinner	130	2	<1	1690	2	na	27
lunch entrée	90	1	0	1120	2	na	18
Sierra Chicken, dinner entrée	410	12	3	1240	2	na	72
lunch entrée	310	9	2	930	2	na	54
Cowboy Pork Chops, dinner entrée	400	14	5	1600	1	na	67
lunch entrée	200	7	3	800	0	na	34
Sides: Seasonal Rice Pilaf	200	<1	0	1600	43	na	4
Fresh Seasonal Vegetables	90	4	1	350	9	na	3
Fresh Steamed Asparagus	80	5	1	55	5	na	4
Grilled Fontina Chicken Sandwich	680	26	8	1330	52	na	59

Caveats:

• Big steaks (and big burgers) are *big* in calories:

LongHorn Porterhouse	1200	85	35	2180	1	na	106
Outlaw Ribeye, 18oz	1070	79	39	1640	0	na	90
Bacon & Cheddar Burger	880	44	18	1230	53	na	33

• Get the salad dressing on the side - or expect this:

Grilled Chicken & Strawberry Salad							
w/vinaigrette	950	60	10	860	58	na	9

• Limit the "unlimited" bread - the meals are large enough:

Baked Bread, loaf w/o butter	510	5	1	590	96	na	19

• Don't get it loaded:

Loaded Baked Potato	430	17	11	150	57	na	14

• All the desserts are huge:

Chocolate Stampede (serves 2)	2180	131	77	760	229	na	22
Caramel Apple Goldrush	1640	71	36	940	237	na	13

Luby's®

Tips:

- While walking through the serving line of this cafeteria, look for the "heart" icon. Select any one of these entrées and any two of the heart sides and your meal will be under 650 calories.

- FYI - most meals include a roll (see below).

- Limited nutrition information is available at Lubys.com.

Suggestions:

	Calories	Fat (g)	Sat+Trans Fat (g)	Sodium (mg)	Carbohydrates (g)	Fiber (g)	Protein (g)
Blackened Tilapia	270	11	na	na	5	2	na
Roasted Turkey w/o skin or gravy	280	3	na	na	0	0	na
Chipotle Lime Chicken	290	17	na	na	12	3	na
Baked Ham	300	11	na	na	6	0	na
Lemon Basil Tilapia	330	12	na	na	0	0	na
Lemon Dill Salmon w/o sauce	330	14	na	na	3	0	na
Pan Grilled Filet	330	12	na	na	19	2	na
Grilled Chicken Breast, 8oz w/o skin	340	16	na	na	1	0	na
Lemon Pepper Salmon	340	16	na	na	4	0	na
Lemon Basil Salmon	360	20	na	na	1	0	na
Cuban Grilled Tilapia and sauce, w/o rice	375	18	na	na	12	2	na
Grilled Summer Tilapia	480	12	na	na	30	4	na
Mixed Melons or Pineapple, 1c serving	75	0	na	na	23	2	na
Steamed Broccoli	50	2	na	na	8	5	na
Lemon Roasted Asparagus	50	4	na	na	3	2	na
Spinach	60	2	na	na	7	4	na
Blue Lake Green Beans	60	3	na	na	5	3	na
Roasted Cauliflower	60	5	na	na	4	2	na
Cauliflower, Peas and Carrots	70	2	na	na	10	6	na
Skillet Fried Cabbage or Buttered Asparagus	70	4	na	na	7	4	na
Fresh Green Beans	75	3	na	na	10	4	na
Sauteed Mushrooms	90	4	na	na	10	1	na
Normandy Vegetables	90	3	na	na	14	7	na
Carrots	100	2	na	na	20	5	na
Roasted Mixed Vegetables	100	5	na	na	14	4	na
Stir Fry Zucchini or Squash Saute (avg)	120	5	na	na	15	6	na
White Roll	130	3	na	na	23	1	na
Whole Wheat Roll	170	5	na	na	23	1	na

Caveat:

- Keep in mind that beverages and desserts can easily double the calories of your tray contents. Though not included in the Smart Meals, count another 165-330 calories for buttered corn, peas, beans or rice (more for mashed potatoes). Refer to the *General Tips to Eat Out Healthy* chapter for more guidance.

Marble Slab Creamery®

Tips:

• "Tasty Creations" involve blending mix-ins into ice cream. If you must have one, start with plain nonfat frozen yogurt or reduced-fat ice cream and add fruit.

• For more nutrition information, go to MarbleSlab.com

Suggestions, per small:	Calories	Fat (g)	Sat+Trans Fat (g)	Sodium (mg)	Carbohydrates (g)	Fiber (g)	Protein (g)
Nonfat Frozen Yogurt:							
No-Sugar-Added Vanilla	80	0	0	80	16	0	4
Orange Smoothie Sorbet	90	0	0	0	22	0	0
Vanilla	100	0	0	55	21	0	4
Chocolate	110	0	0	55	22	0	4
Reduced-Fat Ice Cream:							
Strawberry	190	9	6	1	23	0	3
Vanilla or Amaretto	210	10	7	0	24	0	3
Cheesecake	210	10	6	0	27	0	3
Chocolate Swiss	215	10	6	1	27	1	3

Caveats:

• Here are the stats for the other ice creams:

Most other flavors ice cream, small	230	13	8	5	25	<1	3
Peanut Butter, Choc Peanut Butter, or							
Pistachio ice cream, small	260	17	9	45	24	1	5

• Get your ice cream in a cup. The cones can double the calories:

Plain Waffle Cone, regular-size	130	3	0	10	23	0	2
Dark Chocolate-Dipped Waffle Cone	200	8	5	10	30	1	3
dipped w/Butterfinger®	270	11	7	45	41	1	3
dipped w/Heath® Bar	280	12	7	60	39	2	3
White Chocolate-Dipped Waffle Cone	210	8	5	15	32	0	3
w/sprinkles	220	8	5	15	35	0	3

• Think before order a "Tasty Creation." These mixtures of ice cream and decadent sweets can break the calorie bank. Here are the stats for the *small* size mixed with ice cream (twice as much for the medium-size):

Small cup mixed w/fruit	280	15	9	40	34	1	3
Small cup w/toppings other than fruit,							
chocolate or nuts	330	18	11	55	40	1	5
Small cup mixed w/chocolate or nuts	420	23	13	50	49	2	6

Marie Callender's®

Tips:

- Ask for pancakes without the butter - and request sugar-free pancake syrup. That dollop of butter has 90 calories while regular syrup contains 50 calories per tablespoon. Sugar-free syrup contains just 10-20 calories.

- For more nutrition information, go to Mariecallenders.com

Suggestions:
Mini Menu:

	Calories	Fat (g)	Sat+Trans Fat (g)	Sodium (mg)	Carbohydrates (g)	Fiber (g)	Protein (g)
Pancakes w/o butter or syrup	300	14	4	280	35	1	8
French Toast w/o butter or syrup	290	13	6	380	37	1	7
1 egg, bacon, toast, jam, hashbrowns	560	25	7	1310	68	4	16
Beef Barley Soup, cup	170	7	3	1150	17	2	7
bowl	250	11	4	1730	25	4	11
Souper Sandwich: Turkey w/o mayo							
and Chicken Noodle Soup	640	23	8	2210	74	2	36

Caveats:

- Nix the potatoes. A full order of hashbrowns contains 480 calories and 18g fat. An order of fries has 380 calories and 20g fat.

- Breakfasts are big. Bacon & Eggs (with hashbrowns and toast) contain over 1000 calories and 39g fat. A slice of quiche has about 1000 calories and 80g fat. The "Oh My" Omelette has 1700 calories. "Oh My" is correct!

- And, lunch is just as big. Sandwich and fries range from 1020 to 1750 calories. Yes, even the Roasted Turkey Croissant and Spicy Grilled Chicken Sandwich!

- No-Sugar-Added Pies are still high in calories (that's because most of the calories are in the pie crust, not the fruit). Regular fruit pies contain an average of 565 calories and 31g fat while the No-Sugar-Added Pies contain about 465 calories and 30g fat.

- If you want pie, stick with the simple fruit pies such as Apple, Strawberry, and Peach. While all pies are high in calories, the cream pies contain an extra 100 calories - or more per slice! The highest calorie pies include Pecan at 920 calories and White Chocolate Raspberry Pie at 940 calories.

- If you must have a sweet, opt for a single cookie (160-210 calories). The Triple Chocolate Brownie Sundae has 1580 calories!

McAlister's Deli®

Tips:

• Sandwiches and wraps are served with your choice of side. Select the fresh fruit cup so you don't break your calorie budget.

• "Choose Two" includes half of any salad, spud, sandwich, wrap or panini, or a cup of soup. Select from those listed below.

• For more nutrition information, go to McAlistersDeli.com.

Suggestions:

	Calories	Fat (g)	Sat+Trans Fat (g)	Sodium (mg)	Carbohydrates (g)	Fiber (g)	Protein (g)
Fresh Fruit Cup (varies by season)	80	0	0	10	11	1	1
Cup of Soup: French Onion Soup	80	3	1	870	11	1	1
Country Vegetable Soup	90	1	0	970	17	3	3
Chicken Noodle Soup	110	2	0	1280	15	1	8
Southwest Roasted Corn Soup	120	4	1	900	20	4	3
Vegetarian Chili	130	1	0	990	28	15	8
Chicken Chili	150	3	0	490	20	4	20
Golden Lentil Soup	210	3	2	830	35	9	12
1/2 Salad w/o dressing, choose from:							
Garden Salad	150	9	6	245	9	1	7
Savannah Chopped Salad	220	10	4	295	20	2	16
1/2 Chipotle Dressing	85	0	0	280	20	0	0
1/2 Sandwiches, choose from:							
New Yorker	245	8	4	1215	25	2	22
The Veggie	265	6	3	975	41	8	11
Memphian™	275	12	3	1235	24	2	20
Turkey Melt	280	13	4	1050	24	2	18
Greek Chicken Pita	285	14	4	815	25	2	15
Ham Melt	295	14	4	980	23	2	16
Grilled Sweet Chipotle Chicken	310	11	4	850	37	1	18
French Dip	325	12	6	805	32	2	18
The Big Nasty®	335	10	5	1070	35	2	27
1/2 Spuds, choose from:							
Grilled Chicken	280	6	4	435	35	3	20
Veggie Spud	295	10	3	455	39	3	13

Caveat:

• Some menu items are considerably higher than most:

Caesar Salad w/grilled chicken & dressing	700	51	12	1890	24	2	35
Spud Max™	730	28	16	1440	72	6	40
Tuscan Tomato Soup in bread bowl	740	61	37	1190	42	12	16
BLT Sandwich	910	64	10	1520	61	2	24
Grilled Chicken Club	1000	56	16	2020	79	7	50
McAlisters Club™	1030	56	16	3140	79	7	54
Colossal Carrot Cake	1170	73	31	700	117	4	11

McDonald's®

Tips:

• Order grilled chicken (instead of crispy chicken) on wraps, salads, and sandwiches to save 70-160 calories.

• Request coffee drinks to be prepared with nonfat milk and sugar-free flavorings. The savings are huge! A small vanilla latte has 230 calories and 7g fat while the small *nonfat* latte with *sugar-free* vanilla syrup contains 80 calories and no fat.

• Combo meal is served with medium Soft Drink (210 calories) entrée and medium French Fries (380 calories and 19g fat).

• Looking for fruits and veggies? Choose from Apple Dippers, Salad, Fruit Smoothies, and Fruit 'n Yogurt Parfait.

• For more nutrition information, go to McDonalds.com

Suggestions:

	Calories	Fat (g)	Sat+Trans Fat (g)	Sodium (mg)	Carbohydrates (g)	Fiber (g)	Protein (g)
Egg McMuffin®	300	12	5	820	30	2	18
Fruit & Maple Oatmeal	290	5	2	160	57	5	5
w/o brown sugar	260	5	2	115	48	5	5
Apple Dippers wi/lowfat caramel dip	100	<1	0	35	23	0	0
Fruit 'n Yogurt Parfait w/granola	160	2	1	85	31	1	4
Snack Size Fruit & Walnut Salad as served	210	8	2	60	31	2	25
Grilled Chicken Snack Wraps (avg)	250	8	4	670	27	1	16
Premium Grilled Chicken Classic SW	350	9	2	820	42	3	28
Salads w/o dressing:							
Bacon Ranch Salad w/grilled chicken	230	9	4	700	10	3	30
SW Salad w/grilled chicken	290	8	3	650	28	7	27
Asian Grilled Chicken Salad	270	9	1	590	21	6	28
Newman's Own® Lowfat (LF) Dressing:							
LF Italian	50	3	0	390	7	0	1
LF Balsamic Vinaigrette	35	4	0	420	3	0	0
LF Sesame Ginger Dressing	90	3	0	410	15	1	1
Kid's Hamburger Meal w/fries, diet soda	480	20	5	680	60	5	15
Iced Coffee w/SF vanilla syrup, small	60	5	4	70	8	0	1
Nonfat Cappuccino, small	60	0	0	85	9	0	6
Nonfat Latte, small	90	0	0	115	13	0	9
Vanilla Reduced-Fat Ice Cream Cone	150	4	2	60	24	0	4
Fruit Smoothies (avg flavors), small	215	<1	<1	35	49	2	2

Caveat:

• Buyer beware. McDonald's® nutrition information references just 150 calories for a 3.2oz Vanilla Reduced-Fat Ice Cream Cone. Sounds good, but I've found that many servers generously fill the cone with way more 3.2 oz. For just 150 calories, be sure the tip of the swirl is only an inch or two above the cone.

Mimi's Cafe®

Tips:

• There are many "Fresh and Fit" options (650 calories or less) at every meal. Keep in mind that nutrition info includes only what's listed with the meal - not the bread basket and butter.

• Request fat-free balsamic or lowfat citrus vinaigrette on any of the salads (at under 100 calories).

• Go to MimisCafe.com for more nutrition information.

Fresh & Fit Meal Suggestions:

	Calories	Fat (g)	Sat+Trans Fat (g)	Sodium (mg)	Carbohydrates (g)	Fiber (g)	Protein (g)
Mimi's Protein Breakfast w/ground turkey	410	16	5	580	3	0	56
Egg White Omelette (avg of varieties)	170	6	2	615	7	1	22
Oatmeal Breakfast	645	7	1	550	133	16	22
Marinara Chicken Ciabatta Sandwich, fruit	610	7	2	1600	102	6	40
Veggie Burger w/fresh fruit	395	7	2	1535	71	7	14
Sweet & Sour Chicken	550	20	4	255	64	7	31
Broiled Chicken & Fruit Plate	425	7	3	110	52	5	40
Grilled Veggie Flatbread	475	10	2	840	83	18	20
Turkey Breast, brown rice, veggies	505	11	3	945	58	6	38
Salmon, brown rice, fresh vegetables	475	21	4	235	36	5	35
Petite Filet, asparagus, baby greens	255	8	3	260	16	3	30
Filet of "Soul" w/fresh vegetables	275	9	2	410	7	0	39
Petite Chocolate Mousse	130	8	5	10	13	1	1

Caveats:

• The Bread Basket includes slices of Carrot Raisin Nut Loaf and Pumpkin Loaf. And, a Muffin is served with every Entrée Salad! (Really...do we need it?) Most of the bakery goods are caloric:

Honey Bran Muffin	385	10	5	435	72	9	9
Nature Valley Granola Muffin	360	4	1	310	66	4	3
Lowfat Blueberry Muffin	440	4	0	1025	101	2	8
Other Muffins, avg	525	23	6	515	74	1	7
Mimi's Famous Carrot Raisin Nut Loaf	905	54	6	1020	102	6	12
one slice	150	9	1	170	17	1	2
Pumpkin Loaf	670	17	8	665	121	3	11

• Nearly all the sandwiches, meals, and desserts contain 1000 calories or more, including these:

Turkey Pesto Ciabatta	1235	71	20	1670	82	5	45
French Fries	460	23	4	790	59	5	5
Honey Dijon Pork Chops w/vegetables	765	36	11	575	37	0	68
Mashed Potatoes	365	21	13	865	42	4	4
Mimi's Chopped Cobb Salad	810	55	20	1850	22	7	46
Balsamic Vinaigrette	630	64	9	675	16	0	1
Triple Chocolate Brownie w/ice cream	1950	87	43	1075	280	6	25

Moe's® Southwest Grill

Tips:

- Streak! Order a "Streaker" and the item is prepared without shell or tortilla to save 290 calories (large tortilla) or 390 calories (shell).

- Get the Junior. Junior Burritos have about *half* the calories and fat of the larger burrito.

- Consider the meat. Tofu is the lowest calorie protein. Fish, pork, and steak add another 20-25 calories on a junior or salad. Chicken and ground beef are the highest in fat and calories (40-50 calories more than tofu on a junior or salad). Choosing no protein (only beans and rice) will knock off another 50-100 calories.

- The whole grain tortilla contains an extra 4g fiber as well as 40 more calories than the regular flour tortilla.

- Calculate the exact nutrition for your favorite combo at Moes.com.

Suggestions:

	Calories	Fat (g)	Sat+Trans Fat (g)	Sodium (mg)	Carbohydrates (g)	Fiber (g)	Protein (g)
Chicken Enchilada Soup, cup (bowl = X3)	180	11	5	860	13	2	9
Joey Jr Burrito, avg all proteins	395	13	5	710	48	5	21
Homewrecker Jr Burrito, avg all proteins	490	19	8	900	55	7	24
Art Vandalay Jr Burrito w/tofu	480	19	8	910	55	8	20
w/o meat	425	15	7	768	54	7	16
"Streaker" Close Talker Salad, avg all protein	435	21	7	1230	28	12	33
"Streaker" Personal Trainer Salad:							
w/tofu	410	21	6	1260	29	12	26
w/o meat	295	13	5	970	27	12	16
"Streaker" Joey Burrito:							
w/o meat	360	10	5	850	46	10	18
w/tofu	470	18	6	1140	48	11	28
w/fish, steak, pork, or chicken (avg)	500	16	7	1170	46	10	39
Funk Meister on corn taco, 1	260	12	4	525	20	5	17
Pulled Pork Rice Bowl (or w/other meats)	660	24	11	1660	75	10	42
Marinated Tofu Bowl	700	23	6	1580	82	14	32

Caveats:

- Skip the Chips (which are served with each meal). A basket with Pico de Gallo has 675 calories and 26g fat. Count on 720 calories with Guacamole and 810 calories with Queso.

- Share the rest. An order of Fajitas is around 1000 calories, while the Nachos are closer to 1500 calories. A Cheese-only Quesadilla contains 500 calories (yet 30g fat!) while the Chicken Club Quesadilla has 1120 calories.

Morton's® The Steakhouse

Tips:

- No nutrition information is available at Mortons.com; the information below was obtained from interviews with restaurant managers.

- All menu items are large - even the sides are "sharable." Feel free to make a meal with an leaner appetizer or smaller steak, then add one of the sides listed below.

- Steaks are seasoned, then grilled. Au Jus (beef broth) is then added, not butter. Request no seasoning or Au Jus to cut sodium.

Suggestions:

- Appetizers - Tuna Tartare, a 2-3oz portion, is served with avocado, tomato, and a small amount of Thai cream sauce. An order of Broiled Sea Scallops Wrapped in Bacon contains three large scallops (weighing a total of 3-5oz); remove the bacon to save calories. Colossal Shrimp Cocktail contains four large 2-2.5oz shrimp (for a total of 8-10oz).

- Salads - Order the Sliced Beefsteak Tomato Salad without the usual blue cheese crumbles. Ask for the Tomato Onion Vinaigrette instead of the Creamy Blue Cheese dressing.

- Steaks - Go with the smallest 8oz Filet Mignon under the "Slightly Smaller" Steak list. The next smaller steak is the 12oz New York Strip Steak or the 14oz Filet Mignon.

- Seafood - Chilean Sea Bass (12oz) is served with a Pineapple Salsa/Relish. The Broiled Salmon Fillet (12oz) is served with a white wine butter sauce on the side, but you can ask for it without the sauce. Another leaner option is the Lobster Tail as long as it's not doused in butter. Instead of dipping the lobster into the butter, dip your fork into the melted butter, then into the meat for a taste with every bite.

- Side Dishes - Choose from Steamed Fresh Jumbo Asparagus (without the Hollandaise sauce), Grilled Jumbo Asparagus, or Sauteed Fresh Spinach & Mushrooms (ask the server to request as little oil as possible).

- Dessert - Order the Fresh Raspberries or Mixed Berries without the creamy Sabayon Sauce.

Caveat:

- A large round Onion Loaf Bread (served with butter) is delivered to all tables, unless requested otherwise.

Nathan's® & Arthur Treacher's®

Tips:

- Make it simple and small. Since everything is high in fat and calories (even the Grilled Chicken), cut a few calories by ordering diet soda and leaving off sauces and dressings. While no nutrition information is available for the Grilled Chicken sandwich or the Grilled Chicken Caesar Wrap without sauce, order it plain and you'll probably save about 100 calories.

- Keep it small. Large Fries, Onion Rings, and Sodas contain about 40% more calories than the regular-size.

- For more nutrition information, go to NathansFamous.com.

Suggestions:

	Calories	Fat (g)	Sat+Trans Fat (g)	Sodium (mg)	Carbohydrates (g)	Fiber (g)	Protein (g)
Nathan's®:							
King-size Pretzel	180	1	0	940	38	1	6
Hot Dog	300	18	7	690	24	<1	11
Corn Dog on a Stick	380	21	5	730	39	1	7
Pretzel Dog	390	16	6	970	49	1	12
Grilled Chicken Sandwich w/mayo	555	32	5	1160	40	3	27
Chicken Cheesesteak Supreme	600	19	9	1720	70	3	40
Grilled Chicken Caesar Wrap	700	34	11	1340	60	1	38
Arthur Treacher's®:							
Fish Sandwich	440	18	3	715	50	3	18
Corn on the Cob w/butter	140	2	0	20	34	2	5

Caveats:

- Don't make it a meal. That regular order of French Fries adds 465 calories and 34g fat, while the small order of Onion Rings adds 545 calories and 45g fat. And, a small 16oz Lemonade is another 200 calories.

- Avoid the cheese. The smallest Hamburger with Cheese has 705 calories and 43g fat. The Supercheese Burger is nearly 1000 calories and the Double Burger with Cheese has close to 1200 calories. Nathan's® Cheesesteak Supreme contains 850 calories and 45g fat. If you think the regular-size French Fries at 465 calories is a lot, when you turn the order into Cheese Fries, you've just added another 100 calories.

- All those little bites add up. Count on about 80 calories for one Chicken Wing, 115 calories per Hot Dog Nugget, and 130 calories per Mozzarella stick. And, that's without the sauce!

- Share dessert. While Apple Pie contains just 315 calories and 19g fat, the funnel cake contains 580 calories and 29g fat.

Noble Roman's® Pizza

Tips:

- An Individual Pizza has about the same calories and fat as three slices of Large Pizza.
- Nutrition information is available online for all the varieties of pizza.
- For more nutrition information, go to NobleRomans.com

Suggestions:

	Calories	Fat (g)	Sat+Trans Fat (g)	Sodium (mg)	Carbohydrates (g)	Fiber (g)	Protein (g)
Breakfast Burrito	410	20	5	1145	42	2	15
Grilled Chicken Wrap	440	12	3	1915	44	2	37
Pizza Stuffer®	420	18	6	1040	48	4	19
Spaghetti with Meat Sauce	490	13	4	1150	72	3	20
Fettucine Alfredo	530	16	10	1260	78	2	22
Cheese pizza, large slice	225	8	4	575	29	1	9
Pepperoni pizza, large slice	250	10	5	675	29	1	10

Caveats:

- Count the extras:

	Calories	Fat (g)	Sat+Trans Fat (g)	Sodium (mg)	Carbohydrates (g)	Fiber (g)	Protein (g)
Bar-B-Que Wing, 1	60	5	1	170	3	0	4
Hot-N-Spicy Wing, 1	60	5	1	85	<1	0	5
Breadstick	105	5	1	185	18	1	5
Tangy Tomato Sauce Dip	25	1	0	170	5	1	1
Spicy Cheese Dip	100	8	4	500	4	0	3
Buttery Garlic Dip	120	14	3	110	0	0	0

- Individual Pizzas range from 620 calories (Cheese) to 820 calories (The Works).

Dr. Jo says

It's your body and you're footing the restaurant charge...so order your food the way you want. Request less oil to be used in your stir-fry, ask for pancakes without that blob of butter, get the salad dressing on the side...

And, please don't make *all* the changes suggested in this book or your food will be tasteless and boring. Make the changes that are "no big deal" for you!

Noodles & Company®

Tips:

• Start with a noodle, salad, or soup base. Then add a protein, if desired. These dishes are available in either small- or regular-size. Sandwiches are also available.

• For more nutrition information, go to Noodles.com.

Suggestions:

	Calories	Fat (g)	Sat+Trans Fat (g)	Sodium (mg)	Carbohydrates (g)	Fiber (g)	Protein (g)
Noodle Bases, small-size (or ½ regular):							
Bangkok Curry	240	7	5	430	40	4	4
Japanese Pan Noodles	320	8	1	1100	55	3	7
Spaghetti	340	9	3	570	53	3	13
Pad Thai	410	9	2	1030	76	2	7
Indonesian Peanut Saute	420	9	2	930	74	4	9
Pasta Fresca	410	13	5	610	58	3	14
Mushroom Stroganoff	410	17	9	550	51	3	15
Salad Bases, small-size (or ½ regular):							
The Med Salad	160	6	2	500	22	2	4
Chinese Chop Salad	190	11	1	440	19	3	2
Caesar Salad	200	15	4	530	10	1	6
Soup Bases, small-size (or ½ regular):							
Chicken Noodle Soup	180	5	2	1200	22	<1	12
Thai Curry Soup	230	9	6	950	35	2	3
Add Protein: Sauteed Shrimp	80	1	0	360	<1	0	17
Chicken Breast	110	3	<1	370	0	0	23
Organic Tofu	180	11	2	310	6	1	16
Parmesan-Crusted Chicken Breast	200	10	3	820	8	<1	20
Extras: Ciabatta Roll	120	1	0	310	24	1	5
Flatbread	200	5	<1	400	35	1	6
Cucumber Tomato Salad	110	0	0	920	24	2	1
Tossed Green Salad w/fat free Asian	45	0	0	420	11	1	0
w/balsamic dressing	60	6	1	140	4	1	0
Sandwiches:							
The Veggie Med	300	9	2	920	45	4	9
The Med	330	10	2	970	41	2	20
Spicy Chicken Caesar w/o dressing	330	9	2	770	40	1	21

Caveats:

• The highest calorie menu item is the regular-size Bacon, Mac & Cheeseburger at 1260 calories and 58g fat.

• Skip the treat - there are no low-cal options. Cookies have about 360 calories and 9g fat. The Rice Krispy Treat has 550 calories and 18g fat!

O'Charley's

Tips:

• Ask to skip the "brushing." Proteins, rolls, and more are brushed with margarine before serving - an extra 50 calories on a roll.

• For more nutrition information, go to OCharleys.com.

Suggestions:

	Calories	Fat (g)	Sat+Trans Fat (g)	Sodium (mg)	Carbohydrates (g)	Fiber (g)	Protein (g)
550 Calories or Less (w/broccoli & tomato):							
Mushroom & Bleu Cheese Sirloin	460	30	11	2880	13	4	36
Buschetta Chicken	470	16	5	1790	25	5	56
Grilled Shrimp on bed of rice	290	7	2	1220	32	1	22
Cedar Planked Tilapia, entrée only	280	11	5	410	2	1	42
Grilled Atlantic Salmon, 6oz entrée only	370	22	5	190	2	1	38
Grilled Top Sirloin, 7oz entrée only	430	28	11	920	1	0	43
Cedar Planked Salmon, entrée only	530	32	6	940	2	1	57
Add sides: Broccoli	140	10	4	1130	10	5	5
Baked Potato, plain	240	5	1	720	50	6	8
Rice Pilaf	190	5	2	790	30	1	4
Fresh Asparagus	80	6	3	380	4	2	2
Yeast roll w/o margarine	130	2	0	110	25	0	4

Caveats:

• Sides matter. Compare the sides listed above with these:

Broccoli Cheese Casserole, side	270	16	5	830	20	4	10
French Fries, side	520	33	7	940	53	4	5
Smashed Potatoes, side	400	14	6	810	47	5	4
Loaded Baked Potato, side	590	40	14	1180	52	6	17

• These may sound healthy, but they are high in fat and calories:

Grilled Turkey Burger	890	54	17	1710	54	3	47
California Chicken Salad w/balsamic	940	55	14	860	66	8	45
Grilled Baja Chicken meal	990	37	11	3540	99	11	64
Teriyaki Sesame Chicken meal	1030	25	7	3740	151	5	46

• Desserts and Brunch can be disastrous:

Cinnamon Sugar Donuts, 10 w/dip	1130	54	12	1160	139	1	11
Mini Cinnamon Sugar Donuts	510	25	7	500	63	0	5
Brownie Lover's Brownie	1600	73	42	1310	216	7	23
Mini Brownie Lover's Brownie	530	24	14	430	71	2	8
O'Charley's® Overloaded Brunch Platter	1690	103	31	2080	116	4	47

• The Lunch Combos may be "good to both your taste buds and your wallet," but they will blow your calorie budget. Most combos are over 1000 calories. The leanest variety (Half Club Sandwich with House Salad and light dressing) adds up to 730 calories. Oh, did you want rolls and a drink with that?

Old Chicago®

Tips:

- Think thin. Order the Thin Crust pizza and you'll save at least 100 calories a slice (and about half the fat) over the deep dish.

- Which size? A ⅛ slice of the large deep dish pizza has about the same calories and fat as a ⅙ slice of the medium. A slice of individual-size deep dish pizza contains about ¾ the calories of the large or medium slice.

- Go veggie. The lowest calorie (and fat) pizzas are cheese, vegetarian, or Hawaiian; meat adds 100-235 calories per slice.

- Pick the veggies; skip the dip. Sandwiches and Stromboli are served with fries (320 calories, 11g fat), coleslaw (180 calories, 11g fat), or 30 calorie veggies (skip the 240 calories of ranch dressing).

- Sub chicken. Ask for your burger to be prepared with a grilled chicken breast instead and save 165 calories and 21g fat.

- For more nutrition information, go to OldChicago.com.

Suggestions:

	Calories	Fat (g)	Sat Fat (g)	Sodium (mg)	Carbohydrates (g)	Fiber (g)	Protein (g)
NY Thin Crust Style Pizza, one 16" slice:							
cheese or Vegetarian 7	310	14	7	490	30	2	18
Malibu Veggie	285	12	5	470	31	2	14
Hawaiian	380	16	8	940	34	2	26
Thai Pie	410	20	9	785	36	2	22
Chicago Style Deep Dish Pizza:							
Malibu Veggie Pizza, lg or med slice	355	14	6	455	45	3	14
Cheese Calzone, lunch	350	10	4	625	56	3	12
Grilled Chicken "Burger"	465	11	2	830	41	2	46
Grilled Chicken Wrap sandwich	585	21	5	1700	62	7	36
½ Asian Salad w/dressing (no garlic toast)	460	12	1	940	65	3	21

Caveats:

- The other pizzas are much higher in calories and fat:

	Calories	Fat (g)	Sat Fat (g)	Sodium (mg)	Carbohydrates (g)	Fiber (g)	Protein (g)
NY Thin Crust Style Pizza, one 16" slice (⅛):							
Chicago Seven or Classic	410	23	11	830	30	2	23
Double Deckeroni or Meat Me	490	30	13	1255	30	2	28
Chicago Style Deep Dish Pizza, lg or med slice:							
Cheese	460	25	10	485	43	2	18
Vegetarian 7 or Hawaiian	505	27	10	690	46	3	22
Double Deckeroni or Meat Me	655	38	15	1100	44	3	27

- Most of the menu is high-calorie. These include: Starters (840-1150 calories), other Strombolis and Calzones (840-1535), Entrée Salads (735-1075) and dinner Pastas (800-1540 calories).

Olive Garden®

Tips:

• An olive branch on the menu designates six menu items as "Garden Fare lowfat entrées."

• At dinner, feel free to order the luncheon portion. The smaller portion size will save you about 30% of the calories and fat.

• All meals come with choice of either salad or soup. Choose the soup for fewer calories, fat, and sodium (see caveat below). Want salad? Ask for the dressing and croutons on the side - and use them sparingly. A lowfat Italian dressing is also available.

• Olive Garden® offers a variety of mini desserts ranging from 210-290 calories. Other desserts contain 510-1000+ calories.

• Request the breadsticks to be served unbuttered.

• For more nutrition information, go to OliveGarden.com

Suggestions:

	Calories	Fat (g)	SatFat (g)	Sodium (mg)	Carbohydrates (g)	Fiber (g)	Protein (g)
Garden-Fresh Salad, 1 serving w/o dressing	120	4	<1	550	17	3	4
Minestrone Soup, 1 serving	100	1	0	1020	18	3	4
Pasta e Fagioli (soup), 1 serving	130	3	1	680	17	6	9
Zuppa Toscana (soup), 1 serving	170	4	2	960	24	2	10
Venetian Apricot Chicken, dinner	400	7	2	1290	34	6	51
lunch portion	290	5	2	1010	34	6	29
Seafood Brodetto, dinner	480	16	3	2250	35	7	47
Capellini di Mare, dinner	650	18	5	1830	82	7	41
Shrimp Primavera, dinner	730	12	2	1620	110	14	46
lunch portion	510	9	2	1130	79	12	30
Capellini Pomodoro, dinner	840	17	3	1250	141	19	31
lunch portion	480	11	2	970	78	11	17
Herb-Grilled Salmon, dinner	510	26	6	760	5	2	64
Linguine alla Marinara, dinner	430	6	1	900	76	9	18
lunch portion	310	4	1	670	55	5	12
Cheese Ravioli w/marinara, lunch	530	18	9	1160	64	6	26
Ravioli di Portobello, lunch	450	19	11	960	53	8	18

Caveat:

• Olive Garden® offers an unlimited soup, salad, and breadstick lunch that may seem "light" but just one serving of each these items adds up to 750 calories and 3510mg sodium!:

Garden-Fresh Salad w/dressing	350	26	5	1930	22	3	5
Chicken & Gnocchi Soup, 1 serving	250	8	3	1180	29	2	16
Breadstick w/butter spread	150	2	0	400	28	2	6
	750	36	8	3510	79	7	27

On the Border®

Tips:

- Share. Just about every entrée contains more than 1000 calories. And, that's before the drinks and chips.

- Skip the basket of chips. Chips and Salsa contain 430 calories and 22g fat. A cup of queso adds another 270 calories.

- Pick rice or beans - not both. Black beans are the best choice.

- For more nutrition information, go to OnTheBorder.com.

Suggestions:

	Calories	Fat (g)	Sat Fat (g)	Sodium (mg)	Carbohydrates (g)	Fiber (g)	Protein (g)
Citrus Chipotle Chicken Salad w/fat-free mango citrus vinaigrette	290	4	2	840	42	11	25
Achiote Chicken Tacos	650	12	2	1690	98	6	37
Chicken Salsa Fresca, as served	520	9	3	2410	60	12	50
Jalapeno-BBQ Salmon, as served	590	21	6	1220	45	24	54
Tomatillo Chicken, as served	850	24	6	1650	109	7	50
Taco Al Carbon w/red-chile tomatillo salsa (w/o rice, beans, or condiments)	890	19	5	2565	124	4	34
Create Your Own Combo: Chicken Tostada, Chicken Soft Taco, black beans (no rice)	580	19	8	2000	65	13	41
Grilled Fish Tacos w/creamy red sauce w/black beans only, no rice	780	34	11	1770	65	16	56

Fajita Suggestions:

served w/black beans, guacamole, 2 tortillas, red salsa (no rice, cheese, sour cream):

	Calories	Fat (g)	Sat Fat (g)	Sodium (mg)	Carbohydrates (g)	Fiber (g)	Protein (g)
Chicken Fajita Grill w/El Diablo veggies	850	30	5	2365	85	16	55
w/o tortillas	610	26	3	1765	47	16	49
Grilled Veg w/Mushrooms Fajita	770	29	5	2275	106	20	25
w/o tortillas	530	21	3	1675	68	20	19

Caveat:

- Quit the "Clean Plate Club" and refrain from finishing the whole meal. Knowing the outrageously high nutritional count for these menu items might help:

	Calories	Fat (g)	Sat Fat (g)	Sodium (mg)	Carbohydrates (g)	Fiber (g)	Protein (g)
Luncheon Little Bordurrito w/chicken and side salad w/o dressing	1010	55	13	2370	92	10	39
Dos XX® Fish Tacos w/red chili sauce w/rice and refried beans	2170	130	32	4200	183	11	67
Grande Chicken Taco Salad w/o dressing	1190	74	28	2160	80	13	53
Classic Chimichanga Chicken w/o sauce	1300	79	24	2340	103	4	46
Create own combo w/Chicken Tortilla Soup, 1 Soft Taco, Mexican rice, black beans	1030	35	14	3190	132	15	53
Border Brownie Sundae w/ice cream	1310	72	34	420	161	7	16

Orange Julius®

Tips:

- Most Premium Fruit Smoothies are blended with orange sherbet or lowfat frozen yogurt. Light Premium Fruit Smoothies are blended with ice, nonfat milk, and SPLENDA® instead. Berry Banana Squeeze and Raspberry Crush Smoothies are dairy-free.

- Stick with small sizes. Large-size Julius® Fruit Drinks and soda have *double* the calories (a medium contains 25-33% more). The medium Light Fruit Smoothies have roughly *twice* as many calories as the small (three times more in the large)!

- For more nutrition information, go to OrangeJulius.com.

Suggestions:

	Calories	Fat (g)	Sat+Trans Fat (g)	Sodium (mg)	Carbohydrates (g)	Fiber (g)	Protein (g)
Light Premium Fruit Smoothies, small:							
Strawberry or Pineapple	115	0	0	50	28	2	1
Berry Pom or Tropical	135	0	0	50	34	2	1
Julius® Fruit Drinks, small:							
Orange, Peach, or Pineapple	235	0	0	30	62	1	0
Mango or Pomegranate	255	0	0	35	69	1	0
Lemon, Strawberry, or Raspberry	290	0	0	35	78	1	0
Premium Fruit Smoothies, small:							
Raspberry Crush	160	0	0	0	41	4	1
Berry Banana Squeeze	220	0	0	10	55	2	0
Mango Passion	230	0	0	110	54	1	5
Peaches/Cream or Pomegranate/Berries	245	0	0	105	60	1	5
Chicken Fajita Pita	370	11	4	1190	49	7	21
Steak Fajita Pita	400	14	5	1210	51	6	23
Grilled Chicken Sandwich	370	16	3	810	32	1	24

Caveats:

- Topped hot dogs are not "Top Dogs." A simple Relish Dog (with relish, chopped onions, and brown mustard) has 420 calories and 27g fat). The Triple Cheese Dog has 540 calories and 38g fat.

- Stick with the Fajita Pitas (listed above). The other Pitas contain an average of 455 calories and 24g fat. The Iron Grilled Sandwiches have an average of 560 calories!

- Say no to Nachos. The regular order has 540 calories while an order of Prime Nachos contains 690 calories.

- Think before you drink. The other Julius® Fruit Drinks (not listed above) contain 5-14g fat (mostly saturated fats) and range from 340-700 calories. The highest is the Cool Mocha. The Fruit Smoothies not listed above, range from 270-370 calories.

Outback Steakhouse®

Tips:

- Think different. Consider pairing the appetizer portion of tuna or shrimp with some steamed veggies. Or sharing the Mediterranean Chicken Flatbread.

- Pick veggies for your sides. For just 50-100 calories, choose from Fresh Green beans, Steamed Veggies, Grilled Asparagus, or Broccoli. Just be sure to request "no butter."

- For more information, go to OutbackSteakhouse.com.

Suggestions:

	Calories	Fat (g)	Sat+Trans Fat (g)	Sodium (mg)	Carbohydrates (g)	Fiber (g)	Protein (g)
Seared Ahi Tuna, small	360	24	3	2565	24	2	16
Grilled Shrimp on the Barbie	290	17	3	520	7	2	26
Mediterranean Chicken Flatbread (share!)	690	37	13	2050	53	4	40
Aussie Chicken Cobb Salad, grilled	510	27	12	935	17	3	49
w/Tangy Tomato dressing	620	27	12	1390	44	4	50
Meal Suggestions* (see note below):							
Simply Grilled Tilapia w/steamed veggies	320	8	3	2005	13	7	46
8oz Mahi w/rice garnish & steamed veggies	390	12	6	1040	19	8	51
Grilled Chicken on Barbie w/mixed veggies	400	8	3	885	21	7	58
6oz Sirloin w/broccoli, Tangy tomato salad	400	11	6	550	30	7	46
2 Lobster Tails w/broccoli, tomato salad	410	8	2	960	32	8	52
Grilled Chicken Sandwich w/broccoli	440	12	5	700	43	6	40
5oz Filet & Grilled Shrimp w/broccoli	480	26	9	870	17	6	45
7oz Salmon w/Seasonal Veggies	490	27	6	665	14	7	43

* Request "no butter" on veggies and "no croutons" on salad

Caveats:

- Onions are outrageous! The Bloomin' Onion® has 1965 calories, 160g fat. A cup of Creamy Onion Soup has 330 calories and 25g fat while French Onion Soup has 465 calories and 30g fat.

- Skip these veggies. The (side) Wedge Salad adds another 430 calories, 46g fat. A small cup of Potato Soup has 410 calories, 24g fat (30% more in the bowl). And, the Spinach Artichoke Dip appetizer contains 1140 calories and 77g fat in an order!

- Caution with the dressing. The Tangy Tomato dressing doesn't add many calories to the Aussie Cobb salad (above); the other dressings nearly double the calories of a salad!

- If you must have a burger, select the Outbacker Burger at 600 calories - the other burgers contain more than 1000 calories!

- Size matters. While the 6oz Outback Special® Steak has 250 calories (13g fat), a 20oz Porterhouse Steak contains 1010 cals!

P.F. Chang's®

Tips:

- Share. Online nutrition information is "per serving." Then there are notations that appetizers contain 4-6 servings, entrées serve 2-4 people and big bowl of soups contain 5 servings. I know... confusing. All nutrition info below is per *total portion served*.

- Follow the same recommendations as mentioned with PeiWei® (P.F. Chang's is the parent company) to reduce fat and calories.

- For more nutrition information, go to PFChangs.com.

Suggestions:

	Calories	Fat (g)	Sat Fat (g)	Sodium (mg)	Carbohydrates (g)	Fiber (g)	Protein (g)
Soup, Sides & Starters:							
Hot and Sour Soup, cup	80	3	1	1000	9	0	5
Egg Drop Soup, cup	60	3	0	640	8	0	1
Shanghai Cucumbers, small side	60	3	0	1115	5	2	3
Spinach Stir-Fried w/garlic, small side	80	4	2	450	8	5	6
Garlic Snap Peas, small side	100	3	0	160	10	3	3
Vegetable Dumplings, steamed	270	0	0	480	48	0	12
Pot Sticker Sauce, 2oz	50	2	0	610	7	0	1
Lunch Bowls (add choice of soup above):							
Buddha's Feast, stir-fried on brown rice	580	12	2	2100	96	10	22
Asian Grilled Salmon on brown rice	640	12	2	1150	88	6	44
Entrées (add choice of rice below):							
Cantonese Shrimp	430	20	4	1900	20	4	42
Asian Grilled Salmon w/asparagus	690	12	4	1430	76	2	64
Vegetarian Fried Rice	920	20	4	2760	152	4	20
Lo Mein with Shrimp	680	18	3	3340	90	6	36
Singapore Street Noodles	900	18	3	3470	126	9	33
Rice: White Rice steamed	220	0	0	0	49	1	4
Brown Rice steamed	190	2	0	0	40	3	4

Caveats:

- Many dishes sound lean, but are not (rice not included, unless noted):

Norwegian Salmon steamed w/ginger	660	38	6	1210	24	6	62
Ginger Chicken with Broccoli	820	33	6	4370	54	6	84
Moo Goo Gai Pan	740	39	6	2470	39	3	54
Beef with Broccoli	870	36	9	4719	63	6	72
Beef A La Sichuan	910	36	9	3250	75	3	66
Chengdu Spiced Lamb	710	36	9	2220	33	3	69
Almond & Cashew Chicken on rice, lunch	1120	42	6	4170	132	6	50

- Share dessert or order a mini (160-300 calories). Check this out:

Mini Great Wall	160	7	3	150	22	1	2
The Great Wall of Chocolate™	1532	54	18	1065	183	9	12

Panda Express®

Tips:

• Panda's Wok Smart™ menu includes entrées with 250 calories or less per single serving. Don't forget to add in your side.

• Order the Panda Bowl (one entrée plus a side of mixed veggies, steamed rice, fried rice, or chow mein). The Mixed Veggies are considerably lower in calories and fat (refer to caveat below). Two and three entrée meals are also offered - choose wisely.

• For more nutrition information, go to PandaExpress.com.

Suggestions:

	Calories	Fat (g)	Sat+Trans Fat (g)	Sodium (mg)	Carbohydrates (g)	Fiber (g)	Protein (g)
Fortune Cookie, 1	30	2	0	8	7	0	1
Mixed Veggies, entrée	35	0	0	260	7	3	2
Mixed Veggie, side	70	<1	0	530	13	5	4
Hot & Sour Soup	100	4	<1	930	12	1	4
Veggie Spring Roll, 2	160	7	1	540	22	4	4
Broccoli Beef, entrée	130	4	1	710	13	3	10
String Bean Chicken Breast, entrée	170	7	2	740	13	3	15
Garlic Lover's Chicken Breast, entrée	180	7	2	790	12	2	17
Kobari™ Beef, entrée	210	7	2	840	20	2	15
Potato Chicken, entrée	220	11	2	780	19	3	11
Mushroom Chicken, entrée	220	13	3	760	9	1	17

Caveats:

• A side of rice or noodles (chow mein) is large:

Steamed Rice, side	380	0	0	0	86	0	7
Chow Mein, side	500	23	4	980	61	4	18
Fried Rice, side	530	16	3	820	82	1	12

• While there are many Wok Smart™ entrées (listed above), the others range from 260-690 calories! Here are some:

King Pao Chicken	280	18	4	800	12	2	18
Mandarin Chicken	310	16	4	740	8	0	34
Eggplant & Tofu	310	24	4	570	20	3	7
Honey Walnut Shrimp	370	23	4	470	27	2	14
Sweet & Sour Chicken Breast	380	17	3	320	40	1	15
Orange Chicken	420	21	4	620	43	0	15
Beijing Beef™	690	40	8	890	57	4	26

• Count the extras:

Sweet & Sour Sauce, 1.8oz	70	0	0	115	21	0	0
Mandarin Sauce, 1.8oz	160	0	0	340	40	0	0
Chicken Egg Roll, 1	200	12	4	390	16	2	8
Chicken Potsticker, 3	220	11	3	280	23	1	7
Cream Cheese Rangoon, 3	190	8	5	180	24	2	5

Panera Bread®

Tips:

• If you want a muffin, order the muffie (a smaller version with 220-320 calories). Muffins have 440-590 calories.

• Sandwiches, salads, and soups are served with your choice of baguette (180 calories), potato chips (160 calories), Baked Lays® chips (130 calories), or an apple (80 calories).

• "You Pick Two" allows choice of two: cup of soup, half sandwich, and half salad. This is often a healthier option than a full sandwich (full sandwiches have 600-990 calories).

• For full portions, multiply the info for the half sandwiches and salads by two. (Soup bowls are 1½ X more than a cup).

• For more nutrition information, go to PaneraBread.com.

Breakfast Suggestions:

	Calories	Fat (g)	Sat+Trans Fat (g)	Sodium (mg)	Carbohydrates (g)	Fiber (g)	Protein (g)
Breakfast Power Sandwich	340	15	8	820	31	4	23
Egg & Cheese on Ciabatta	390	15	7	710	43	2	19
Asiago Cheese Bagel SW w/egg, cheese	480	18	11	900	54	2	24
Jalapeno & Cheddar Bagel w/smoked ham	500	17	9	1290	57	2	28
Strawberry Granola Parfait	310	11	4	100	44	3	9

"You Pick Two" Suggestions:

	Calories	Fat (g)	Sat+Trans Fat (g)	Sodium (mg)	Carbohydrates (g)	Fiber (g)	Protein (g)
Cup of Soup: Lowfat Chicken Noodle	80	2	1	960	15	2	6
Lowfat Garden Vegetable w/pesto	100	4	1	620	18	8	3
Vegetarian Black Bean	170	2	1	880	35	6	9
½ Sandwich: Turkey Breast on Country	210	2	0	820	33	2	16
Tuna Salad on Honey Wheat	260	8	2	580	33	3	14
Smoked Ham & Swiss on Rye	290	8	5	930	32	2	22
Mediterranean Veggie	300	6	2	700	48	5	11
Smokehouse Turkey® Panini	360	13	6	1250	34	2	26
Napa Almond Chicken Salad Sandwich	340	13	2	600	45	2	15
Bacon Turkey Bravo®	400	14	5	1400	42	2	26
½ Salad: Classic Cafe Salad	80	5	1	140	9	2	1
Thai Chopped Chicken Salad	200	7	1	670	18	2	17
Asian Sesame Chicken Salad	200	10	2	410	15	2	15
BBQ Chopped Chicken Salad	250	11	2	380	25	3	16
Light Ranch, Thai or Asian vinaigrette, ½	40	2	1	190	4	0	0

Caveat:

• Most bakery goods (bagels, cookies, and pastries) contain about 350-500 calories. Those that are higher include: Bear Claw (550 calories), Chocolate Chip Scone (610 calories), Cinnamon Roll (630), Cobblestone (650), and Pecan Roll (740 calories).

Papa John's® Pizza

Tips:

• While the Thin Crust pizza has fewer calories and carbs, the fat content is higher than the original crust pizza.

• The Spinach Alfredo sounds high-fat, but it's not.

• Both the Crushed Pepper and the Special Seasoning packets have negligible calories, but the Special Seasoning packet contains 410mg sodium.

• For more nutrition information, go to PapaJohns.com.

Suggestions, per slice:

	Calories	Fat (g)	Sat+Trans Fat (g)	Sodium (mg)	Carbohydrates (g)	Fiber (g)	Protein (g)
Garden Fresh Pizza, large, original crust	280	9	4	700	39	2	11
large, thin crust	220	11	4	360	24	2	8
medium, original crust	200	7	3	500	27	2	8
Spinach Alfredo, large, original crust	280	10	5	690	36	1	11
large, thin crust	220	12	5	350	21	1	8
medium, original crust	200	8	4	500	26	1	8
Cheese, large, original crust	290	10	5	720	37	2	11
large, thin crust	230	12	5	380	22	1	9
medium, original crust	210	8	4	530	26	1	8
Hawaiian BBQ Chicken, original crust	350	12	5	1030	46	2	15
large, thin crust	290	13	5	690	31	1	13
medium, original crust	250	8	4	740	33	1	11

Caveats:

• John's Pizza (sausage, pepperoni, and a six-cheese blend) is the highest calorie pizza on the menu. One large original crust slice contains 410 calories and 21g fat. The other specialty pizzas range from 330-380 calories per original crust large slice - but a bit higher in fat than the ones listed above under Suggestions.

• Add on 95 calories for just one Cheesestick, 150 calories for one Breadstick, and 170 calories for one Garlic Parmesan Breadstick. The Pizza Sauce (at 20 calories per container) or Cheese Sauce (40 calories) are both far better choices for dipping than the 150 calorie Special Garlic dip.

• Desserts (Applepie or Cinnapie) contain 120-140 calories per stick.

• Wings contain 85-95 calories (and 6g fat) for just one. A better choice might be the Chicken Strip for 65 calories and 3g fat for each strip. If you need to dip, choose the buffalo sauce (15 calories) or BBQ sauce (45 calories). The other dips (just one tiny container) contain 100-160 calories.

Papa Murphy's® Take 'N' Bake Pizza

Tips:

- The deLite Pizzas are described as "cracker thin." Because of the thinner crust, they are *proportionately* lower in carbs, but higher in fat than the original crust.
- For more nutrition information, go to PapaMurphys.com

Suggestions (average per slice):

	Calories	Fat (g)	Sat+Trans Fat (g)	Sodium (mg)	Carbohydrates (g)	Fiber (g)	Protein (g)
Cheese, deLite crust, large slice	140	7	4	200	13	0	7
Original crust, medium slice	220	9	5	520	24	0	10
Original crust, large slice	240	10	5	570	26	0	11
Hawaiian or any Veggie, deLite Crust, lg	160	7	4	280	15	0	8
Original crust, medium slice	240	8	4	450	22	0	9
Original crust, large slice	265	10	6	620	30	0	13
Other Varieties (other than those listed under caveats):							
deLite crust, large slice	175	9	4	390	14	0	10
Original crust, medium slice	260	11	6	640	25	0	13
Original crust, large slice	290	13	6	720	29	0	13
Salads w/o dressing or croutons, ½ portion:							
Caesar	50	2	1	120	4	3	4
Garden	100	6	3	230	8	3	6
Italian Salad	130	9	4	370	7	3	7
Club Salad	140	8	4	480	6	3	12
Chicken Caesar	140	6	3	500	4	2	18
Low-calorie Italian Dressing, ½ pkt	15	<1	0	330	1	0	0

Caveats:

- Stuffed Pizza, Calzones, and Lasagna are higher in calories:

	Calories	Fat (g)	Sat+Trans Fat (g)	Sodium (mg)	Carbohydrates (g)	Fiber (g)	Protein (g)
Lasagna, ⅛	335	19	10	700	26	2	18
Calzone, ⅛ slice of family size or 1/6 slice of large size (w/o marinara sauce):							
Vegetarian (avg)	390	15	8	920	45	2	18
Other varieties (avg)	440	19	9	1090	46	1	22

- All the extras add up (dips and toppings extra):

	Calories	Fat (g)	Sat+Trans Fat (g)	Sodium (mg)	Carbohydrates (g)	Fiber (g)	Protein (g)
Cheesy Bread, 2 slices, ⅛	220	7	3	480	31	0	7
Marinara sauce, 1 small cup	10	0	0	60	2	0	0
Dessert Pizza, ⅛ pie (avg)	250	6	2	340	43	0	2
Cream Cheese Frosting, ⅛	45	3	2	40	4	0	0
Cookie Dough w/chocolate chips, ⅛ tub	175	11	5	220	34	1	2

- Highest calorie pizza slices include All Meat, Chicken Bacon Ranch, Cowboy, Meat, Murphy's Combo, Gourmet Classic Italian, Papa-Roni, and Papa's Favorite. Each have about 40% more calories and more than 50% more fat than a Cheese Pizza. So, if a cheese slice contains 200 calories and 10g fat, one of these meat pizza slices will have about 280 calories and 15g fat.

Pei Wei® Asian Diner

Tips:

- Share a meal. Online nutrition info is "per serving" with a note of two servings per order. Information below is per *full order*.

- Order the brown rice (instead of white) for a nutritional boost. About two cups of rice are served (340 calories for brown, 400 calories for white). Fried rice has twice as many calories.

- Request "stock velvet." The chef will cook the protein in vegetable broth, rather than oil (a 60-520 calorie savings) though the chef doesn't recommend this for beef dishes.

- Shrimp dishes, generally, contain the least fat and calories. Chicken and beef are often comparable. Interestingly, "vegetables & tofu" are generally highest in calories and fat.

- Most dishes contain large amounts of protein. Dilute calories and boost nutritional value by requesting more veggies. Do this by ordering "beef *and* vegetables," "chicken *and* vegetables"...

- Ask the chef for specific guidance with your dish. "Light oil" and "light sauce" may also be helpful to reduce calories.

- For more nutrition information, go to PeiWei.com

Suggestions:

	Calories	Fat (g)	Sat+Trans Fat (g)	Sodium (mg)	Carbohydrates (g)	Fiber (g)	Protein (g)
Soup, 6 fl oz: Thai Wonton	110	6	2	1030	5	1	10
Hot & Sour	190	8	2	1640	12	2	16
Japanese Teriyaki Bowl w/white rice							
and shrimp (stock velveted)	980	16	3	2860	156	6	40
Dan Dan Noodles w/chicken	780	20	5	3180	106	6	42
Signature Dish (w/o rice), request stock velveted:							
Thai Dynamite w/shrimp	320	16	3	1340	22	2	26
Honey Seared Chicken	660	16	3	860	74	2	48
Ginger Broccoli w/shrimp	440	20	3	2800	32	4	32
Sweet & Sour Chicken	500	6	1	860	70	2	46
Pei Wei Spicy w/shrimp	640	16	3	1560	94	4	26
Sesame Chicken	640	24	2	2820	52	4	50
Mongolian Chicken	920	27	4	2340	114	8	60
Brown Rice	340	3	0	0	74	6	8
White Rice	400	0	0	0	88	2	8

Caveats:

- Noodle & Rice Bowls range from 780-1580 calories, while Signature Dishes with rice add up to 660-1720 calories.

- Salads with dressing contain 780-1120 calories (and 48-50g fat).

Perkin's®

Tips:

• Lighten it up. Request Eggbeaters® for omelettes and scrambled eggs. Ask for sugar-free syrup for pancakes.

• Request fruit instead of fries with the sandwiches to save 530 calories! The Fruit Cup has 40 while Fries contain 570 calories.

• Split an entrée. Most complete meals (including the salads) contain more than 1000 calories.

• Go mini. Mini cookies contain about 80 calories (versus 320 in the regular); mini muffins have an average of 95 calories (550 in the regular Mammoth Muffins).

• Think "No-Sugar-Added (NSA)." A slice of NSA Wildberry Pie contains 360 calories (vs an average of 565 in the other fruit pies and 765 in the cream pies). The NSA Blueberry Muffin has 360 calories while the other Mammoth Muffins have about 550.

• For more nutrition info, go to PerkinsRestaurants.com.

Suggestions:

	Calories	Fat (g)	Sat+Trans Fat (g)	Sodium (mg)	Carbohydrates (g)	Fiber (g)	Protein (g)
Border Gr'd Chicken Omelette w/toast, fruit	400	8	2	1290	43	5	38
Short Stack Pancakes, 3 w/o butter, syrup	410	15	5	1250	57	0	12
sugar-free syrup	25	0	0	95	6	0	0
Florence Benedict w/fruit	420	11	5	1250	47	3	35
Mini Muffins (avg)	95	4	1	110	12	1	2
Energizer Wrap w/salsa & fruit cup	680	19	7	2560	77	7	51
Salmon Dijon w/rice and veggies	660	32	7	1080	46	3	48
Island Tilapia w/rice and broccoli	450	6	2	1060	50	5	50
Top Sirloin w/baked potato, butter, broc, roll	770	34	13	470	67	8	50
Sauteed Spinach or Asparagus (avg)	60	4	<1	45	4	2	3
Steamed Broccoli w/o butter	80	5	4	50	6	3	3
Carrots, Mashed Potatoes or Corn (avg)	140	8	2	270	17	2	2
Blueberry Muffin, No-Sugar-Added	360	18	3	540	60	15	9
Wildberry Pie slice, No-Sugar-Added	360	15	6	440	50	5	7

Caveats:

• Most complete breakfast meals are over the top. Here's the rundown for some full breakfasts (including butter & syrup):

Benedicts w/hashbrowns, fruit (avg)	1350	69	26	3770	140	9	45
Omelettes w/hashbrowns, pancakes	1770	80	27	4630	205	9	59

• A plain Hamburger and fries contain 1060 calories and 62g fat. Want to guess the calories in the other burgers? More than 1200 calories. The Tangler contains 1500 calories and 100g fat!

Piccadilly®

Tips:

• For more nutrition information, go to Piccadilly.com.

Suggestions, a la carte:

	Calories	Fat (g)	Sat+Trans Fat (g)	Sodium (mg)	Carbohydrates (g)	Fiber (g)	Protein (g)
Soup (8oz) and Salads w/o dressing:							
Tomato, Cucumber, & Onion Salad	40	0	0	575	10	1	1
Vegetable Soup	45	0	0	555	9	2	2
Picadilly Fruit Salad	70	0	2	10	18	2	1
Spinach Salad	95	5	1	185	7	3	7
Chicken Noodle or Tomato Mac Soup	105	1	0	930	21	1	4
Spiced Beets	145	0	0	945	34	3	1
Watermelon	170	1	0	5	43	2	3
Entrées: Salmon Pattie	230	9	3	390	24	1	13
Chicken & Dumplings	285	10	4	900	7	0	39
Chicken Teriyaki w/Polynesian rice	660	16	6	2340	79	3	48
Turkey & Dressing	375	14	2	2345	43	3	21
Ham Steak	105	6	1	850	1	0	12
Parmesan Crusted Tilapia	350	9	4	760	27	2	41
Mediterranean Style Tilapia	240	8	2	950	8	3	36
Tilapia w/shrimp cream sauce	280	6	3	210	10	1	46
Chicken Florentine	465	9	3	2105	44	5	52
Blackened Boneless Chicken Breast	295	14	8	195	3	1	40
Sides:							
Green Beans	35	2	1	925	5	1	1
Greens, Turnip w/diced turnip	60	2	1	635	11	4	2
Black Beans & Rice	80	0	0	675	17	2	2
Buttered Okra	80	6	4	385	6	2	2
Yellow Squash & Zucchini	85	5	3	410	11	2	1
Buttered Baby Carrots	85	6	4	570	8	3	1
Broccoli Florets	90	7	4	535	6	2	3
French Style Baked Yellow Squash	95	4	2	385	14	2	3
Baby Lima Beans	105	6	4	495	10	3	3
Mashed Potatoes	115	4	2	175	19	2	2
Green Bean Supreme	115	7	1	575	16	2	1
Black-Eyed Peas	195	2	1	730	32	5	12
Roasted New Potatoes	200	7	1	515	31	4	4
Bread: Soft Roll	210	8	3	340	30	1	6
Mexican Corn Bread	215	13	2	350	20	2	4

Caveat:

• These are shocking - especially the chicken:

	Calories	Fat (g)	Sat+Trans Fat (g)	Sodium (mg)	Carbohydrates (g)	Fiber (g)	Protein (g)
Italian Boneless Chicken Breast	820	62	10	3995	25	0	41
Chocolate Cream Pie	695	48	22	330	66	3	5
Red Velvet Cake	835	54	10	380	83	1	6

Pizza Hut®

Tips:

- Some stores offer Fit 'n Delicious® Pizzas (listed below) prepared on a multi-grain crust. Nutritionally, it contains about the same calories, carbs, and fiber as the Thin 'N Crispy®, but with fewer fat grams.

- A large slice of Thin'N Crispy has about 60 calories fewer calories than a slice of Hand Tossed pizza (about 30 calories savings per slice when ordering the medium pizza).

- Choose lean toppings. The leanest pizzas are listed below. If you want more protein, select just one choice (sausage or pepperoni) rather than many (e.g. Meat Lover's®). The Meat Lover's® pizzas contain about 100 calories more per slice than those listed below.

- For more nutrition information, go to PizzaHut.com.

Fit 'n Delicious® Suggestions:

Per medium slice:

	Calories	Fat (g)	Sat+Trans Fat (g)	Sodium (mg)	Carbohydrates (g)	Fiber (g)	Protein (g)
Chicken, Onion & Green Pepper	180	5	2	510	23	1	11
Chicken, Mushroom & Jalapeno	170	5	2	720	22	1	11
Ham, Red Onion & Mushroom	160	5	2	550	23	1	8
Ham, Pineapple & Red Tomato	160	5	2	550	24	1	7
Green Pepper, Onion & Tomato	150	4	2	400	24	2	6
Tomato, Mushroom & Jalapeno	150	4	2	610	23	2	6

Other Suggestions:

Cheese, Ham & Pineapple, Veggie Lover's®, or Pepperoni & Mushroom (avg/slice):

	Calories	Fat (g)	Sat+Trans Fat (g)	Sodium (mg)	Carbohydrates (g)	Fiber (g)	Protein (g)
Thin 'N Crispy®, medium	180	7	4	540	23	1	9
Hand-Tossed, medium	210	7	4	540	27	1	10
Thin 'N Crispy®, large	250	10	5	730	30	1	11
Hand-Tossed, large	300	10	5	800	39	2	14

Pepperoni, Italian Sausage & Mushroom, or Hawaiian Luau (avg/slice):

	Calories	Fat (g)	Sat+Trans Fat (g)	Sodium (mg)	Carbohydrates (g)	Fiber (g)	Protein (g)
Thin 'N Crispy®, medium	210	10	4	615	22	1	9
Hand-Tossed, medium	235	10	5	610	26	1	11
Thin 'N Crispy®, large	290	14	6	840	30	1	13
Hand-Tossed, large	340	14	6	890	39	2	15

Caveats:

- A large slice of Pan Pizza or Stuffed Crust Pizza contains 40 calories (and 3-5g extra fat) *more* than a large slice of Hand-Tossed - 100 calories more than a Thin'N Crispy® slice.

- Go Veggie. Meat Lover's® Personal Pan Pizza contains 830 calories and 46g fat; Veggie Lover's® has 550 calories, 20g fat.

Pollo Tropical®

Tips:

• For a smaller meal, opt for a bowl of Caribbean Chicken Soup (240 calories) or one of the regular-size TropiChop® meals listed below (330-580 calories).

• For a larger meal (600-700 calories), select a complete meal (from below) consisting of chicken on the grill and two sides. But, skip the 90 calorie roll accompaniment.

• Spice it up with salsa. Whether regular or spicy, it's 5 calories or less per plastic cup. Guacamole has just 45 calories a serving.

• For more nutrition information, go to PolloTropical.com.

Suggestions:

	Calories	Fat (g)	Sat+Trans Fat (g)	Sodium (mg)	Carbohydrates (g)	Fiber (g)	Protein (g)
Caribbean Chicken Soup, small or ½ large	120	2	0	650	21	3	9
Guava Pork BBQ Sandwich	460	14	5	550	52	3	32
Chicken on the Grill:							
¼ Dark Chicken w/o skin	180	9	3	250	0	0	24
¼ White Chicken w/o skin	230	7	2	510	0	0	41
Boneless Chicken Breasts, 2	230	4	1	330	0	0	51
Sides, regular:							
Balsamic Tomatoes	170	13	2	1240	13	3	2
Black Beans	200	6	1	860	40	15	14
Red Beans	240	4	1	1080	39	12	13
Yellow Rice w/vegetables	240	4	1	620	48	3	5
Kernel Corn	240	7	2	40	37	10	6
Boild Yuca w/o mojo	260	0	0	640	67	4	1
TropiChop® meals, regular size:							
Chicken w/yellow rice & veggies	330	5	1	780	51	3	23
Chicken w/white rice & black beans	530	10	2	1460	90	10	31
Vegetarian	580	12	3	1200	110	16	18
Pork w/yellow rice & veggies	490	18	6	930	54	4	30
Flan	210	9	5	550	26	0	8

Caveats:

• Take the skin off the chicken to save about 100 calories from fat.

• The highest calorie item on the menu is a salad! The Caribbean Chicken Cobb Salad has 1190 calories and 55g fat. Next highest item is the Fajitas at 1130 calories and 58g fat.

• Sweet sauces (such as BBQ, Pineapple Rum, and Sweet & Sour Sauce) have about 50 calories per mini container, while Mojo has 80. Curry Mustard and Cilantro Garlic average 155 calories!

• Desserts (except flan) and TropiChillers® average 320 calories.

Popeyes®

Tips:

- Popeyes® serves mostly fried chicken. Naked Tenders (chicken strips) are seasoned and fried, but not breaded so they absorb less fat than the chicken pieces.
- More nutrition information is available at Popeyes.com.

Suggestions:

	Calories	Fat (g)	Sat+Trans Fat (g)	Sodium (mg)	Carbohydrates (g)	Fiber (g)	Protein (g)
Naked Tenders, 3 pieces	220	10	4	720	2	0	30
Louisiana Travelers, 6 piece nuggets	230	14	7	350	14	1	11
Corn on the Cob, 1 ear	190	2	<1	0	37	4	6
Mashed Potatoes, regular	110	4	2	590	18	1	3
Green Beans, regular	40	2	0	420	6	2	2
Cajun Rice, regular	170	5	2	530	25	1	7

Caveats:

- Both the mild and spicy varieties have about the same calories and grams of fat, though the mild is slightly higher in sodium:

Chicken Leg, mild	160	9	4	460	5	1	14
Chicken Wing, mild	210	14	4	610	8	1	13
Chicken Thigh, mild	280	21	8	640	7	1	14
Chicken Breast, mild	440	27	12	1330	16	2	35

- Since fried chicken is high in calories and fat, feel free to remove the breading and skin before eating. I won't tell Mom.

- Don't dip. Cocktail Sauce has 30 calories and the Spicy BBQ sauce has 45. But, Ranch, Spicy Honey Mustard, and Tartar Sauces contain 100-150 calories each.

- Combos could easily be over 1000 calories since it includes a regular side (70-310 calories), biscuit (260 calories and 15g fat), and regular drink (230 calories).

- Food is fried in a mix of beef tallow, partially hydrogenated beef tallow, and partially hydrogenated soybean oil - all contribute to the higher amounts of saturated fat.

- Red Beans & Rice sounds like a healthy side, but a regular serving contains 230 calories and 14g fat (4g saturated fat). Cole Slaw is right up there with 220 calories and 15g fat. That's about as much as the regular order of Cajun Fries with 260 calories and 14g fat - or the Onion Rings (6) at 280 calories and 19g fat.

- Desserts (pies and cheesecake) contain 280-410 calories each.

Potbelly™ Sandwich Shop

Tips:

- Stick with the Skinny or the Original sandwiches. Order the multigrain wheat bread to double the fiber content.

- Add low-calorie stuff (lettuce, mustard, onion, tomato, and pickles). Ordering cheese, mayo, hot peppers, and oil will add 230-380 calories to a sandwich!

- For more information, go to Potbelly.com.

Suggestions:

	Calories	Fat (g)	Sat+Trans Fat (g)	Sodium (mg)	Carbohydrates (g)	Fiber (g)	Protein (g)
Irish Oatmeal w/brown sugar & raisins	230	1	0	15	55	3	3
Egg & American Cheese on thin-cut bread	410	20	8	950	39	3	19
Bowl Soup: Garden Vegetable Soup	105	0	0	1100	24	3	3
Chicken Noodle Soup	140	2	0	1645	17	0	10
Salads w/o dressing:							
Farmhouse Vegetarian Salad	200	12	7	480	9	4	13
Chickpea Veggie Salad w/bleu cheese	280	13	7	705	23	7	17
Chicken Salad Salad	460	22	5	650	47	7	22
Uptown Vegetarian Salad	400	22	7	460	40	9	11
Uptown Grilled Chicken Salad	510	25	8	1065	42	9	28
Farmhouse Grilled Chicken Salad	435	24	11	1505	11	4	39
Nonfat Vinaigrette	50	0	0	400	12	0	0
Sandwich, multigrain w/o cheese or any toppings:							
SKINNY T-K-Y	270	4	0	1050	41	4	20
SKINNY Ham	305	8	2	1270	39	4	20
SKINNY Little Tuna	355	11	1	760	40	1	26
ORIGINAL Turkey Breast	395	5	1	1550	57	6	29
ORIGINAL Roast Beef	405	6	2	1480	55	6	31
ORIGINAL Smoked Ham	445	12	3	1885	54	6	29
ORIGINAL Grilled Chicken	445	12	3	1885	54	3	29
Mayo on ORIGINAL or SKINNY, Add:	100	1	2	70	0	0	0
Hot Peppers	50	5	1	420	2	0	0
Oil	25	3	0	0	0	0	0

Caveats:

- Avoid the BIG sandwiches. They range from 560-1305 calories - not counting mayo, cheese, or any other topping!

- Get the dressings on the side. Except for the Nonfat Vinaigrette, they have 250-365 calories.

- Sweet tooth? Choose the Mini Oatmeal Chocolate Chip Cookie (100 calories); other desserts have 435-550 calories. Smoothies, Shakes, and Malts average 470, 655, and 775 calories respectively.

Qdoba®

Tips:

• Go Naked. Naked Burritos® and Naked Taco Salads™ contain everything in the burritos and taco salads, without a tortilla or tortilla bowl. Fat-free Picante Ranch Dressing is offered.

• Make leaner choices. Skip the rice and chips. Say no to cheese and ground beef. Opt for pork (it's the leanest protein option).

• Pile on the pico or salsa for low-calorie flavor.

• Use Qdoba's online nutrition calculator at Qdoba.com.

Suggestions:

	Calories	Fat (g)	Sat+Trans Fat (g)	Sodium (mg)	Carbohydrates (g)	Fiber (g)	Protein (g)
Taco Base: Crispy Taco Shells, 3	180	9	0	75	24	3	0
Soft Tortillas, 3	270	6	3	600	45	0	6
Burrito Base: Large Flour Tortilla	300	7	3	750	50	3	8
Naked Salad Base: Lettuce only	15	0	0	10	3	2	1
Fat-Free Picante Ranch dressing	45	0	0	540	11	1	0
Cilantro Lime dressing	90	8	1	490	6	1	0
Main Ingredient: Pulled Pork	160	5	2	390	10	0	19
Shredded Beef	190	8	4	560	5	0	24
Grilled Chicken	190	10	3	540	1	0	25
Grilled Veggies & Guacamole	190	15	2	400	12	6	2
Additions: Beans for burrito (avg)	200	2	0	370	35	17	12
Beans for tacos and salads (avg)	135	0	0	240	21	10	7
Pico de Gallo or Salsa (avg)	15	0	0	300	3	1	<1
Mango Salsa	30	0	0	95	7	1	0
Roasted Chili Corn	60	<1	0	135	11	1	1
Tortilla Soup w/pork and salsa	155	6	2	1040	13	2	11
10" Breakfast Burrito w/potato, egg, pico	455	19	5	910	53	4	20

Caveats:

• Avoid the higher calorie additions. On a burrito, ground beef adds 240 calories, rice adds another 330, cheese adds 180, and sour cream adds 60 calories.

• Share the quesadilla and nachos. The Quesadilla with just cheese contains 740 calories and 43g fat. Nachos with only Queso adds up to 750 calories and 42g fat. To calculate the other additions, refer to the burrito ingredients above. So, a quesadilla with cheese and pork contains about 930 calories.

• Control the chips. A small basket contains 280 calories and 13g fat (there's twice as much in the large). Add another 190 calories for the queso and 170 calories in the guacamole. The empty taco shell, used for the salads, contains 390 calories and 22g fat.

Quizno's®

Tips:

• Skimp on the dressing and cheese. All small Subs and Torpedoes™ include about 100 calories of dressing (and sometimes as much as 210 calories). Cheese adds another 45-110 calories. Why not request the dressing on the side?

• Think small, very small. Flatbread Sammies (260-395 calories) and Bullets (385-505 calories) have fewer calories - though many are very high in fat due to added cheese and dressing.

• Small salads are roughly half the size of the regular-size.

• For more nutrition information, go to Quiznos.com.

Suggestions:

	Calories	Fat (g)	Sat+Trans Fat (g)	Sodium (mg)	Carbohydrates (g)	Fiber (g)	Protein (g)
Subs: Honey Bourbon Chicken, small	320	6	3	790	48	4	16
regular size	530	10	5	1370	78	6	29
Turkey Ranch & Swiss, small	420	18	5	1140	44	4	20
The Traditional, small	430	20	7	1260	43	4	21
Harvest Chicken Sub, small	370	11	3	880	54	4	17
Torpedo™: Pesto Turkey	690	22	5	2100	94	5	31
Bullets™: Pesto Turkey	380	13	3	1250	48	3	18
Flatbread Sammies: Cantina Chicken	280	7	2	640	36	2	12
Roadhouse Steak	270	6	1	1060	39	1	14
Veggie	340	20	5	740	29	3	9
Fresh Farmers Market Salads, reg-size w/o dressing:							
Harvest Chicken	220	6	2	415	33	4	11
Chicken Caesar	130	5	4	640	6	2	19
Cobb	260	12	7	730	5	2	19
Mediterranean Chicken	180	7	4	1010	13	4	25
Fat-Free Balsamic Vinaigrette	130	0	0	750	29	0	0
Acai Vinaigrette	230	17	3	425	15	0	1

Caveats:

• While Quizno's® promotes many subs are under 500 calories, most didn't end up on the suggested list because the fat content is very high (due to dressing and cheese)!

• Even the small isn't so small. Small subs average 570 calories and 31g fat - but can be as high as 770 calories and 47g fat (Double Cheese Cheesesteak). Except for one Torpedo™ above, the rest have 825-980 calories. The Sammies not listed contain almost 340-395 calories and 19⁺g fat (even the Veggie is high)!

• Since the small-size is so high in calories, save calories by sharing a regular-size sub. Surprisingly, the large size often has more than *twice* the fat and calories of the small size.

Red Lobster®

Tips:

• All fresh fish is available in half-portions (or luncheon size). "Lighthouse Menu" items are half-portions and simply prepared.

• For more nutrition information, go to RedLobster.com.

Suggestions:

	Calories	Fat (g)	Sat+Trans Fat (g)	Sodium (mg)	Carbohydrates (g)	Fiber (g)	Protein (g)
Garden Salad w/o dressing	90	3	0	105	13	na	na
Balsamic Vinaigrette, 1oz	80	6	1	190	4	na	na
Shrimp Cocktail w/cocktail sauce	120	<1	0	580	9	na	na
Manhattan Clam Chowder, bowl	160	2	1	1420	25	na	na
Lobster, 1¼# steamed	230	2	0	840	0	na	na
Lighthouse Salmon w/fresh broccoli	270	9	2	310	6	na	na
Lighthouse Tilapia w/fresh broccoli	210	3	1	230	9	na	na
Lighthouse Rainbow Trout w/broccoli	220	10	3	380	6	na	na
Garlic-Grilled Jumbo Shrimp	370	9	2	2160	40	na	na
Grilled Scallops, Shrimp & Chicken, dinner	600	13	3	3190	42	na	na
Maple-Glazed Chicken, luncheon portion	410	7	2	1430	55	na	na
Rock Lobster Tail	90	1	0	490	0	na	na
Snow Crab Legs, 1#	180	2	0	1580	0	na	na
Fish, oven-broiled, dinner	320	2	0	470	10	na	na
lunch	150	1	0	150	3	na	na
Broiled Seafood Platter	300	10	3	1880	9	na	na
Fresh Asparagus, seasonal	60	3	2	270	5	na	na
Fresh Broccoli	45	<1	0	200	6	na	na
Wild Rice Pilaf	180	3	1	650	34	na	na
Home-Style Mashed Potatoes	210	10	6	620	27	na	na
Baked Potato	220	1	0	730	47	na	na
Fresh Fish, lunch/half portion: Sole	140	2	0	860	6	na	na
Cod, Corvina, Haddock, Halibut, Perch,							
Monchong, Red Rockfish, Walleye (avg)	180	2	0	470	7	na	na
Flounder, Grouper, Lake Whitefish, Tilapia,							
Mahi Mahi, Snapper, Tuna, Wahoo (avg)	210	2	0	330	7	na	na
Barramundi, Pompano, Rainbow Trout,							
Salmon, Sea Bass (avg)	240	6	2	340	6	na	na

Caveats:

• Boiled/Steamed Lobster and Crab are naturally low in fat and calories. Resist dipping heavily - each cup of melted butter contains 350 calories and 38g of fat.

• Count on 150 calories (8g fat) for each Cheddar Bay Biscuit - before the butter is added.

• The Traditional Lobserita® contains 890 calories!

Red Robin®

Tips:

• Make it simple, such as the sandwiches listed below...request no mayo, dressing, cheese, fried egg, or crispy onion straw topping.

• Add a fruit or vegetable for a side (instead of French Fries at 435 calories and 18g fat).

• For more nutrition information, go to RedRobin.com.

Suggestions:	Calories	Fat (g)	Sat+Trans Fat (g)	Sodium (mg)	Carbohydrates (g)	Fiber (g)	Protein (g)
Simply Grilled Chicken, plain	410	7	na	1020	51	2	37
Keep It Simple Burger, plain	570	24	na	990	51	2	37
Garden Burger w/dijon spread	480	13	na	1755	74	5	9
Vegan Boca® Burger w/dijon spread	460	11	na	1870	62	10	36
Grilled Turkey Burger, plain	500	22	na	720	49	2	29
Grilled Salmon Burger w/dijon sauce	570	22	na	1405	52	2	32
Sides: Steamed Broccoli	30	0	na	30	6	3	3
Melon Wedge	60	0	na	30	15	2	2
Simply Grilled Chicken Salad w/o dressing	555	21	na	980	45	7	47
add balsamic vinaigrette or light ranch, 2oz	100	10	na	515	5	0	0

Caveats:

• Some menu items with chicken sound lean, but are not. These include Whiskey River BBQ Chicken Wrap (1120 calories and 62g fat), Southwest Grilled Chicken Salad (855 calories and 52g fat), or Southwest Chicken Pasta (1170 calories and 46g fat).

• The Mountain High Mudd Pie has 1370 calories and 61g fat!

Rita's®

Tips:

• For more nutrition information, go to RitasIce.com.

Suggestions:	Calories	Fat (g)	Sat+Trans Fat (g)	Sodium (mg)	Carbohydrates (g)	Fiber (g)	Protein (g)
Italian Ice, kids	200	0	0	20	50	0	0
Sugar-Free Ice, regular	130	0	0	35	46	0	0
Custard, kids	230	12	8	150	28	0	4
Slenderita™, kids	160	0	0	180	34	1	6

Caveats:

• A *regular*-size of any of the other items ranges from 390 calories (Gelati w/Italian Ice) to 780 calories for the Ritaccino™.

Romano's Macaroni Grill®

Tips:

- The website doesn't include fat content; numbers below were calculated using a commonly used scientific formula.
- Most entrées, not discussed below, range from 800-1200 calories.
- For more nutrition information, go to MacaroniGrill.com

Suggestions:

	Calories	Fat (g)	Sat+Trans Fat (g)	Sodium (mg)	Carbohydrates (g)	Fiber (g)	Protein (g)
Warm Spinach & Shrimp Salad	340	11	5	1210	17	6	43
Grilled Chicken Spiedini w/sides	490	26	3	1140	24	10	39
Jumbo Shrimp Spiedini w/sides	300	10	3	960	22	9	31
Pollo Caprese, as served	550	14	5	1660	45	5	60
Pan-Seared Branzino w/sides	570	34	3	920	29	5	37
Build Your Own Pasta:							
Pasta (capellini, regatoni, spaghetti), avg	340	5	1	320	67	4	8
Pomodoro (tomato basil)	190	13	1	860	15	4	4
Arrabbiata (spicy red sauce)	230	14	2	820	21	4	5
Broccoli, mushrooms, spinach or tomatoes	5-25	0	0	0 - 80	2	1	1
Shrimp	180	14	1	360	0	0	13
Roasted Chicken	290	17	2	560	3	0	31

Lunch Combination Suggestions:

	Calories	Fat (g)	Sat+Trans Fat (g)	Sodium (mg)	Carbohydrates (g)	Fiber (g)	Protein (g)
Caesar Salad w/dressing, side	110	10	2	190	3	2	3
Fresh Greens w/dressing, side	80	7	1	70	3	1	2
Sausage & Kale Soup	200	12	3	1010	13	5	10
Roasted Turkey Sandwich, half	310	14	5	960	26	2	19
Carmela's Chicken	410	11	6	760	55	4	22
Whole Wheat Fettuccine	430	14	5	670	45	9	32
Capellini Pomodoro	440	24	1	860	48	6	7

Caveats:

- Peasant bread and olive oil is served with every meal.

	Calories	Fat (g)	Sat+Trans Fat (g)	Sodium (mg)	Carbohydrates (g)	Fiber (g)	Protein (g)
Peasant Bread, loaf	480	8	0	2150	89	4	8
Olive Oil, 1Tbsp	120	14	2	0	0	0	0

- Check out these calorie shockers:

	Calories	Fat (g)	Sat+Trans Fat (g)	Sodium (mg)	Carbohydrates (g)	Fiber (g)	Protein (g)
Bibb & Blue Salad w/dressing	680	56	15	2070	22	4	22
Spicy Herb-Roasted Mussels, tapas	1240	72	12	2750	92	5	57
Parmesan Fries	800	55	19	1730	61	4	16
Mama's Trio	1530	91	34	3600	96	9	82

- Flatbreads and Pizzas range from 840 (Margherita) to 1230 (Smoky Shrimp) calories. Therefore, count on about 100 calories per piece.

Round Table Pizza®

Tips:

- Total fat was not available online. Suggestions, below, were evaluated based on total calories and saturated fats.

- For more nutrition information, go to RoundTablePizza.com.

Suggestions:

	Calories	Fat (g)	Sat+Trans Fat (g)	Sodium (mg)	Carbohydrates (g)	Fiber (g)	Protein (g)
Salad w/o dressing or croutons, individual or ½ family size:							
Garden salad	45	na	0	100	7	na	na
Caesar salad	60	na	1	170	5	na	na
Artisan Flatbread, ¼ indiv or ⅛ family (avg)	225	na	4	510	21	na	na
RT Veggie Sandwich	630	na	11	1740	65	na	na
Large Original Crust Pizza Slice (avg):							
Geneviere's Garden Delight or Hawaiian	220	na	4	550	25	na	na
Cheese	230	na	5	500	24	na	na
Gourmet Veggie	240	na	5	620	26	na	na
Large Thin Crust Pizza Slice (avg):							
Geneviere's Garden Delight or Hawaiian	185	na	4	525	20	na	na
Cheese	190	na	5	420	18	na	na
Gourmet Veggie	200	na	5	540	20	na	na
Large Pan Crust Pizza Slice (avg):							
Geneviere's Garden Delight or Hawaiian	300	na	5	715	40	na	na
Cheese	300	na	6	670	25	na	na
Gourmet Veggie	320	na	5	810	41	na	na

Caveats:

- Choose your dip carefully. While the pizza sauce has just 30 calories per 2oz container, the creamy garlic/ranch dipping sauce has 200 calories! Ouch!

- Before you slice, consider that a full loaf of the garlic bread contains 420 calories. Garlic Bread with cheese has 600 calories. Garlic Twists contain 170 calories each.

- Interestingly, all menu items are in a narrow calorie range of 710-990 calories. Here are the averages:

	Calories	Fat (g)	Sat+Trans Fat (g)	Sodium (mg)	Carbohydrates (g)	Fiber (g)	Protein (g)
Sandwiches, other than Veggie	740	na	14	2020	58	na	na
Pastas, individual portion or ½ family	860	na	18	2165	71	na	na
Individual Flatbread, whole (avg all)	895	na	14	2025	84	na	na
Pizzas varieties not listed above:							
Original Crust Pizza, 3 slices	830	na	17	2120	80	na	na
Pan Crust Pizzas, 2 slices	720	na	14	1740	80	na	na

- Reconsider dessert:

	Calories	Fat (g)	Sat+Trans Fat (g)	Sodium (mg)	Carbohydrates (g)	Fiber (g)	Protein (g)
Dessert Pizza	210	na	2	250	32	na	na
Cinnamon Twists	180	na	0	290	34	na	na

Rubio's®

Tips:

• Look for HealthMex® Tacos and Burritos. All the items have less than 30% of the calories from fat.

• Choose grilled seafood like wild salmon, ono, or shrimp.

• Make special requests. Hold the cheese, sour cream, chipotle, or white sauce to save about 100 calories *each*. Use salsa instead (just 5 calories). Request "No-Fried" Pinto Beans or Black Beans instead of Chips (150 calories fewer). Ask for salsa on your salad instead of dressing. Tasty-good and few calories.

• Stick with the corn tortilla. Nutrition information for tacos (below) is with corn tortillas. When prepared with flour tortillas, add another 50 calories and 5g fat (subtract 2g fiber) per taco.

• Tacos can be ordered Single or as a Two Taco Plate with pinto beans *and chips*. Instead, request beans (pinto or black) *and rice* instead to save 140-150 calories and 12-13g fat per plate.

• For more nutrition information, go to Rubios.com.

Suggestions:

	Calories	Fat (g)	Sat Fat (g)	Sodium (mg)	Carbohydrates (g)	Fiber (g)	Protein (g)
Chicken Tortilla Soup, a la carte	200	6	3	1340	24	3	13
Tacos on corn tortillas w/o chips:							
HealthMex® Grilled Ono Taco	150	2	0	90	21	3	13
two taco plate w/beans and rice	530	7	2	1180	89	15	30
Chile-Lime Wild Salmon or Grilled Ono	230	9	2	215	26	4	13
two taco plate w/beans and rice	700	21	4	980	97	17	30
Health-Mex® Grilled Chicken Taco	130	1	0	340	22	3	10
two taco plate w/beans and rice	490	5	1	1230	89	16	24
Classic Grilled Steak Taco	200	8	3	340	22	4	12
two taco plate w/beans and rice	620	18	6	1230	91	16	28
Classic Grilled Chicken Taco	250	12	4	380	23	4	13
Street Taco Plate, 3 tacos w/black beans & rice:							
w/chicken	480	9	2	1110	67	11	33
w/carnitas or steak, avg	505	14	4	1080	66	10	29
HealthMex® Burritos on whole wheat tortilla w/chips:							
w/grilled ono	560	12	3	1550	74	9	40
w/grilled veggie	490	9	3	1260	80	11	13
w/grilled chicken	490	9	3	1260	80	11	13
Balsamic & Roasted Veggie Salad	310	11	4	950	29	7	20
Balsamic Vinaigrette, 1oz	45	3	1	190	4	0	0

Caveat:

• Some plates are huge! Consider these approximate calories: Quesadilla (1200), Nachos (1300), Cabo Plate (1400 calories).

Ruby Tuesday®

Tips:

- Look on the menu for "Fit & Trim" (F&T) meals which are under 700 calories (when served as described on menu). The luncheon ("Petite Plate") F&T portions are smaller than the dinner F&T plates. Cut calories and fat further by choosing a side other than mashed potatoes.

- For more nutrition information, go to RubyTuesday.com.

Lunch Suggestions (served as described on menu):

	Calories	Fat (g)	Sat+Trans Fat (g)	Sodium (mg)	Carbohydrates (g)	Fiber (g)	Protein (g)
White Bean Chicken Chili only	230	8	na	1420	29	8	16
Petite F&T Spaghetti Squash Marinara	180	9	na	665	17	5	5
Petite F&T Grilled Chicken Salad only	355	13	na	1005	26	5	33
add Balsamic Vinaigrette dressing	40	2	na	530	5	0	0
Petite F&T Zucchini Cakes meal	430	22	na	1385	49	6	9
Petite F&T Sliced Sirloin meal	395	24	na	995	19	4	27
Petite F&T Chicken Fresco meal	430	25	na	1205	25	4	29
Petite F&T Jumbo Shrimp Scampi meal	370	25	na	1095	23	6	17
Petite F&T Grilled Salmon meal	465	32	na	655	24	6	25

Dinner Suggestions (served as described on menu):

	Calories	Fat (g)	Sat+Trans Fat (g)	Sodium (mg)	Carbohydrates (g)	Fiber (g)	Protein (g)
F&T Barbeque Grilled Chicken meal	585	23	na	1655	41	6	55
F&T Jumbo Lump Crab Cake meal	395	29	na	1035	20	4	17
F&T Creole Catch meal	560	29	na	815	34	8	47
F&T Grilled Salmon meal	660	39	na	805	34	8	46
F&T Petite Sirloin meal	610	36	na	1630	31	6	43
Veggie Options:							
Baked Potato, plain	260	2	na	105	52	10	9
Creamy Mashed Cauliflower	140	8	na	715	14	3	3
White Cheddar Mashed Potatoes	225	14	na	430	21	2	3
Fresh Grilled Zucchini	40	2	na	560	4	1	1
Fresh Grilled Green Beans	45	2	na	385	5	2	2
Fresh Steamed Broccoli	85	6	na	185	7	3	3
Sugar Snap Peas	115	6	na	165	8	3	3
Roasted Spaghetti Squash	55	3	na	70	6	2	1
Desserts: Berry Good Yogurt Parfait	160	3	na	125	28	1	5

Caveats:

- The burgers are big. The Turkey Burger contains 700 calories and Ruby's Classic Burger has 930 calories; the rest are over 1000 calories (not counting the fries). Even the Grilled Chicken Sandwich alone contains 925 calories.

- Watch the extras. Each Garlic Cheese Biscuit contains 110 calories and 5g fat. And, each cupcake has about 300 calories.

Ruth's Chris® Steak House

Tips:

• No nutrition information is available at RuthsChris.com. Information below was obtained from interviews with restaurant managers.

• Choose one treat. Most menu items are both high in fat and calories. If you choose to indulge, consider indulging with just one menu item, then trim the calories from all the other menu items you order.

Suggestions:

• Appetizers - Crabtini or Shrimp Cocktail (order both with cocktail sauce rather than the much-higher-calorie remoulade sauce). The Crabtini is tossed in a vinaigrette but can be made without, if requested. The Ahi Tuna is a 6oz portion.

• Salads - Most salads are filled with high-fat/high-calorie ingredients such as fried onion, pecans, cheese, bacon, and croutons. Best bets include the Steakhouse Salad (ask for it without croutons) or Sliced Tomato and Onion (cut out or limit the bleu cheese crumbles). Each rounded tablespoon of blue cheese contains 50 calories and 5g fat. Ask for the oil-based vinaigrette dressing on the side.

• Signature Steaks - All the steaks are USDA Prime Cut; these tend to be the most marbled (highest in fat and calories). The smaller and leaner cuts include the Petite Filet (8oz) or Filet with Broiled Shrimp (Filet is 6oz). Clarified butter is poured on all steaks prior to serving - ask for without.

• Entrées - Fresh Lobster is very low in calories and fat. A small lobster may only have 200 calories and a few grams of fat. That is, as long as you don't dip it in butter. Each tablespoon of butter contains 100 calories and 12g fat!

• Vegetables - All of the potato options are prepared with a lot of added fat. Leanest veggie choices are Broccoli (without the cheese sauce) or Fresh Asparagus (request without the hollandaise sauce). Baby Spinach or Broiled Tomatoes are moderate in added fats, but can be requested without.

• Dessert - Order the Fresh Seasonal Berries (skip the cream) or ask for a single scoop of Sorbet.

Caveat:

• It's easy to overindulge at Ruth's Chris® Steak House if you order a full meal without any of the special requests noted above. But the staff is very accommodating.

Schlotzsky's®

Tips:

• Select a small sandwich. Many are in the 340-500 calorie range; the medium-size sandwiches contain 50% more calories.

• Combo meals include chips and a fountain drink. Baked chips contain 140 calories, Original Kettle Chips have 190 calories, and the other chips have 220 calories. The combo with a small sandwich also comes with a small fountain drink (250 calories).

• Almost every sandwich contains cheese, mayo, and/or dressing. To cut calories and fat, ask for these to be omitted. Light mayo, mustard, and fat-free spicy ranch dressing are lower calorie options.

• For more nutrition information, go to Schlotzsky.com.

Suggestions:

	Calories	Fat (g)	Sat+Trans Fat (g)	Sodium (mg)	Carbohydrates (g)	Fiber (g)	Protein (g)
Salad w/o dressing: Garden	45	1	0	390	11	3	2
Pasta Salad	70	3	0	290	12	1	0
Grilled Chicken Caesar Salad	505	17	6	1760	42	2	49
Fat-Free Raspberry Vinaigrette, 6 Tbsp	100	0	0	225	23	0	0
Small Sandwich: Fresh Veggie	340	10	5	750	50	4	14
Chicken Breast	340	3	0	1480	53	3	22
Smoked Turkey Breast	350	6	1	1070	52	2	20
Turkey & Guacamole	370	8	1	1115	52	5	21
Chipotle Chicken	370	7	1	1175	51	3	21
Dijon Chicken	380	7	1	1660	53	5	25
Chicken & Pesto	380	8	1	1260	51	3	23
Angus Corned Beef	390	9	2	1560	53	4	27
Homestyle Tuna	400	12	2	1065	48	3	25
Sante Fe Chicken	430	10	4	1590	54	3	27
8" Pizza: Fresh Veggie	570	20	7	1480	75	4	23
BBQ Chicken & Jalapeno	705	16	8	2590	109	3	41
Grilled Chicken & Pesto	650	19	7	1880	76	4	42
Wrap: Asian Chicken Wrap	540	11	2	2270	81	4	29
Homestyle Tuna Wrap	480	18	4	1390	55	4	26
Parmesan Chicken Caesar Wrap	600	23	7	2035	62	5	38
Soup, cup (multiply X 1.5 for bowl):							
Vegetable Beef Soup	60	3	1	570	7	1	3
Chicken Noodle Soup	85	2	1	1020	12	1	6
Vegetarian Vegetable Soup	100	1	0	1040	22	5	2
Cookie (average for all flavors)	160	8	4	170	22	1	2

Caveat:

• The medium-size Deluxe Original-Style Sandwich contains 960 calories and 46g fat. The Carrot Cake has 720 calories, 42g fat.

Sizzler®

Tips:

• Pair one of the leaner proteins listed below with steamed broccoli or vegetable medley.

• At the salad bar, fill up with veggies, fruits, and beans. Lettuce has just 10 calories per cup. Plain veggies add 5 calories per spoon, while beans add another 25 calories. And, fruit contains just 15-30 calories per spoon.

• Soups are generally low in calories. Except for the creamy soups such as Broccoli Cheese or Clam Chowder, most soups average about 80 calories per 6oz bowl.

• For more nutrition information, go to Sizzler.com

Suggestions:

	Calories	Fat (g)	Sat+Trans Fat (g)	Sodium (mg)	Carbohydrates (g)	Fiber (g)	Protein (g)
Salad, 1 small serving spoon:							
Cucumber Tomato Salad	25	1	0	370	4	1	1
Three Bean Salad	25	1	0	70	5	1	1
Asian Chopped Salad	30	2	0	15	3	1	1
Spinach Cranberry Salad	45	3	0	25	6	1	1
Carrot Raisin Salad	100	6	1	70	12	2	1
Waldorf Salad	130	8	1	45	16	2	1
Dressing, 1oz or 2Tbsp:							
Lowfat Italian dressing	40	3	1	270	3	0	0
Balsamic Vinaigrette or Italian, avg	85	8	1	315	3	0	0
Petite Steak, 6oz	300	16	6	820	1	0	35
Grilled Salmon w/rice pilaf	530	20	6	915	40	1	47
Grilled Shrimp Skewers w/rice pilaf	460	16	7	1210	42	2	33
Hibachi Chicken, single	180	4	0	1130	7	0	28
Hibachi Chicken, double	340	8	0	1900	9	0	56
Lemon Chicken, single	170	6	0	900	0	0	28
Lemon Chicken, double	320	10	0	1670	0	0	56
Sides: Broccoli	50	0	0	40	7	3	4
Vegetable Medley	80	4	3	70	9	3	3
Sweet Potato mashed	115	1	0	510	25	4	2
Sweet Potato whole	210	0	0	80	47	8	5
Baked Potato	265	4	1	15	51	4	6
Rice Pilaf	225	4	2	740	39	1	5
Fresh Baked Roll	160	1	0	65	33	0	5

Caveats:

• Think before you pour. Most salad dressings contain more than 100 calories per two tablespoons.

• Big Appetite Trio is BIG indeed! It has 1100 calories, 50g fat!

Smokey Bones Bar & Grill

Tips:

- For more nutrition information, go to SmokeyBones.com.

Suggestions (a la carte):	Calories	Fat (g)	Sat+Trans Fat (g)	Sodium (mg)	Carbohydrates (g)	Fiber (g)	Protein (g)
Soup: Brunswick Stew, bowl	260	7	2	1500	43	7	9
Roasted Chicken Noodle Soup, bowl	110	4	1	1430	15	1	3
$5 Lunch Salads w/o dressing:							
Steak & Spinach	480	19	8	2560	37	4	38
Nutty Grilled Chicken	510	20	6	810	56	4	23
Southwest Chicken	470	22	7	1260	44	8	33
Entrées only:							
Pork Tenderloin w/teriyaki	320	8	3	1160	10	0	48
w/spicy chipotle	330	8	3	660	14	0	47
7oz Top Sirloin w/mushroom sauce	420	14	4	610	4	1	66
Sliced Smoked Turkey Breast	420	20	6	2360	23	2	38
Hand Pulled Pork	480	30	9	630	16	1	34
Salmon w/teriyaki (instead of butter)	570	37	9	1090	9	0	45
Smokehouse Chicken	680	33	14	2420	28	2	68
Sides: Steamed Broccoli	70	4	3	110	5	3	3
Cinnamon Apples	200	4	<1	90	43	3	0
Mashed Potatoes w/gravy	200	8	3	1110	30	3	0
BBQ Baked Beans	260	1	0	670	55	4	5
Fire Roasted Corn	280	15	9	410	32	4	5
Sandwich: Pulled Pork Sammy	560	23	8	810	54	2	31
Sweet Shots: Banana Pudding	120	3	2	160	21	0	2
Strawberry Cheesecake	190	10	6	180	16	2	4
Keylime	190	13	7	135	16	0	2
Bread Pudding	210	4	2	310	39	0	5
Chocolate Cake	250	8	4	130	46	1	2

Caveats:

- Entrée-size Salads are larger than those listed above. Nutrition info above does not include dressing (and nutrition info doesn't list them), so get dressing on the side and do the "Dip 'N Stab."

- Check these out: ½ BBQ Roasted Chicken (800 calories, 51g fat), Flatbreads (905 calories, 52g fat). Basic Nachos (1740 calories, 71g fat), Chocolate Layer Cake (1450 calories, 42g fat).

- Burgers start at 900 calories (and that's the Avocado Turkey Burger). The others have 1180-1590 calories (fries not included)!

- Those ribs will stick to your ribs...and around your waist. A full rack of ribs contains an average of 2025 calories and 149g fat!

Smoothie King®

Tips:

- Smoothies aren't light snacks. Here are the average calories of the small 20oz smoothies for each category: Trim Down (325); Shape Up (345, except for the Hulks); Stay Healthy, Get Energy, and Snack Right (390); Indulge (565); and Hulks (940). For the 32oz smoothie, multiply by 1.5 (X 2 for 40oz).

- Make it Skinny. Most smoothies are sweetened with turbinado (raw sugar) and honey. Ask for it without the turbinado and save about 100 calories. Some have just 50 calories of turbinado, while most of the Indulge Smoothies have 200 calories worth!

- For more nutrition information, go to SmoothieKing.com.

Lower-Cal Suggestions (20oz):	Calories	Fat (g)	Sat+Trans Fat (g)	Sodium (mg)	Carbohydrates (g)	Fiber (g)	Protein (g)
Slim-N-Trim Orange-Vanilla™	215	1	0	260	46	0	7
*Slim-N-Trim Vanilla™	255	1	0	260	53	3	7
*Celestial Cherry High™	260	0	0	10	64	3	1
*Coffee, Mocha	260	2	0	225	43	1	17
Cherry Picker®	275	1	0	235	66	2	4
Lean1™, strawberry	275	6	1	320	35	5	20
Lean1™, vanilla or chocolate	285	11	1	320	27	6	22
*Pineapple Pleasure®	280	0	0	20	67	3	1
*MangoFest™	285	0	0	10	72	1	0
Vanilla Shredder™	285	2	0	590	30	0	36
*Slim-N-Trim Chocolate™	300	2	0	165	57	3	15
Island Impact® or *Peach Slice™	315	0	0	105	73	1	3
Chocolate Shredder™	310	3	0	315	36	1	39
Blueberry Heaven®	325	1	0	260	73	2	7
*Island Treat®	335	0	0	10	82	6	2
*Yogurt D-Lite®	335	4	2	370	59	0	13
Raspberry Collider™	340	0	0	100	86	4	1
*Coffee, vanilla or caramel	345	1	0	235	68	0	14

   * Save 100 calories if ordered "Skinny."

Caveats:

- Bulk up or pudge up? Many of the Indulge and Hulk Smoothies are loaded with peanut butter, ice cream, and turbinado. Even Fit n' Crunchy Bowls average 440 calories and 8g fat.

- Careful. Some Smoothies offer "choice of fruit" and the calories might not be calculated into the nutrition information.

- The website offers promises of weight loss, muscle building and health yet also states, "These statements have not been evaluated by the Food and Drug Administration."

Sonic®

Tips:

- Low-Cal Diet Lime Limeade or Low-Cal Diet Cherry Limeade are tasty low-calorie options to regular soda. In addition, 1% milk is also available.
- Some of the sandwiches may not be available at every restaurant.
- For more nutrition information, go to SonicDriveIn.com.

Suggestions:

	Calories	Fat (g)	Sat+Trans Fat (g)	Sodium (mg)	Carbohydrates (g)	Fiber (g)	Protein (g)
Low-Cal Diet Limeade, medium	15	0	0	15	3	0	0
Jr. Breakfast Burrito	340	21	7	930	24	0	12
Apple Slices w/caramel dipping sauce	110	0	0	60	28	2	0
Jr. Burger	310	15	6	610	30	3	15
Grilled Chicken Wrap	390	14	4	1420	39	2	28
Grilled Chicken Sandwich w/mayo	400	19	3	960	32	3	28
Veggie Burger w/ mustard or ketchup	505	14	4	1330	76	8	19
Jr. Banana Split	200	6	5	80	35	1	2
Jr. Sundae (Oreo®, M&Ms®, others)	200	9	7	120	26	0	3
Vanilla Dish	240	13	9	150	26	0	4
Vanilla Cone	250	13	9	150	31	0	4

Caveats:

- Want dessert? Here are the stats for these regular-size sweets:

Strawberry or Pineapple Sundae, avg	425	21	15	230	54	0	6
Hot Fudge, Chocolate or Caramel Sundae	510	24	18	290	67	0	6
Banana Split	490	18	13	210	76	2	6

- Most specialty drinks are very high in calories. Check out the average number of calories for these 14oz drinks (the next size up contains about 50% more):

Limeade, small	140	0	0	30	38	0	0
Slushes, small	190	0	0	30	52	0	0
Floats/Blended Floats w/diet soda, reg	260	14	10	170	29	0	4
Iced Latte, avg all flavors, 14oz	270	8	5	130	46	0	3
Floats/Blended Floats w/soda, regular	330	14	0	170	49	0	4
CreamSlush® Treat, regular	375	15	11	175	57	0	4
Java Chillers, regular	520	24	17	300	65	0	7
Shakes, regular	540	27	19	320	67	0	8
Malts, regular	565	28	20	330	70	0	8
SONIC Blast®, regular	710	37	26	415	83	<1	11

- Avoid the combo meals. Medium-size offerings include Tator Tots (200 calories), Fries (330 calories) or Onion Rings (440 calories) plus a medium drink (160-190 calories).

Sonny's BBQ®

Tips:

• Pick the beans. Sandwiches are served with either fries (360 calories and 17g fat) or Bar-B-Q Beans (150 calories and 2g fat).

• Stick with the bun. Sandwiches are offered on either a bun or garlic bread. Choose the bun and save 160 calories and 11g fat.

• All dinners are served with two sides and choice of garlic bread or cornbread. Pick your options from the choices below.

• For more nutrition information, go to SonnysBBQ.com.

Suggestions (a la carte):

	Calories	Fat (g)	Sat+Trans Fat (g)	Sodium (mg)	Carbohydrates (g)	Fiber (g)	Protein (g)
Salads w/o dressing:							
Backyard Garden Salad	30	<1	<1	10	6	2	2
Big Salad w/Charbroiled Chicken	310	7	2	700	34	6	36
Big Salad w/Sliced Smoked Turkey	250	5	2	1060	34	6	23
Lo-Cal or Fat-free Dressings, 2Tbsp (avg)	45	1	0	300	6	0	0
Sliced Pork only, lunch	300	19	9	110	<1	0	30
dinner portion	440	29	13	160	<1	0	45
Bar-B-Q-Chicken only, ¼ chicken	270	13	10	280	0	0	38
½ chicken only	540	27	19	560	0	0	74
Charbroiled Chicken only, lunch	130	3	1	450	1	0	23
dinner portion	260	5	2	900	2	0	56
Smoked Turkey only, lunch	80	1	2	810	1	0	16
dinner portion	120	2	2	1210	2	0	23
Sides: Broccoli	40	0	0	55	8	5	5
Southern Green Beans	100	5	1	470	11	4	3
Corn on the Cob	140	2	<1	20	34	2	5
Bar-B-Q Beans	150	2	<1	640	25	5	8
Baked Potato	260	<1	<1	15	60	4	6
Baked Sweet Potato	290	<1	<1	120	68	11	7
Sauces, 2Tbsp: Mustard Bar-B-Q	25	<1	0	350	4	0	0
Mild or Smokin" Bar-B-Q	45	1	0	435	8	0	0
Sweet Bar-B-Q	60	0	0	460	14	0	0
Sandwich on bun: Smoked Turkey	280	4	4	1200	39	1	22
Catfish	360	8	5	1050	52	2	19
Charbroiled Chicken	380	6	2	1030	40	1	46
Pulled Chicken	490	17	10	740	39	1	29

Caveats:

• Both Garlic Bread (180 calories and 7g fat) and Cornbread (260 calories and 9g fat) contribute to the total calories of your dinner.

• Desserts contain about 350 calories...except for the Double Chocolate Brownie Bliss at 1470 calories! You call that bliss?

Souplantation & Sweet Tomatoes®

Tips:

• It's easy to overeat with so many choices, so plan ahead.

• Nutrition information for all menu items is available at Souplantation.com. Note: not all items are available every day.

Suggestions:

• Salad Bar - Design your own salad with plenty of fruits, veggies, and beans. To reduce excess calories, avoid cheese and creamy salad dressings.

• Tossed Salads - For 150 calories or less per cup, choose: Azteca Taco w/turkey, Field of Greens w/citrus vinaigrette, Honey Minted Fruit Toss, or Strawberry Fields w/carmelized walnuts. Others average around 215 calories, but as much as 360!

• Prepared Salads - Each of these have 120 calories or less per ½ cup: Aunt Doris' Red Pepper, Herb Thai, or Oriental Ginger Slaw; Poppyseed Coleslaw; Carrot Raisin; Mandarin Shells w/almonds; Southern Dill Potato; Southwestern Rice & Beans; Summer Barley w/black beans; Tomato Cucumber Marinade; or Sweet Marinated Vegetables. Other salads average 200 calories (but as much as 350 calories) per ½ cup serving.

• Hot Pasta - For under 250 calories (per cup) consider these: Curried Pineapple & Ginger, Oriental Noodle & Green Beans, Balsamic Vegetables, and Tuscany Sausage w/capers & olives. Others average 330 calories (the highest has 420 calories).

• Bakery - Pieces under 150 calories include: 96% Fat-Free or No-Sugar-Added Muffins; Strawberry Buttermilk, Wildly Blue Blueberry, or Tangy Lemon Muffins; Lowfat Cornbread; Bruschetta or Quattro Formaggio Focaccia. Others contain an average of 180 calories each, but some have as much as 250 calories.

• Soups at 120 calories or less include: Asian Ginger Broth, Lowfat Chicken Tortilla, Classical Minestrone, Old Fashion Vegetable, Ratatouille Provencale, Spicy Navajo Vegetable, Sweet Tomato Onion, Tomato Parmesan & Vegetables, Vegetable Medley, X-Treme Spice Vegetable Chili w/energy boost. Other soups average 220 calories.

• Desserts - For under 80 calories, select ¾ cup Sugar-Free Mousse, a small cookie, or ½ cup Fat-Free Apple Medley or Banana Royale. Count on about 100 calories in ½ cup gelatin and 150 calories in ½ cup frozen yogurt or pudding (before toppings!). Most of the other desserts (per piece or ½ cup) averages over 300 calories!

Caveats:

• The highest calorie foods include butter, bacon, sausage, cheese, cream, and nuts. Therefore, some of the highest calorie menu choices include BBQ Smokehouse w/bacon & peanuts, Buffalo Chicken, Canadian Cheese w/smoked ham Soup, Creamy Vegetable Chowder, Broccoli Alfredo, Nutty Mushroom Pasta, Spicy Italian Sausage & Peppers, Pumpkin Walnut Cobbler, French Quarter Praline Muffin, and Apple Walnut Cake.

• Watch out for the little extras. A tablespoon of flavored butter adds 90 calories.

Starbucks®

Tips:

• Order your coffee "Skinny." Your drink will be prepared with nonfat milk (2% is the standard), sugar-free syrup, and no "whip" (whipping cream).

• Customize. Ask for fewer pumps of flavoring (about 25 calories each). Typical: 2 pumps for Tall, 3 pumps for Grande, 4 pumps for Venti. Hold the whip to save 80-120 calories.

• Go short. It's not on the menu, but an 8oz short size is available just for the asking - with ⅔ the calories of the tall.

• For more nutrition information, go to Starbucks.com.

Suggestions:

	Calories	Fat (g)	Sat+Trans Fat (g)	Sodium (mg)	Carbohydrates (g)	Fiber (g)	Protein (g)
Smoothie, avg. of 3 flavors	270	3	na	na	51	6	16
Petite Lemon Square or Van. Scone, avg	130	6	na	na	19	na	1
Other Petite Sweets (avg)	180	10	na	na	22	na	1
Spinach Feta Egg White Breakfast Wrap	280	10	na	na	33	6	18
Turkey Bacon & White Cheddar SW	320	7	na	na	43	3	18
Starbucks® Perfect Oatmeal	140	3	na	na	25	4	5
nut medley topping	100	9	na	na	2	<1	2
dried fruit topping	100	0	na	na	24	2	<1
brown sugar topping	50	0	na	na	13	0	0
Roasted Vegetable Panini	350	12	na	na	48	4	13
Ham & Swiss Panini	360	9	na	na	43	2	28
Tarragon Chicken Salad Sandwich	480	13	na	na	46	6	32
Turkey & Swiss Sandwich	390	13	na	na	36	2	34
Bistro Boxes: Chicken & Hummus	270	8	na	na	29	6	16
Sesame Noodles	350	11	na	na	50	6	15
Chipotle Chicken Wraps	380	15	na	na	35	6	26
Deluxe Fruit Blend	90	0	na	na	23	2	<1
Caffe Latte, nonfat tall	100	0	na	na	15	0	10
Cappuccino, nonfat tall	60	0	na	na	9	0	6
Iced Skinny Flavored Latte	60	0	na	na	9	0	6
Iced Caffe Latte, nonfat tall	70	0	na	na	10	0	6
Skinny Flavored Latte, nonfat tall	90	0	na	na	14	0	9
Skinny Caramel Machiato, nonfat tall	100	1	na	na	16	0	8

Caveats:

• A grande Double Chocolaty Chip Frappuccino® Blended Beverage has 500 calories while the Peppermint Mocha Frappuccino® Light blended beverage has just 150 calories.

• All Bistro Boxes are under 500 calories. Except for those listed above, the other Boxes are very high in fat (45-53% of calories).

Steak 'N Shake®

Tips:

- Steak 'N Shake® is famous for its Steakburgers, but keep to the Single or just a couple of Shooters. Cheese adds 50 calories.

- Request "no Frisco sauce or mayo" on burgers to save calories.

- Order a la carte. Regular Fries contain 440 calories and 21g fat, while the 22oz soda has 170 calories.

- Cholesterol-free eggs are available for a slight upcharge.

- For more nutrition information, go to SteakNShake.com

Suggestions:

	Calories	Fat (g)	Sat+Trans Fat (g)	Sodium (mg)	Carbohydrates (g)	Fiber (g)	Protein (g)
Breakfast Shooter w/bacon	170	9	4	420	13	0	9
Perfect Start Oatmeal	340	11	1	260	57	6	7
Yogurt Parfait	210	4	3	95	38	1	7
Apple and Caramel	120	2	1	75	27	2	18
Vegetable Soup, bowl	130	3	<1	1740	24	3	3
Chicken Gumbo Soup, bowl	140	4	0	1860	22	3	7
Steakburger Shooter, plain	130	6	2	210	12	0	6
A-1, BBQ, Ketchup & Mustard (avg)	140	6	2	290	15	<1	6
Buffalo Shooter	130	7	3	380	13	0	6
Steakburger Shooter, plain w/cheese	150	8	4	349	13	9	7
Single Steakburger	280	11	5	310	30	<1	12
with cheese	330	16	8	570	31	<1	15
Grilled Chicken Sandwich	400	15	2	980	51	<1	25
Turkey Club Sandwich	420	16	4	1270	45	2	24
Grilled Chicken Salad	270	10	4	860	30	3	26
Apple Pecan Salad w/gr. chicken	330	8	1	640	39	6	21
Red. Fat Berry Balsamic Vinaigrette, 1oz	50	2	0	160	12	0	0
Lite Ranch, 1oz	70	7	1	240	<1	0	0

Caveats:

- A simple cup of Chili contains 440 calories and 24g fat (the bowl contains twice as much). Chili Deluxe has 1220 calories!

- Keep the sandwiches simple. The chicken sandwiches not mentioned above contain about 530 calories and 26g fat. Classic Melts have an average of 700 calories and 45g fat.

- Franks range from 380 calories to 620 calories for the Chili Cheese. All are very high in fat.

- Craving a milkshake? Ask for the kid's size - though it still contains around 455 calories. Fruit flavors are around 365 calories while the chocolate and nut flavors have 500-630 calories. Skip the whipped cream for a bit of a calorie savings.

Subway®

Tips:

• Skip the mayo, oil, and cheese (see the caveat below) to save about 200 calories on a 6" sub (nutrition information below doesn't contain these). Mustard is a low-calorie option.

• For more fiber, choose 9 Grain Wheat Bread (4g fiber) or Honey Oat (5g fiber) versus just 1-2g for the other choices. If you're watching calories, the 9 Grain bread has 50 fewer calories - and less carbohydrate than the Honey Oat. The Mornin'Flatbread contains 30 calories more than the 9 Grain Wheat Bread, but contains just 1g fiber.

• Want more protein? Order "Double Meat." With the selection of turkey, you'll get 9 more grams of protein for just 50 calories.

• All breakfast egg sandwiches are available with egg whites for a 40 calorie savings over whole eggs.

• For more nutrition information, go to Subway.com.

Suggestions:

	Calories	Fat (g)	Sat+Trans Fat (g)	Sodium (mg)	Carbohydrates (g)	Fiber (g)	Protein (g)
Apple Slices	35	0	0	0	9	2	0
Yogurt Dannon Light & Fit®	80	0	0	80	16	0	5
Veggie Delite®, 6" sub on 9 grain wheat	230	3	<1	310	44	5	8
on flatbread	240	5	1	450	42	3	8
Turkey &/or Ham, 6" 9 grain sub (avg)	280	4	1	820	46	5	18
on flatbread (avg)	295	7	2	965	44	3	17
Rst Beef, Chicken, or Club® 6", 9 grain (avg)	320	5	2	740	46	5	23
on flatbread (avg)	325	7	2	885	44	3	22
Sweet Onion Teriyaki, 6" sub on 9 grain	380	5	1	900	59	5	26
on flatbread	390	7	2	1050	57	3	25
Egg Muffin Melt - egg/cheese on Eng muffin	170	6	2	460	24	6	12
when ham, steak or bacon is added	200	7	3	585	25	6	14
Sunrise Melt	230	8	3	810	26	6	18
6" Omelet SW w/egg & cheese on 9 grain	360	12	5	890	44	5	19
w/ham	390	13	5	1150	45	5	24

Caveats:

• Nutrition info at Subway.com (and above) does NOT include:

Light mayonnaise, 1 Tbsp	50	5	1	100	<1	0	0
Mayonnaise, 1 Tbsp	110	12	2	80	0	0	0
Olive Oil Blend, 1 tsp	45	5	0	0	0	0	0
Cheese: Swiss	50	5	3	30	0	0	4
Cheese: other varieties	50	4	2	125	0	0	4

• At 530 calories and 30g fat, the 6" Tuna Sub is one of the highest fat subs on the menu.

T.G.I. Friday's®

Tips:

• "Right Portion, Right Price" menu items are all under 750 calories - yet, often the fat content is very high.

• Turn an appetizer into dinner. The flatbread and skewers listed below might fit your calorie budget - as long as you don't order anything else!

• For more nutrition information, go to TGIFridays.com.

Right Portion, Right Price Suggestions:

	Calories	Fat (g)	Sat+Trans Fat (g)	Sodium (mg)	Carbohydrates (g)	Fiber (g)	Protein (g)
Spinach Florentine Flatbread	410	23	10	1280	31	3	19
Japanese Hibachi Tapa-tizer Skewers:							
Black Angus Sirloin	620	18	5	1700	73	4	35
Grilled Chicken	750	20	4	3110	105	6	38
Mediterranean Tapa-tizer Skewers:							
Black Angus Sirloin	620	27	9	1360	49	4	36
Grilled Chicken	660	20	5	1570	74	4	47
Balsamic Glazed Chicken Caesar Salad	500	28	7	1870	25	5	40
Lowfat Balsamic Vinaigrette, 3oz	130	5	0	430	22	0	0
Dragonfire Chicken	670	15	5	2160	99	11	40
Dragonfire Salmon	590	23	4	2090	57	7	40
Jack Daniel's® Chicken (add choice of sides)	620	8	2	3120	79	1	62
Petite Sirloin only (add choice of sides)	370	24	11	1450	2	0	38
Broccoli	50	<1	0	370	10	5	3
Fruit Cup	80	0	0	0	19	2	0
Mandarin Oranges	100	0	0	0	25	2	0
Ginger-Lime Slaw	90	5	1	220	11	0	0
Mashed Potatoes	290	14	6	940	30	4	5
Roasted Vegetable Medley	100	6	1	490	12	3	2

Caveats:

• Some items in the moderate calorie range are very high in fat. The Shrimp Key West has 750 calories and 55g fat. Southwest Wedge Salad has 460 calories, but 38g fat!

• Almost everything else on the menu is over 1000 calories. Sizzling Chicken meals average 1100 calories. Friday's® Fusion Skewers average 1385 calories. Count on 1250 calories and 68g fat for the Baby Back Ribs. Most of the salads not mentioned above are over 1000 calories with dressing. The Turkey Burger with fries? 1230 calories and 60g fat! (But lower than the Jack Daniel's® Burger at 1360 calories and 74g fat).

• Still thinking about dessert? The Oreo® Madness contains 510 calories - the others range from 780-2020 calories.

Taco Bell®

Tips:

• Order any menu item "Fresco-style." Items are prepared without cheese or sour cream. Salsa is added instead for great flavor.

• Chicken is usually the leanest choice of meats. Choose "steak" rather than "beef" to save calories and fat.

• More nutrition information is at TacoBell.com

Suggestions:

	Calories	Fat (g)	Sat+Trans Fat (g)	Sodium (mg)	Carbohydrates (g)	Fiber (g)	Protein (g)
Crunchy Taco	170	10	4	330	12	3	8
Fresco Crunchy Taco	150	7	3	350	13	3	7
Grilled Steak Soft Taco	250	14	4	550	19	2	11
Fresco Grilled Steak Soft Taco	150	4	2	520	19	2	9
Chicken Soft Taco	180	6	3	460	18	2	14
Fresco Chicken Soft Taco	150	4	1	480	18	2	12
Soft Taco, beef	200	9	4	540	19	3	10
Fresco Soft Taco, beef	180	7	3	560	20	3	8
Burrito Supreme®, chicken	400	12	5	1060	51	7	21
Fresco Burrito Supreme®, chicken	350	8	3	1060	50	7	18
Burrito Supreme®, steak	390	13	5	1100	51	7	17
Fresco Burrito Supreme®, steak	340	8	3	1100	50	7	15
Bean Burrito	370	10	4	980	56	10	13
Fresco Bean Burrito	350	8	3	1090	56	12	13
Guacamole, side	35	3	0	85	2	1	0
Mexican Rice	120	4	0	200	20	1	2
Pintos 'n Cheese	170	6	3	580	20	8	9
Gordita Supreme®, chicken	280	10	4	410	29	2	17
Gordita Supreme®, steak	270	11	4	450	29	2	14
Gordita Nacho Cheese, chicken	270	11	2	470	30	1	15
Gordita Nacho Cheese, steak	260	11	2	510	30	1	12
Chicken Taquitos	320	11	5	770	37	3	18
Steak Taquitos	310	11	5	810	37	3	15

Caveats:

• Volcano Nachos are the highest calorie item on the Taco Bell® menu at 980 calories. And, believe it or not...the next two highest are salads: Chicken Ranch Taco Salad (910 calories) and Chipotle Steak Taco Salad (900 calories). Fiesta Taco Salad contains 770 calories - save 290 calories by omitting the fried shell.

• Think before you drink. While the 16oz sodas (small) contain around 200 calories, the small-size Fruitista Freeze® contains an average of 240 calories.

Taco Bueno®

Tips:

• Ask for Bueno Choice™ (BC) options. These menu choices will be prepared with pico de gallo instead of cheese and/or sour cream, for a savings of about 45 calories and 5g fat.

• Get black beans, rather than refried beans (at ⅓ the calories).

• Fill up with soup. A bowl of Chicken Tortilla Soup has just 240 calories (or 150 calories without the tortilla strips and cheese).

• For more nutrition information, go to TacoBueno.com.

Suggestions:

	Calories	Fat (g)	Sat+Trans Fat (g)	Sodium (mg)	Carbohydrates (g)	Fiber (g)	Protein (g)
Taco Bueno Choice™ Options:							
BC Crispy Chicken Taco	150	6	na	460	12	1	11
BC Crispy Beef Taco	170	9	na	440	12	1	10
BC Soft Chicken Taco	180	6	na	710	19	1	12
BC Chicken Fajita Taco	190	6	na	690	20	1	14
BC Soft Beef Taco	200	9	na	680	19	1	11
BC Steak Fajita Taco	210	9	na	590	21	1	13
BC Vegetarian Black Bean Burrito	440	10	na	780	71	10	15
BC Chicken Tortilla Soup, bowl	150	6	na	1380	11	2	17
Other Options: Chicken Taco Rollup™	180	7	na	540	18	1	11
Chicken Soft Taco	180	8	na	610	19	1	10
Flame-Grilled Chicken Fajita Taco	210	8	na	600	19	1	15
Black Bean Burrito	490	15	na	730	70	9	18
Breakfast: Potato Egg Breakfast Taco	230	10	na	550	24	1	9
Bacon Egg Breakfast Taco	240	13	na	690	18	1	12
Potato Egg Breakfast Burrito	460	22	na	680	47	3	17

Caveats:

• It all adds up. A small taco has about 250 calories while a burrito contains 350-770 calories. A Chilada® contains around 500 calories. Cheese Nachos add another 570 calories and 35g fat.

• Avoid the salads, unless you're willing to make some compromises. The Nacho Salads (chicken or beef) contain an average of 735 calories and 46g fat. The Chicken Taco Salad has 840 calories and 57g fat; the Beef Taco Salad has 1040 calories and 75g fat. The shell alone has 480 calories! Skip the cheese and save 80-160 calories.

• Mucho indeed! A single Muchaco has 390 calories, while the beef has 500 calories. The Mucho Nachos (chicken or beef) contain more than 1500 calories and 90g fat (that's as much fat as an entire stick of butter).

Taco Cabana®

Tips:

• Think before you combo. Combo meals provide a 20oz drink (go diet) and the choice of beans, rice, or chips. Best choices: Black Beans (80 calories, 0g fat), Borracho Beans (140 calories, 3g fat), or Rice (120 calories and <1g fat).

• For more nutrition information, go to TacoCabana.com.

Suggestions:

	Calories	Fat (g)	Sat+Trans Fat (g)	Sodium (mg)	Carbohydrates (g)	Fiber (g)	Protein (g)
Breakfast Taco (potato, bacon, chorizo), avg	215	10	4	510	21	1	10
Breakfast Burrito (potato, bacon, chorizo), avg	415	19	7	1023	44	2	19
Crispy Chicken Taco (stewed)	160	7	3	430	13	2	11
Chicken Breast Fajita Soft Taco	190	4	2	650	21	1	14
Carne Guisada Soft Taco	190	6	2	330	21	1	12
Black Bean Soft Taco	200	4	2	630	34	2	6
Steak Fajita Soft Taco	200	6	3	650	21	1	12
Chicken Soft Taco (stewed)	210	7	3	720	23	2	13
Black Bean Burrito	450	8	4	1720	82	5	14
4 Under 400 Bowls (w/o shell):							
Vegetarian Bowl w/o shell	280	15	8	760	22	4	14
Chicken Taco Bowl w/o shell	330	12	6	1500	25	4	28
Chicken Fajita Bowl w/o shell	370	8	4	1640	47	4	26
Steak Fajita Bowl w/o shell	390	11	5	1630	47	4	23
Personal-size Fajita Plates:							
Chicken Fajita meal w/borracho beans	740	20	9	2450	98	13	38
Steak Fajitas meal w/borracho beans	760	24	10	2450	98	12	34
¼ White Flameante Chicken Dinner							
w/borracho beans	800	23	8	2660	87	9	62
Carne Guisada Plate w/rice, beans, tortillas	840	28	11	1650	94	9	45

Caveats:

• Skip the shell and chips. That fried tortilla shell has 390 calories and 27g fat. A combo order of chips has 180 calories and 16g fat.

• Stick with Pico de Gallo or Salsa for flavor with negligible calories. Guacamole adds 110 calories and 9g fat while Queso adds 200 calories and 15g fat. Shredded Cheese added to a "Plate" piles on an extra 110 calories and 9g fat.

• A large flour tortilla has 240 calories. Once you stuff and roll your favorite meat into a Burrito, it contains 630 calories or more.

• Plates are huge. Super Tex-Mex Plate has 1490 calories, 76g fat.

• Cheese is fattening. While a personal Quesadilla has 710-860 calories (39-50g fat), the regular-size Quesadilla has 1250[+] cals.

Taco John's®

Tips:

• Pick the chargrilled chicken or beans. Ground beef items are always higher in calories and fat. Crunchy Chicken is over the top high!

• Cut the cheese. Order menu items without cheese to save about 20 calories on small tacos and 50-60 calories on chili, refried beans, and burritos.

• Spice it up with salsa. Two tablespoons have just 10 calories!

• For more nutrition information, go to TacoJohns.com.

Suggestions:

	Calories	Fat (g)	Sat+Trans Fat (g)	Sodium (mg)	Carbohydrates (g)	Fiber (g)	Protein (g)
Jr. Breakfast Burrito w/bacon	200	9	3	620	21	1	10
Fruit & Nut Oatmeal	280	8	0	150	51	8	8
w/o cinnamon sugar	260	8	0	150	45	6	8
Crispy Taco	170	10	4	290	11	2	9
Chicken Softshell Taco	190	6	3	680	21	1	14
Softshell Taco	220	10	5	580	23	2	11
w/o cheese	190	8	3	540	23	2	9
Chili w/o crackers	200	11	5	1130	16	4	12
w/o crackers or cheese	150	6	2	1040	16	4	9
Refried Beans w/o cheese	260	3	1	970	45	15	15
Bean Burrito	370	11	5	1090	53	7	14
w/o cheese	310	7	2	1000	52	7	11
Combination Burrito (beef and bean)	410	16	8	1120	47	5	18
Taco Burger w/o cheese	250	9	3	530	29	2	12

Caveats:

• Caution with the salad. Even the lightest salad, the Chicken Taco Salad without dressing, contains 500 calories and 27g fat. Much of the calories is in the fried shell. A portion of salad dressing adds another 70 to 140 calories. Season your salad with salsa instead.

• It all adds up. A "small" combo meal with just two Crispy Tacos, Potato Ole's®, and soda contains almost 1000 calories and 47g fat (600 from the soda and potatoes). Just one Churro adds another 200 calories and 9g fat.

• Say no to Nacho Cheese. Nachos have 380 calories and 23g fat. A side of Nacho Cheese has 110 calories and 9g fat.

• "Super" often translates to super high in calories. Regular Super Nachos contain 800 calories and 48g fat while the Super Potato Oles® have 1030 calories and 65g fat.

Taco Time®

Tips:

• For more nutrition information, go to TacoTime.com.

Suggestions (per item):

	Calories	Fat (g)	Sat+Trans Fat (g)	Sodium (mg)	Carbohydrates (g)	Fiber (g)	Protein (g)
Breakfast Burritos:							
Egg & Cheese Burrito	370	16	7	580	40	7	16
Egg & Tators Burrito	430	19	8	760	48	8	17
Egg & Chicken Burrito	470	19	8	900	49	8	26
Salads w/o dressing:							
Regular Chicken Taco	310	13	4	680	22	2	25
Chicken Tostado Delight	450	19	7	2050	35	4	30
Tacos:							
Soft Chicken Taco	360	9	5	860	40	7	28
Pork Street Taco	300	11	2	240	28	5	19
Soft Junior Taco	310	13	6	800	28	6	18
Super Soft Chicken Taco	530	16	8	2180	59	6	34
w/whole wheat tortilla	530	16	8	2160	60	10	34
Burritos:							
Crisp Pinto Beans	360	14	4	1910	47	5	13
Soft Pinto Beans	370	10	5	2100	54	10	14
Crisp Chicken	380	17	6	540	33	2	22
Soft Ground Beef	430	16	7	1090	43	8	23
Chicken & Black Bean	480	16	6	1270	54	9	30
Beef, Bean & Cheese	490	17	7	2310	55	11	26
Soft Veggie	520	17	7	2530	73	12	19
Big Juan	580	16	8	2550	70	11	34
Other Favorites:							
Chicken Enchilada	230	5	3	610	17	1	23
Refritos with chips	230	7	4	2620	29	5	11

Caveats:

• Skip the Combo. It includes a 22oz drink (220 calories) and small Mexi-Fries® (270 calories and 18g fat).

• Stay away from the Cheddar and Stuffed Fries. A small order of Cheddar Fries contains 350 calories and 25g fat. There are 320 calories and 20g fat in the small Stuffed Fries. The large order is twice as loaded in calories.

• Many of the menu items are very high in sodium, even many of the ones listed above. Be sure to balance the rest of the day with lower sodium choices.

• While all deserts contain 210-260 calories, the Crustos and Empanada contain around half the fat of the Churros.

Texas Roadhouse

Tips:

- No nutrition information is currently available at the company website. Information below is from interviews with restaurant managers.

- For detailed menu information, go to TexasRoadhouse.com.

Suggestions:

- Grilled BBQ Chicken (½ pound) and Half Oven Roasted Chicken are on the menu. Unfortunately, both of these entrées are large portions. Eat half and take the other half home for another meal. The entrées come with two sides (see below).

- Select the smaller 6oz Sirloin or Dallas Fillet® Steaks. These are raw weights and will cook to about 4½ oz. Another smaller beef option is the Sirloin Kabob (7oz raw weight).

- Grilled Salmon and Grilled Shrimp are available - just ask for the garlic lemon pepper butter sauce "on the side." Rather than dousing the entrée with the butter, dip your fork into the butter and then into the fish for a taste with every bite. FYI there are five shrimp in the Grilled Shrimp appetizer and ten shrimp in the entrée portion.

- The Grilled Chicken Salad is dressed with calorie-ladened cheese, eggs, and croutons. Feel free to order it plain - and ask for the nonfat ranch dressing.

- Opt for the BBQ Chicken Sandwich (made with a 7oz breast) instead of a half-pound burger. Feel free to substitute one of the lower-calorie sides instead of fries with a sandwich.

- Sides that are most likely lower in calories include Apple Sauce and Fresh Vegetables (ask for "no butter"). The Green Beans are prepared with bacon. Order the Baked Potato or Sweet Potato plain.

Caveats:

- Rolls are served with the meal - typically four to a table. Feel free to grab one (or none) and send the rest back.

- Don't "smother" your steak. Resist the menu suggestion to cover your steak with sauteed mushrooms, sauteed onions, and choice of brown gravy or jack cheese. Do you really need the extra calories?

- Skip the Ribs and Combo meals. Do I need to tell you why?

- Desserts are family-size. They don't call it a "Big Ol' Brownie" for nothing!

The Capital Grille®

Tips:

• All menu items are sold a la carte and portions are big (sharable).

• More nutrition information can be found at TheCapitalGrille.com.

Suggestions:

	Calories	Fat (g)	Sat+Trans Fat (g)	Sodium (mg)	Carbohydrates (g)	Fiber (g)	Protein (g)
Appetizers, add sauce listed below:							
Oysters on the half shell	100	2	<1	500	9	0	10
Shrimp Cocktail	120	<1	0	680	0	0	28
Cold Shellfish Platter, luncheon	230	3	1	1140	2	0	50
dinner portion	340	4	1	1560	11	0	65
Cocktail + Mignonette Sauce, add	65	0	0	680	15	0	1
Salads w/o dressing:							
Field Greens/Tomatoes/Herbs, luncheon	30	0	0	30	5	na	3
dinner portion	45	0	0	30	5	na	3
North Atlantic Lobster Salad, luncheon	140	3	2	540	60	0	24
Chopped Salad w/chilled shrimp, luncheon	420	12	6	580	35	8	43
Chopped Salad, dinner	300	8	5	460	70	<1	18
Vinaigrette, average, 2Tbsp (get on side)	140	14	2	80	3	0	0
Luncheon Entrées (a la carte):							
Filet Mignon, 8oz	370	21	11	490	3	0	44
8oz Sliced Filet w/onions & mushrooms	450	22	11	730	16	0	46
Lobster & Crab Stuffed Shrimp	325	20	9	1165	5	1	31
Dinner Entrées (a la carte):							
Filet Mignon, 10oz	470	26	13	590	3	0	54
Broiled Fresh Lobster, per pound	150	1	0	570	3	0	33
Sesame Seared Tuna w/ginger rice	450	3	<1	460	36	0	71
Sides (per order, though serves 2):							
Fresh Asparagus	110	7	4	160	5	na	6
Sauteed Spinach	160	5	5	1050	18	12	12
Haricots Vert w/fennel & tomatoes	120	2	<1	580	19	9	7
Mashed Potatoes, luncheon (or ⅓ dinner)	230	16	11	430	18	na	3
Desserts: Seasonal Fruit Sorbet	160	0	0	15	41	0	1
Fresh Berries in vanilla cream	200	12	7	20	17	na	5
Fresh Strawberries Capital Grille	290	10	6	85	43	na	7

Caveats:

• Some sides are outrageous. A *luncheon* side of Housemade Chips or Shoe String Fries contains 510-620 calories. A *full* order of Parmesan Truffle Fries has 950 calories and Shoe String Fries has 1870 calories! Lobster Mac 'n Cheese has 1560 calories!

• Watch the extras (butter, dressing, sauces...). Lobster contains just 150 calories per pound, but a 2oz cup of drawn butter adds 460 calories, 50g fat! A cup or crock of soup contains 440-590 calories.

The Original Pancake House®

Tips:

- Pancakes aren't]. Plain pancakes have just 290-540 calories, but the toppings can make this dish fattening (see the caveat below).

- Want meat? Choose Canadian Bacon or Ham. The other meats range from 360-530 calories.

- Choose eggs over an omelet. Two Eggs have just under 200 calories. A Veggie Omelet has 600 calories, the Cheese Omelet contains 930 calories, and The Irish Omelet has nearly 1400 calories - not counting the pancakes served with the omelets.

- Ask for nonfat milk. Oatmeal and the other cereals are served with heavy whipping cream - just one tablespoon has 50 calories of nearly pure fat (mostly saturated)! OMG!

- Find out more about the menu at OriginalPancakeHouse.com.

Suggestions:

	Calories	Fat (g)	Sat+Trans Fat (g)	Sodium (mg)	Carbohydrates (g)	Fiber (g)	Protein (g)
Eggs, 2 scrambled	180	13	5	175	2	0	12
2 poached	149	10	3	300	0	0	12
Ham	140	3	2	1020	8	0	20
Canadian Bacon	180	8	3	1600	2	0	23
Pancakes w/o butter or syrup:							
Dollar	290	7	2	820	49	2	9
Potato	305	5	1	405	57	2	8
Buckwheat	340	6	1	910	63	3	9
Buttermilk	380	9	2	1095	65	2	12
Wheat Germ	420	12	4	965	65	4	14

Caveats:

- Watch the extras. Most pancakes are served with 150 calories of butter and 140 calories of maple syrup (or other flavored syrup or compote). Request "no butter" and use the syrup sparingly. Whipped cream and chocolate syrup (on the Chocolate Chip Pancakes) adds on another 350 calories. Nearly 800 calories of pecans are added to the Pecan Pancakes or Waffles!

- Avoid the 49er Flapjacks. Even without the butter and syrup a plate contains 540 calories and 28g fat.

- Skip the "Specialties of the House." Dutch Baby contains 990 calories while the Apple Pancakes contains 1620 calories.

- Cross off the Crepes. The Fresh Fruit Crepes are the lowest in calories - at close to 500 calories and 22g fat. The others range from 580-1070 calories!

Tony Roma's®

Tips:

- More nutrition information can be found at TonyRomas.com.

Suggestions (a la carte, unless noted):

	Calories	Fat (g)	Sat+Trans Fat (g)	Sodium (mg)	Carbohydrates (g)	Fiber (g)	Protein (g)
Chicken Tortellini Soup, cup	110	6	2	495	9	na	6
Mahi, grilled or blackened (avg)	260	2	0	1395	6	1	53
Tuscan Pesto Mahi Mahi	495	24	8	1585	12	2	57
Cajun Mahi, rice, roasted vegetables	480	6	1	2265	47	6	60
Harvest Valley Chicken, rice, vegetables	620	7	1	3560	76	4	63
Mojo Chicken w/wild rice	490	4	0	3760	50	2	62
Chicken Spinach Stack w/rice	595	18	7	3910	40	2	69
Broccoli w/herb butter	145	12	5	150	6	2	3
Wild Rice Blend	145	0	0	600	32	1	5
Mashed Sweet Potatoes	145	1	0	50	32	3	1
Salads w/o dressing:							
Asian Salad w/grilled chicken	355	3	0	2010	46	5	35
Asian Salad w/grilled salmon	475	17	3	1010	45	5	35
Grilled Chicken & Fire Roasted	400	15	6	1695	15	6	41
Orchard Harvest Chop	225	8	2	580	36	3	4
Salad Dressings, 1.5oz (3Tbsp):							
Italian Fat-free	15	0	0	735	5	0	0
Apple Citrus Vinaigrette	40	0	0	450	10	0	0
Balsamic Fig Dressing	90	0	0	285	24	0	0
Balsamic Vinaigrette	90	8	1	285	6	0	0
Pulled Pork BBQ Sandwich	570	31	11	3085	46	2	25
Flat Iron Steak, 8oz	490	35	18	1395	2	0	40

Caveats:

- Skip the appetizers. The lowest calorie item is the Roasted Vegetable Tuscan Flatbread at 635 calories. The Onion Loaf has 1200 calories and Roma's Sampler has 2465 calories, 135g fat.

- Caution with the fish toppings. While the Pineapple Salsa, Mojo Glace, and Tomato Pesto Salad toppings have under 40 calories, the others are much higher. The Sweet Thai Chili Sauce has 110 calories; Kickin' Sauce, Garlic Scampi Butter, and Shrimp Piccata add another 250[+] calories.

- Rethink ribs. A full slab of Pork Ribs contains 844 calories and 38g fat while the Beef Ribs contain 2290 calories and 189g fat! A side of Barbecue Sauce has 20-30 calories per tablespoon.

- Burgers average 925 calories. Fries add another 405 calories!

- The Flat Iron Steak (above) is the lowest calorie/fat steak on the menu; skip the toppings. Both the Bacon Chimichurri and the Crispy Onion & Bistro Sauce add on about 500 calories more!

Uno® Chicago Grill

Tips:

• Make special requests. Ask for steamed vegetables without butter or sauce, salad dressing on the side, broiled instead of fried meats, no crunchy fried noodles/toppings/croutons/nuts...

• Please note, most of the nutrition information at Unos.com (and at the kiosk in the restaurant lobby) is per "serving" - with a note that menu items contain anywhere from 1.5 - 3 servings! Nutrition information below is based on the entire menu item.

Suggestions (a la carte):

	Calories	Fat (g)	Sat+Trans Fat (g)	Sodium (mg)	Carbohydrates (g)	Fiber (g)	Protein (g)
Veggie Soup	145	2	0	930	27	5	4
House Salad	180	10	2	190	20	4	4
Chopped Power Salad	540	14	3	1220	64	10	46
Chopped Honey Citrus Chicken Salad	570	29	3	1220	45	7	40
LF Blueberry Pomegranate Vinaigrette	120	6	1	220	16	0	0
8oz Sirloin	400	14	5	1320	0	0	66
Lemon Basil Salmon	480	34	5	740	0	0	42
Steamed Broccoli	70	6	1	360	5	3	3
Roasted Seasonal Vegetables	80	5	0	160	10	3	2
Seasonal Steamed Vegetables	100	7	2	90	9	3	2
Whole Grain Brown Rice	180	6	1	100	32	1	3
Veggie Burger	400	16	2	2260	44	8	26
Roasted Vegetable & Feta Wrap	420	20	6	920	26	12	22
Chicken Tikka Marsala	560	24	5	1600	48	4	46

Caveats:

• Some seemingly healthful choices are very high in fat - because of added cheese and dressings such as mayo and pesto:

Herb-Rubbed Breast of Chicken	520	42	5	1260	2	0	20
Eggplant Panini	640	46	11	1490	42	13	27
Grilled Chicken Wrap	700	40	9	1380	58	12	40
Turkey Panini	780	47	11	1830	48	14	46
Chicken Milanese	860	58	10	2240	42	6	56

• The breadstick is not included in the information above. Add:

Breadstick	210	13	4	460	18	1	6

• While the menu states an individual deep dish pizza serves *one*, the nutrition info online is per *one-third* pizza! Here are the stats for the *whole* individual-size pie:

Thin Crust Pizza: Eggplant, Spinach & Feta	870	33	11	1680	114	12	27
Cheese & Tomato Deep Dish Pizza	1740	120	36	2490	117	6	63
Chicago Classic Deep Dish Pizza	2310	165	54	4650	120	6	99
Harvest Vegetable on Five-Grain Crust	1620	102	30	1940	129	12	60

Wawa®

Tips:

• Choose Junior rolls for lower calorie sandwiches. Select roast
beef, ham, or turkey - all are the leaner meats. The meats lowest
in sodium (yet, not low sodium) include Roast Beef, then
Premium Oven Roasted Turkey. Regular Turkey has nearly
three times more sodium! Yikes!

• Nutrition calculator is
available at Wawa.com.

Suggestions:

	Calories	Fat (g)	Sat+Trans Fat (g)	Sodium (mg)	Carbohydrates (g)	Fiber (g)	Protein (g)
Breakfast Jr Hoagie w/egg	260	9	2	760	33	1	12
Breakfast Jr Ciabatta w/egg	300	8	2	760	42	1	14
Add Bacon	25	2	1	125	0	0	2
Add Turkey	40	1	0	480	2	0	6
Add Cheese (avg)	55	4	3	70	1	0	4
Pancakes w/syrup	450	10	3	510	87	1	5
Turkey, Ham or Roast Beef (avg) on:							
Junior Roll	200	3	0	750	31	1	13
Junior Ciabatta	240	2	0	750	40	1	15
Add cheese (other than American), avg	55	5	3	130	0	0	3
White Bread	260	4	0	1320	35	2	23
Kaiser Roll	290	4	1	1210	38	2	24
Whole Wheat Bread	300	5	0	1240	39	6	25
Rye Bread	300	4	0	1460	45	2	23
Shorti Roll	300	4	1	1330	43	2	24
Whole Wheat Shorti Roll	340	6	0	1170	47	4	26
Shorti Ciabatta	360	4	0	1520	55	1	27
Add cheese (other than American), avg	110	9	5	260	0	0	6
Salsa Chicken Toasted Flatbread, plain	560	19	10	1650	58	5	40
Chicken Florentine Toasted Wrap	390	16	5	1320	37	6	33
Jalapeno Turkey Toasted Wrap	400	18	5	1170	35	6	28
Southwest Turkey Toasted Wrap	420	19	6	1140	39	6	27

Caveats:

• Skip sandwiches on the Classic Roll. Not only does the bread
add another 100 calories more than the highest sandwich listed
above, there's more meat, cheese, and condiments.

• Avoid the mayo. Mayo on the smaller sandwiches adds 70
calories, but 140 on the larger sandwiches. Egg, chicken, and
tuna salad can add an extra 100-400+ calories (depending on the
size of the bread or roll) more than the leaner meat.

• Muffin mania! Muffins contains 610-800 calories and 29-41g
fat. The Cream Filled Coffee Cake Muffin is the highest.

Wendy's®

Tips:

- Ask for a substitute for the fries. This may include the Garden Side Salad, Caesar Side Salad, Apple Slices, Baked Potato and Small Chili. Great way to increase your fruit and veggie intake.

- Pour Chili on top of the plain Baked Potato for a filling meal with just 460 calories, 6g fat, 21g protein, and 12g fiber!

- Garden Sensations® Salads are available in half-size portions.

- Combo meals include medium Fries (420 calories and 21g fat) and medium Soda (240 calories).

- Go to Wendys.com for more nutrition information.

Suggestions:

	Calories	Fat (g)	Sat+Trans Fat (g)	Sodium (mg)	Carbohydrates (g)	Fiber (g)	Protein (g)
Apple Slices	40	0	0	0	9	2	0
Small Chili, no cheese or crackers	210	6	3	880	21	6	17
Cheddar Cheese, shredded	70	6	4	110	1	0	4
Saltine crackers, 2	25	<1	0	80	5	0	1
Jr. Hamburger	230	8	3	470	26	1	12
¼ Pound Single Burger	550	28	14	1270	43	2	30
Plain Baked Potato	270	0	0	25	61	7	7
Sour Cream & Chives Baked Potato	320	4	2	50	63	7	8
Buttery Best Spread, 1 packet	50	5	1	0	95	0	0
Grilled Chicken Go Wrap	260	10	4	730	25	1	19
Frosty: vanilla or chocolate (avg)	255	7	5	120	42	0	6
Ultimate Chicken Grill Sandwich	360	7	2	1110	42	2	33
Apple Pecan Chicken Salad w/o dressing	340	11	7	1150	28	5	35
half-size portion	170	6	4	580	15	3	18
Roasted Pecans, 1 packet	110	9	1	60	5	1	1
Pomegranate Vinaigrette, 1 packet	60	3	0	160	8	0	0
BLT Cobb Salad, half size w/o dressing	230	13	6	810	5	1	23
Avocado Ranch Dressing, 1 packet	100	10	2	210	2	0	1
Baja Salad, half size w/o dressing	280	17	7	840	18	6	16
Seasoned Tortilla strips, 1 packet	80	5	2	105	11	1	1
Creamy Red Jalapeno dressing, 1 packet	100	10	2	270	2	0	1
Light Classic Ranch	50	5	1	150	2	0	1

Caveat:

- Garden Sensations® Salads are chock full of fruits, vegetables, and calcium-rich cheese. Nutrition information for the accompaniments (such as nuts, croutons, tortilla strips and dressing) is provided separately - so be sure to add them into your totals. Fully loaded salads (as served) range from 510-730 calories, while half-size salads contain 330-460 calories.

WhatABurger®

Tips:

- Everything is big in Texas and that's true for the food at this Texas-based restaurant chain, as well.

- Most WhatAMeals® include medium Fries (480 calories and 27g fat) and medium Drink (300 calories).

- If you want a burger, fries, and drink, order the smaller Justaburger® kid's meal. While 760 calories with regular soda, if you select a diet beverage such as Minute Maid® Light Lemonade the meal drops to 610 calories.

- For more nutrition information, go to WhatABurger.com.

Suggestions:

	Calories	Fat (g)	Sat+Trans Fat (g)	Sodium (mg)	Carbohydrates (g)	Fiber (g)	Protein (g)
Fruit Chew	80	0	0	10	19	0	1
Pancake, 1 pancake only a la carte	180	3	1	650	35	1	5
Syrup, 1 packet	120	0	0	15	31	0	0
Egg Sandwich	310	17	5	605	25	1	12
Cinnamon Biscuit	320	14	7	640	46	1	3
Cinnamon Roll	340	9	4	390	71	3	7
Breakfast on a Bun® w/bacon	360	21	6	805	25	1	15
Taquito w/bacon & egg	380	21	7	930	27	3	17
Taquito w/potato & egg	430	23	6	870	57	3	15
Garden Salad w/o dressing	50	0	0	15	11	4	1
Grilled Chicken Salad w/o dressing	220	7	2	630	18	4	21
lowfat vinaigrette	40	2	0	885	5	0	0
fat-free ranch dressing	40	0	0	460	10	1	0
Justaburger®	290	15	5	725	26	1	13
WhatABurger Jr.®	300	15	5	730	28	1	13
Chicken Strips, 2	300	16	6	595	22	1	18
Fries, small	320	18	3	230	36	5	3
Grilled Chicken Sandwich	470	19	4	1020	49	3	27

Caveats:

- The signature WhatABurger® (even without cheese or mayo) has 620 calories and 30g fat. The Steak Sauce Double, Green Chili Double, and the Chop House Cheddar Burgers contain over 1000 calories - without the drink and fries!

- Have a sweet tooth? Cookies and Pie range from 210-250 calories. Kid's Shakes and Malts average about 500 calories and 13g fat while the medium Shakes and Malts are close to 1000 calories. Malts are about 50 calories more than the Shakes.

White Castle®

Tips:

• White Castle® is the home of tiny burgers (Sliders) - just a couple might be enough for your calorie budget.

• For more nutrition information, go to WhiteCastle.com.

Suggestions (per one Slider):	Calories	Fat (g)	Sat+Trans Fat (g)	Sodium (mg)	Carbohydrates (g)	Fiber (g)	Protein (g)
Breakfast Sliders:							
Egg Slider	130	5	2	180	12	1	8
Egg & Cheese Slider	160	7	3	320	13	1	9
Sliders:							
Original Slider®	140	6	3	360	13	1	7
Cheeseburger	170	9	5	550	15	1	8
Jalapeno Cheeseburger	160	9	5	460	14	1	8

Caveats:

• It all adds up. Sack Meal 1 contains 4 hamburgers, medium fries, and small drink - for a total of 1150 calories:

Original Sliders®, 4	560	24	12	1440	52	4	28
French Fries, medium	370	25	7	50	33	3	3
Small Drink (avg)	220	0	0	15	60	0	0

• Fish and chicken sound like better choices than ground beef, but not when they are fried. Check out these stats:

Original Slider®, 1	140	6	3	360	13	1	7
Fish Slider, 1	310	22	6	270	18	1	9
Chicken Breast Slider, 1	360	26	7	510	20	1	11

• Different isn't always better. While a medium order of French Fries has 370 calories (25g fat), an order of Sweet Potato Fries has 480 calories (30g fat), and Onion Chips have 670 calories and 50g fat. An order of six Chicken Rings contains 530 calories and 47g fat - and, that doesn't include the dip.

Dr. Jo says

Mayonnaise has 100 calories a tablespoon - and your burger or sandwich could easily have more than that! Get used to the feisty (and low-calorie) taste of mustard instead.

Wienerschnitzel®

Tips:

- Steer clear of the combos. Hot Dogs alone have between 260-620 calories! But, combos often include *two* hotdogs, plus regular Fries (300 calories), and 20oz Soda (about 250 calories w/o ice) - adding up to a grand total of 800-1300 calories per meal.

- Gobble, gobble. The Turkey Hotdogs are slightly lower in calories, saturated fat, and sodium than the Original Hot Dogs.

- Nix the Pretzel Bun. Ordering your hot dog on a Pretzel Bun adds an extra 130 calories more than the standard bun.

- Only limited nutrition information is available at Wienerschnitzel.com.

Suggestions:

	Calories	Fat (g)	Sat Fat (g)	Sodium (mg)	Carbohydrates (g)	Fiber (g)	Protein (g)
Turkey Plain Dog, standard bun	260	na	3	610	28	na	na
w/mustard, relish, kraut or "Deluxe" (avg)	260	na	3	760	30	na	na
Turkey Stadium Dog, standard bun	270	na	3	760	31	na	na
Turkey Chili Dog, standard bun	290	na	3	1000	32	na	na
w/cheese	340	na	5	1260	32	na	na
Turkey Chicago Dog, standard bun	320	na	3	1910	31	na	na
Original Plain Hot Dog, standard bun	270	na	4	740	27	na	na
w/mustard, relish, kraut or "Deluxe" (avg)	270	na	4	970	29	na	na
Original Stadium Dog, standard bun	280	na	4	890	30	na	na
Original Chili Dog, standard bun	300	na	4	1130	31	na	na
w/cheese	350	na	6	1390	31	na	na
Original Chicago Dog, standard bun	330	na	4	2040	41	na	na
Sea Dog	350	na	3	640	38	na	na
Chili Burger	280	na	3	750	29	na	na
Fish Wrap	450	na	5	860	38	na	na
Breakfast Sandwich w/egg, bacon, cheese	300	na	6	830	26	na	na
Small Cone, 4oz plain	210	na	4	150	34	na	na

Caveats:

- The Angus All Beef dogs are bigger (and have more calories) than the Original. But you can save calories by ordering one Angus All Beef Dog, instead two of the Original dogs. The highest calorie hot dog is the Angus All Beef Chili Cheese Dog at 620 calories.

- Most Breakfast Sandwiches have 400-670 calories.

- Keep it simple. Dipping the cone in chocolate nearly doubles the calories! Sundaes average 390 calories, but the Banana Split has 820. Freezes and Shakes average 640 calories; the Chocolate Chip Cookie Dough Freeze has 940 calories!

Zaxby's®

Tips:

• Stick with Grilled Chicken items (Zalads or Sandwich). Most other menu items are fried (Chicken FingerZ, Wings, French Fries, Onion Rings).

• Skip the Honey Mustard Sauce that's added to the Grilled Chicken Sandwich. The sauce contains 220 calories, 20g fat!

• Order the salads prepared with grilled chicken (instead of fried chicken strips) to save 160 calories, 13g fat. Then, trim the salad of additional calories by leaving off the fried onions, croutons, or Texas Toast (see the breakdown below). Reduced-calorie dressings are available.

• When ordering a meal consider that Crinkle Fries contain 360 calories, 16g fat and a medium regular soda has 200 calories.

• For more nutrition information, go to Zaxbys.com.

Suggestions:

	Calories	Fat (g)	Sat Fat (g)	Sodium (mg)	Carbohydrates (g)	Fiber (g)	Protein (g)
House Zalad w/grilled chicken w/o dressing							
request no toast, cheese, or fried onions	345	14	8	1165	7	2	44
add for Texas Toast	150	6	1	270	20	1	3
add for fried onions	110	9	4	145	7	0	0
Caesar Zalad w/grilled chicken w/o dressing	570	26	10	1715	29	4	48
request no croutons	370	15	8	1355	8	2	45
Blue Blackened Zalad w/o dressing	605	29	13	1690	34	3	48
request no Texas Toast or fried onions	345	14	8	1275	7	2	45
Dressings							
Light Vinaigrette, 1 packet	35	0	0	320	8	0	0
Light Ranch dressing, 1 packet	90	8	2	390	3	0	1
Grilled Chicken Sandwich w/o sauce	550	21	6	1350	46	2	43

Caveats:

• Meals are served with Fries (360 calories, 16g fat) and a 22oz Soda (150 calories).

• Salads with fried chicken and regular dressings add up to over 900 calories!

• The Cajun Club™ Sandwich (prepared with blackened chicken, not fried) contains 780 calories and 42g fat. The Kickin'Chicken Sandwich with fried chicken strips has 1070 calories, 55g fat!

• Count on 60-70 calories (3-4g fat) per Wing and 110 calories (4g fat) for each Chicken Finger. Then add about 200 calories and 20g fat for each cup of dipping sauce.

Other Titles By:

Dr. Jo®

inspiring busy people stay healthy, sane, and productive

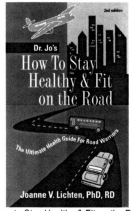

How to Stay Healthy & Fit on the Road

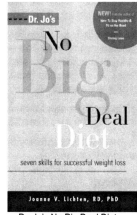

Dr. Jo's No Big Deal Diet

Invite Dr. Jo to speak to
your company, association, or conference.
Topics include:

- **Reboot - how to stay focused, energized, and more productive**

- **What Every Woman Wants - great legs, more energy, and peace of mind**

- **How to Stay Healthy & Fit on the Road**

- **Swimming in a Sea of Priorities**

www.DrJo.com

CPSIA information can be obtained at www.ICGtesting.com
Printed in the USA
LVOW010414101211

258775LV00001B/1/P